Gamma Knife Radiosurgery for Brain Vascular Malformations

Progress in Neurological Surgery

Vol. 27

Series Editor

L. Dade Lunsford Pittsburgh, Pa.

Gamma Knife Radiosurgery for Brain Vascular Malformations

Volume Editors

Ajay Niranjan Pittsburgh, Pa.
Hideyuki Kano Pittsburgh, Pa.
L. Dade Lunsford Pittsburgh, Pa.

60 figures, 25 in color, and 28 tables, 2013

KARGER

Basel · Freiburg · Paris · London · New York · New Delhi · Bangkok · Beijing · Tokyo · Kuala Lumpur · Singapore · Sydney

Ajay Niranjan, MCh, MBA
Hideyuki Kano, MD, PhD
L. Dade Lunsford, MD, FACS
Department of Radiosurgery
UPMC Brain Mapping Center
200 Lothrop Street
Pittsburgh, PA 15213 (USA)

Library of Congress Cataloging-in-Publication Data

Gamma knife radiosurgery for brain vascular malformations / volume editors,
Ajay Niranjan, Hideyuki Kano, L. Dade Lunsford.
p. ; cm. -- (Progress in neurological surgery, ISSN 0079-6492 ; v.
27)
Includes bibliographical references and indexes.
ISBN 978-3-8055-9619-0 (hard cover : alk. paper) -- ISBN 978-3-8055-9620-6
(electronic version)
I. Niranjan, Ajay. II. Kano, Hideyuki. III. Lunsford, L. Dade. IV. Series:
Progress in neurological surgery ; v. 27., 0079-6492
[DNLM: 1. Central Nervous System Vascular Malformations--surgery. 2.
Radiosurgery--methods. W1 PR673 v. 27 2013 / WL 350]

617.4'81059--dc23

2012040349

Bibliographic Indices. This publication is listed in bibliographic services, including Current Contents® and Index Medicus.

www.karger.com
Printed in Germany on acid-free and non-aging paper (ISO 9706) by Kraft Druck, Ettlingen
ISSN 0079–6492
e-ISSN 1662–3924
ISBN 978–3–8055–9619–0
e-ISBN 978–3–8055–9620–6

Contents

Series Editor's Note

In the 40 years since radiosurgery was introduced as an option for the management of vascular malformations, an enormous volume of clinical outcome research has substantiated its role in properly selected patients. Across the world, various technologies are available to perform radiosurgery. The unifying feature of each technology is its ability to conformally deliver a high dose of radiation to a small intracranial volume with precision and selectivity (rapid fall-off of the dose in adjacent normal structures). The Gamma Knife® represents the technology most commonly used and is currently a tool available at more than 300 medical centers.

At our own center, we have recently completed a long-term analysis of almost 1,000 patients who had Gamma Knife radiosurgery for arteriovenous malformations (AVMs) during a 20-year interval. Like other centers, many of whom are represented by reports in this volume, the role of radiosurgery expanded to include carefully selected cavernous malformations and dural vascular malformations. I believe that the current volume of *Progress in Neurological Surgery* will provide additional data that will further define the long-term benefit and risks of radiosurgery for these often complex vascular disorders.

I hope that you will enjoy reading the work of the superb international group of individuals who work with the Gamma Knife in the management of AVMs.

L. Dade Lunsford, MD, FACS
Pittsburgh, Pa.

Niranjan A, Kano H, Lunsford LD (eds): Gamma Knife Radiosurgery for Brain Vascular Malformations.
Prog Neurol Surg. Basel, Karger, 2013, vol 27, pp 1–4 (DOI: 10.1159/000341608)

A Brief History of Arteriovenous Malformation Radiosurgery

Ajay Niranjan · L. Dade Lunsford

Department of Neurological Surgery, University of Pittsburgh, Pittsburgh, Pa., USA

Abstract

Stereotactic radiosurgery was first described by Leksell in Stockholm, Sweden in 1951. In 1967, Leksell introduced the 'Gamma Knife' for clinical use in carefully selected patients. A major role for radiosurgery further emerged in 1972 after its application for brain arteriovenous malformations. Radiosurgery was initially used for high risk or deep seated AVMs that were unsuitable for resection or embolization. Several additional pioneers contributed towards its continued development. Stereotactic radiosurgery is now considered as an important option for patients with brain vascular malformations, including AVMs, cavernous malformations, and dural AV fistulas.

In 1949, Lars Leksell designed his first stereotactic guiding device and described its use in a landmark article [1]. The first stereotactic instrument was designed for use with probes and electrodes. The first attempt to replace electrodes with ionizing radiation began in the early fifties. In 1951, he coined the term 'stereotactic radiosurgery' [2]. He defined radiosurgery as a technique for noninvasive destruction of intracranial tissues or lesions that may be inaccessible or unsuitable for surgery. Leksell began to collaborate with Borje Larsson in the use of cross-fired protons from a 185-MeV cyclotronic accelerator in Uppsala, Sweden [3–5]. In 1967, they arranged for the construction of the first prototype Gamma Knife (unit I). The first Gamma Knife had 179 cobalt sources arranged in a hemisphere array, focused on a target point within the brain. A number of the initial pioneers in radiosurgery in Stockholm worked with Leksell, especially after the construction of the second Gamma Knife in 1975. This unit was placed in the basement of the Radiumhemmet at the Karolinska Hospital in Stockholm.

A general concept in radiobiology is that blood vessels are easily injured by ionizing radiation [6]. This was one of the reasons for the first attempt in 1970 to treat an arteriovenous malformation (AVM) with stereotactic radiosurgery. Gamma Knife radiosurgery was first used by Ladislau Steiner to treat an AVM patient in Stockholm, in March of 1970 [7]. For this first AVM patient, the radiosurgery target was defined by angiography, and feeding arteries were included in the 50% isodose volume. A single radiation isocenter was used and 5,000 rad (50 Gy) was delivered over a period of half an hour. Angiography was repeated 3 weeks, 3 months and 19 months after radiosurgery. The AVM remained unchanged until the last follow-up angiography at which time the feeding vessels were obliterated and the AVM could no longer be visualized. However, this optimal result could not be replicated in 3 subsequent patients treated using a similar technique of irradiating some or all of the feeder vessels. In a fourth patient the entire malformation was small enough to be covered by the radiation field. Angiography 1 year later showed no residual AVM [8]. Further work was done using somewhat different principles. It seemed reasonable that numerous small shunting vessels of AVM should be irradiated as the morphology of these vessels was assumed to differ from the normal vessels. The reaction to radiation seemed to vary with the blood vessel diameter. The idea of irradiating the fine caliber vessels was supported by animal research. Studies of cat basilar artery radiosurgery showed that the small vessels of the neighboring brainstem became obliterated but the basilar artery itself remained patent [9].

After technical modifications and improvements of radiosurgical technique [10], a further series of patients was treated. A Leksell stereotactic frame was attached to a thermoplastic 'shell' which fit the patient's head. Angiography was performed to identify the target. The stereotactic coordinates of the target were calculated. The computer-planned dose distribution was then superimposed upon the stereotactic films. A single radiosurgery dose varying between 5 and 12.5 krad was used. The aim was to irradiate the abnormal shunting vessels and to include as completely as possible the whole cluster of pathological vasculature within the radiation field. Work continued in Stockholm as well as at Buenos Aires, Argentina (Herman Bunge), and Sheffield, UK (David Forster).

During the 1970s and early 1980s, more than 1,000 AVM patients were treated using Bragg peak stereotactic radiation at the Harvard affiliated proton facility in Cambridge, Mass., USA [11, 12]. Helium ion beam was used to perform multisession AVM irradiation at the Lawrence Livermore Laboratory in Berkeley [13–15]. Linear accelerator-based radiosurgery efforts using newer generation linear accelerators began in Paris and Buenos Aires [16], Spain, Italy [17, 18] and the USA [19–21]. Most programs evaluated radiosurgery as an alternative to microsurgical removal, especially for AVMs in high-risk locations.

During the early 1980s, the financial and regulatory approval for the establishment of the next generation Gamma Knife (No. 5) was completed in Pittsburgh. The unit entered clinical operation in Pittsburgh in 1987. AVM radiosurgery using the fifth-generation Gamma Knife began in the USA at the University of Pittsburgh in August of 1987 [22, 23]. During the next 23 years more than 1,200 patients with AVMs underwent Gamma Knife stereotactic radiosurgery at the University of Pittsburgh [24]. By the year 2008, more than 65,000 AVM patients had undergone Gamma Knife radiosurgery worldwide.

The evolution in technologies for the Gamma Knife went hand in hand with the evolution of superior quality brain and body imaging. Computed tomography became integrated in the late 1970s and magnetic resonance imaging in the early 1990s. The resolution, quality and reliability of these imaging tools greatly expanded the indications and potential role of radiosurgery. AVMs became better delineated using multidimensional magnetic resonance imaging, digital-subtraction angiography, and 2- and 3-dimensional angiography. Stereotactic radiosurgery is now considered a highly effective and minimal access approach for patients with AVM.

References

1 Leksell L: A stereotaxic apparatus for intracerebral surgery. Acta Chir Scand 1949;99:229–233.
2 Leksell L: The stereotaxic method and radiosurgery of the brain. Acta Chir Scand 1951;102:316–319.
3 Larsson B, Leksell L, Rexed B, Sourander P, Mair W, Andersson B: The high-energy proton beam as a neurosurgical tool. Nature 1958;182:1222–1223.
4 Leksell L, Larsson B, Andersson B, Rexed B, Sourander P, Mair W: Lesions in the depth of the brain produced by a beam of high energy protons. Acta Radiol 1960;54:251–264.
5 Leksell L, Larsson B, Andersson B, Rexed B, Sourander P, Mair W: Research on 'localized radio-lesions'. VI. Restricted radio-lesions in the depth of the brain produced by a beam of high energy protons. AFOSR TN US Air Force Office Sci Res 1960; 60-1406:1–13.
6 Rubin P, Casarett GW: Clinical radiation pathology as applied to curative radiotherapy. Cancer 1968;22: 767–778.
7 Steiner L, Leksell L, Greitz T, Forster DM, Backlund EO: Stereotaxic radiosurgery for cerebral arteriovenous malformations. Report of a case. Acta Chir Scand 1972;138:459–464.
8 Steiner L, Leksell L, Forster DM, Greitz T, Backlund EO: Stereotactic radiosurgery in intracranial arterio-venous malformations. Acta Neurochir 1974; (suppl 21):195–209.
9 Nilsson A, Wennerstrand J, Leksell D, Backlund EO: Stereotactic gamma irradiation of basilar artery in cat. Preliminary experiences. Acta Radiol Oncol Radiat Phys Biol 1978;17:150–160.
10 Dahlin H, Sarby B: Destruction of small intracranial tumours with ^{60}Co gamma radiation. Physical and technical considerations. Acta Radiol Ther Phys Biol 1975;14:209–227.
11 Kjellberg RN: Stereotactic Bragg peak proton beam radiosurgery for cerebral arteriovenous malformations. Ann Clin Res 1986;18(suppl 47):17–19.
12 Kjellberg RN, Hanamura T, Davis KR, Lyons SL, Adams RD: Bragg-peak proton-beam therapy for arteriovenous malformations of the brain. N Engl J Med 1983;309:269–274.
13 Fabrikant JI, Levy RP, Steinberg GK, Silverberg GD, Frankel KA, Phillips MH, et al: Heavy-charged-particle radiosurgery for intracranial arteriovenous malformations. Stereotact Funct Neurosurg 1991;57: 50–63.
14 Steinberg GK, Levy RP, Fabrikant JI, Frankel KA, Phillips MH, Marks MP: Stereotactic helium ion Bragg peak radiosurgery for angiographically occult intracranial vascular malformations. Stereotact Funct Neurosurg 1991;57:64–71.
15 Fabrikant JI, Levy RP, Steinberg GK, Phillips MH, Frankel KA, Lyman JT, et al: Charged-particle radiosurgery for intracranial vascular malformations. Neurosurg Clin N Am 1992;3:99–139.
16 Betti OO, Munari C, Rosler R: Stereotactic radiosurgery with the linear accelerator: treatment of arteriovenous malformations. Neurosurgery 1989; 24:311–321.
17 Colombo F, Pozza F, Chierego G, Casentini L, De Luca G, Francescon P: Linear accelerator radiosurgery of cerebral arteriovenous malformations: an update. Neurosurgery 1994;34:14–20, discussion 21.
18 Colombo F, Pozza F, Chierego G, Francescon P, Casentini L, De Luca G: Linear accelerator radiosurgery of cerebral arteriovenous malformations: current status. Acta Neurochir Suppl 1994;62:5–9.
19 Friedman WA, Bova FJ: Radiosurgery for arteriovenous malformations. Clin Neurosurg 1993;40: 446–464.

20 Friedman WA, Bova FJ: Linear accelerator radiosurgery for arteriovenous malformations. J Neurosurg 1992;77:832–841.
21 Loeffler JS, Alexander E 3rd, Siddon RL, Saunders WM, Coleman CN, Winston KR: Stereotactic radiosurgery for intracranial arteriovenous malformations using a standard linear accelerator. Int J Radiat Oncol Biol Phys 1989;17:673–677.
22 Dawson RC 3rd, Tarr RW, Hecht ST, Jungreis CA, Lunsford LD, Coffey R, et al: Treatment of arteriovenous malformations of the brain with combined embolization and stereotactic radiosurgery: results after 1 and 2 years. AJNR Am J Neuroradiol 1990; 11:857–864.
23 Altschuler EM, Lunsford LD, Coffey RJ, Bissonette DJ, Flickinger JC: Gamma knife radiosurgery for intracranial arteriovenous malformations in childhood and adolescence. Pediatr Neurosci 1989;15: 53–61.
24 Kano H, Kondziolka D, Flickinger JC, Yang HC, Flannery TJ, Awan NR, et al: Stereotactic radiosurgery for arteriovenous malformations. 3. Outcome predictors and risks after repeat radiosurgery. J Neurosurg 2012, E-pub ahead of print.

Ajay Niranjan, MCh, MBA
Department of Neurological Surgery, University of Pittsburgh Medical Center, Suite B-400
200 Lothrop Street
Pittsburgh, PA 15213 (USA)
Tel. +1 412 647 6250, E-Mail niranjana@upmc.edu

Niranjan A, Kano H, Lunsford LD (eds): Gamma Knife Radiosurgery for Brain Vascular Malformations.
Prog Neurol Surg. Basel, Karger, 2013, vol 27, pp 5–21 (DOI: 10.1159/000341616)

Natural History of Cerebral Arteriovenous Malformations and the Risk of Hemorrhage after Radiosurgery

Chun-Po Yen · David Schlesinger · Jason P. Sheehan

Department of Neurological Surgery, University of Virginia, Charlottesville, Va., USA

Abstract

The annual hemorrhage rate of intracranial arteriovenous malformations (AVMs) varies from 2 to 4%. In a patient with decades of life ahead, the cumulative risk of hemorrhage is significant. AVMs exhibiting characteristics such as deep venous drainage, venous stenosis, associated aneurysms and feeders from perforators are associated with an elevated risk of hemorrhage. We reviewed 1,400 AVM patients who underwent Gamma Knife surgery (GKS) at the University of Virginia between 1989 and 2009. The dose selection was based on the size and location of the nidus. The mean prescription dose was 21.2 Gy (range 5–36 Gy), and the mean maximum dose was 39.4 Gy (range 10–60 Gy). A total of 657 patients suffered 803 hemorrhagic events over 42,495 risk years before GKS. Assuming that these patients were at risk for hemorrhage since birth, the annual hemorrhage rate was 2.0%. If we calculate the hemorrhage rate after the diagnosis of the AVMs, the hemorrhage rate was 6.6%. Following GKS and prior to a radiographic documented obliteration, the annual hemorrhage rate was 2.5%; this rate is very similar to the 2.0% one computed prior to radiosurgery by assuming AVMs to be congenital. Once angiographic obliteration was confirmed after GKS, the hemorrhage rate dropped to zero.

In extrapolating from their experience with cerebral aneurysms, early neurological surgeons had been convinced that cerebral arteriovenous malformations (AVMs) had a propensity to rupture and lead to catastrophic sequelae [1]. As such, neurosurgeons were inclined to offer treatment for many patients with accessible AVMs. Prior to the advent of radiosurgery, microsurgically inaccessible lesions had been managed conservatively. In the ensuing decades, some natural history studies on AVMs became available [2–5]. Over time, neurosurgeons came to realize that some but not all AVMs are prone to rupture, and the prognosis was not usually as dismal as with cerebral aneurysms [5].

Later, several studies revealed that AVMs at different locations or with certain angioarchitectural characteristics behave differently. Thus, all AVMs are not the same and those with a greater risk of rupturing should be treated. Treatment of unruptured but rupture-prone AVMs became more appealing with the emergence of embolization and radiosurgery; these treatment approaches offered a reasonable chance for obliteration and a relatively low rate of procedural complications.

Since the first AVM treated with the Gamma Knife was published in 1972 [6], over 60,000 AVMs have been treated worldwide with radiosurgery. The AVM is not obliterated immediately following radiosurgery. As such, patients are followed closely over the ensuing years. Several large series including some from the University of Virginia have provided a clearer sense of the benefits and risks of stereotactic radiosurgery for AVM patients [7–9]. Pretreatment information from AVM patients provides useful insight into the preradiosurgical hemorrhage risk and the natural history of AVMs. Also, careful follow-up of AVM patients after radiosurgery has led to a thorough understanding of the hemorrhage rate during the latency period before and after obliteration of the nidus.

The first part of this report will focus on the available literature with regard to the natural history of AVMs and the risk factors associated with hemorrhage. The second portion of this report will focus on the hemorrhage rate following radiosurgery.

The Natural History of Arteriovenous Malformations

Even though the prognosis for AVM patients is no longer considered dismal, it is generally accepted that the lifetime risk of hemorrhage remains high, and most AVMs require treatment [10]. As most patients are treated with microsurgery, embolization or radiosurgery, few purely observational studies of AVM patients exist.

In the current literature, 4 major studies were published on the natural hemorrhagic history of untreated AVMs (table 1). In 1986, Crawford et al. [11] published a retrospective study of 217 patients treated conservatively (13 patients did have surgery or embolization at a later point), and, in this study, patients were followed for a mean of 10.4 years. The authors reported a 2% hemorrhage rate. Itoyama et al. [12] reported on 50 patients unsuitable for surgery and noted a similar hemorrhage rate after a mean observation period of 13.4 years. Ondra et al. [4] published their landmark study on 160 patients managed conservatively for an average of 24 years. They reported an annual hemorrhage rate of 4%, and a mortality rate of 1% [4]. Yamane et al. [13] studied 115 patients (including 53 patients with partially treated AVMs) and reported a 4.2% annual hemorrhage rate. Based on these 4 studies, the natural hemorrhage rate of AVMs is widely held to be between 2 and 4%.

In addition to the aforementioned studies, information regarding the hemorrhage risk of AVMs was also provided in series that included a mixture of treated and untreated AVM patients [3, 14, 15]. However, the hemorrhage rates reported by these studies should be viewed more cautiously. Retrospective studies face the difficulty of determining when the patients started to be at risk for hemorrhage. Although AVMs

Table 1. Hemorrhage rates in untreated cerebral AVMs

Authors	Year	Patients n	Follow-up years	Annual hemorrhage rate %	Accumulated mortality rate %	Risk factors associated with hemorrhage (before/after diagnosis)			
						age	size	location	pregnancy
Crawford et al. [11]	1986	217	10.4	2	29	n.a./old	small/n.a.	deep/n.a.	yes
Itoyama et al. [12]	1989	50	13.4	2.1	10	–	small/n.a.	deep/deep	n.a.
Ondra et al. [4]	1990	160	23.7	4	23	–	–	–	–
Yamane et al. [13]	1998	115	6.5	4.2	10	–	small/large	deep/n.a.	–

n.a. = Not associated; – = not stated.

are considered congenital anomalies and theoretically patients are at risk for hemorrhage since their birth, hemorrhage usually occurs in adolescence or young adulthood. It is believed that AVMs are dynamic lesions with ongoing morphological and hemodynamic changes. Unknown factors may play a significant role in causing rupture later in the progression of the vascular malformations. The hemorrhage rates obtained from these studies tend to be lower due to the assumed longer at-risk period [2, 15].

An alternative approach taken by some is to base the calculation of the hemorrhage rate from the time of diagnosis of the AVM until the date of intervention. Such studies frequently consist of a mixture of patients with large and deep AVMs that were left untreated as well as small, superficial AVMs that were successfully treated. Therefore, most of the follow-up data on hemorrhage risks were contributed by patients with large and deep AVMs. Such a selection bias may limit the value of the hemorrhage risk calculations. Also, AVMs tend to exhibit a higher rebleeding rate at least for some period of time following a previous hemorrhage. Including patients during a period of heightened risk for hemorrhage (i.e. hemorrhagic clustering) may overestimate the hemorrhage rates and not be reflective of the 'natural history' of AVMs in several papers [16, 17]. Despite these limitations, such studies do provide valuable insight into AVM behavior; these studies reveal a hemorrhage rate that ranges from 2.4 to 13% (table 2).

Predicting Risk Factors of Arteriovenous Malformation Hemorrhage

As previously noted, not all AVMs have a similar risk of hemorrhage. A number of retrospective studies have compared patients with or without hemorrhage as the presentation symptom. These studies have identified clinical features that affect hemorrhage

Table 2. Hemorrhage rates in series with treated and untreated cerebral AVMs and risk factors of hemorrhage

Authors	Year	Patients n	Follow-up years	Annual hemorrhage rate %	Risk factors associated with hemorrhage after diagnosis	
					related	not related
Graf et al. [3]	1983	191 (120/71)	2/4.8	6/2–3	old age small AVMs[1]	size
Brown et al. [2]	1988	168 (0/168)	8.2	2.2		size
Mast et al. [18]	1997	281 (142/139)	0.7/1.0	13/2	deep vein prior hemorrhage	age size
Stefani et al. [19]	2002	390 (146/244)	3.1	3.2	large AVMs deep location deep draining vein single draining vein deep feeders	prior hemorrhage
Halim et al. [20]	2004	790 (367/423)	2.3/5.4	3.7/1.4	prior hemorrhage	size deep draining vein
Stapf et al. [21]	2006	622 (282/340)	2.3	2.8	old age deep location deep draining vein prior hemorrhage	size aneurysm
Yamada et al. [22]	2007	305 (159/146)	2.4/3.5	6.8/3.1	young age deep location prior hemorrhage	size deep draining vein
Hernesniemi et al. [23]	2008	238 (139/99)	13.5	2.4	large AVMs deep location	draining vein
Da Costa et al. [24]	2009	678 (258/420)	2.9	7.5/4.2	deep draining vein aneurysm prior hemorrhage	age size deep location deep draining vein

For patient number, follow-up and annual hemorrhage rate, when appropriate, data are presented as hemorrhagic cases/nonhemorrhagic cases.
[1] Size was not related to hemorrhage in patients who presented initially with hemorrhage, but small size was a predicting factor in patients with nonhemorrhagic presentation.

risk: young age, smaller size and deep location may increase the risk of hemorrhage [25–28]. Certain angioarchitectural characteristics such as deep venous drainage, venous stenosis, associated aneurysms and feeders from perforators have also been reported to be associated with an increased risk of nidus rupture. The hemorrhage risk related to nidus size has been the subject of debate [26–28]. However, most studies have failed to demonstrate a significant relationship between hemorrhage risk and the AVM volume. It is probable that smaller volume AVMs are less likely to cause focal neurological deficits or headache, and thus are diagnosed only after a more dramatic event such a seizure or a hemorrhage. Other factors such as deep location and its associated features (deep feeders and deep draining veins), unsecured aneurysms, and prior history of hemorrhage are consistently associated with an increased risk of hemorrhage.

Hemorrhage Risk before and after Radiosurgery

Whether radiosurgery reduces the risk of AVM rupture during the latency period remains controversial. Various studies report that AVM hemorrhage risks are [15, 29–31] decreased [16, 30], unchanged [15, 32] or increased [29, 31, 33] after radiosurgery. The incidence of postradiosurgical hemorrhages has been reported to be between 1.7 and 4.8% [15–17, 30, 32, 34, 35]. Since there is no control group in such studies, the best way to compare the postradiosurgical hemorrhage rates would be using the numbers from published natural history studies (e.g. 2–4% annual risk). Using a hemorrhage rate of 2–4%, there does not seem to be significant change of hemorrhage rate following radiosurgery until the AVM is obliterated.

It is widely accepted that radiosurgical obliteration confers a substantial benefit in terms of preventing future hemorrhages. However, the benefit of radiosurgery in terms of reducing hemorrhage in the latency period (i.e. prior to obliteration) remains the subject of much debate. Since it is difficult if not impossible to conduct a randomized control study, it is tempting to compare the postradiosurgical hemorrhage rates to the preradiosurgical rates. Maruyama et al. [16] reported a 54% decreased risk of hemorrhage following radiosurgery. However, as previously mentioned, the major concern is that the preradiosurgical hemorrhage risk could represent an overestimation. It is not clear whether the decrease in hemorrhage rate is just the natural decline of risk after an initial hemorrhage or truly a beneficial effect of radiosurgery.

For example, we can use a simple method to recalculate the hemorrhagic rates in the paper of Maruyama et al. During the preradiosurgical period, there were 42 hemorrhages in 500 patients within a median follow-up of 0.4 years (the mean was not provided and since the authors mentioned most patients were treated soon after hemorrhage, we assumed that the median is close to the mean); the annual hemorrhage is almost 20% (42 events in 200 risk-years) This hemorrhagic rate is extremely high. The authors observed 23 hemorrhages in 458 patients within a median of 2 years after radiosurgery and reported a postradiosurgical hemorrhage rate of 2.5%. The authors utilized alternative statistical methods to define a 'significant' reduction of the hemorrhage rate after radiosurgery. Although they note that the recurrent hemorrhage rate is stable over 3 years following an initial hemorrhagic episode, the patient and event numbers are too small to draw a definite conclusion.

Table 3. Hemorrhage rates in radiosurgery series and risk factors of AVM hemorrhage

Authors	Year	Patients n	Annual hemorrhage rate (birth to radiosurgery) %	Annual hemorrhage rate after radiosurgery %	Risk factors for hemorrhage after radiosurgery	
					related	not related
Pollock et al. [15]	1996	315 (196/119)	2.4	4.8 (within 2 years)	unsecured aneurysm	location size draining vein prior hemorrhage dose
Friedman et al. [32]	1996	199 (121/78)		4.4	unsecured aneurysm large AVMs venous stenosis periventricular location low dose	age prior hemorrhage
Karlsson et al. [36]	2001	1,593		1.8 (within 2 years)	old age large AVMs low dose	location aneurysm prior hemorrhage
Nataf et al. [35]	2004	756 (423/333)	1.8	3.1	unsecured aneurysm large AVMs prior hemorrhage complete coverage low dose	
Maruyama et al. [16]	2005	500 (318/182)	2.0	2.5		
Liscak et al. [37]	2007	330 (207/123)	2.5	2.1		
Kaliswal et al. [34]	2008	160 (103/57)	2.5	1.7		

For patient number, when appropriate, data are presented as hemorrhagic cases/nonhemorrhagic cases.

Most studies examining the natural history of AVMs actually have demonstrated a temporary period of increased risk of hemorrhages once an AVM ruptures [18, 20, 22, 24] In a subsequent study, Maruyama et al. [17] calculated the hemorrhage rate considering AVMs as congenital lesions, and they reported a preradiosurgical hemorrhage rate of 2%. There is no doubt that the 2.5% hemorrhage rate they reported following radiosurgery is similar to their 2% preradiosurgical rate and the natural history. Therefore, whether radiosurgery provides protective effects from AVM rupture before AVM obliteration remains uncertain given the evidence currently available (table 3).

Hemorrhage from Arteriovenous Malformations Confirmed Obliterated on Angiography after Radiosurgery

Magnetic resonance imaging (MRI) is currently the most widely used imaging modality to assess the AVM response after radiosurgery and provides a high positive predictive rate of nidus obliteration [15]. Angiography is still recommended by most neurosurgeons to confirm complete obliteration of the nidus before a patient can be declared 'cured'. Total obliteration of the AVMs after radiosurgery was defined by Lindquist and Steiner [38] as 'complete absence of pathological vessels in the former nidus, disappearance or normalization of afferent and efferent pathological vessels, and a normal circulation time on high-quality rapid serial subtracted angiography'. It is generally accepted that once the nidus is obliterated based on a high-quality angiography, the risk of hemorrhage is essentially eliminated.

Lindquist et al. [39] reviewed 48 patients in whom follow-up cerebral angiography was performed 4–17 years after the AVM had previously been deemed obliterated. They reported 4 patients who had experienced hemorrhage despite documentation of AVM obliteration [39]. The hemorrhage was from a recanalized nidus in 2 patients, a new AVM appearing adjacent to the previously treated nidus in 1 patient and unknown in 1 patient. Maruyama et al. [16, 17] reported 4 patients with hemorrhages 16–51 months after angiographic confirmation of AVM obliteration. Two patients underwent surgery. Histopathology revealed small residual AVM vessels in addition to the occluded AVM. The blood vessels showed typical radiation-related thickening of the intima and dense hyalinization of the vascular lumen. The authors reported that continuous contrast enhancement of the treated nidus on computed tomography (CT) or MRI is a risk factor for hemorrhage despite angiographic obliteration of a nidus. Others have been unable to confirm this finding, and instead note that persistence of contrast enhancement at the target site of radiosurgery may persist for many years after angiographic confirmation of obliteration.

Recurrent AVMs following a complete surgical resection have also been reported [40]. Similar to the cases reported in radiosurgical series, this phenomenon is more common in pediatric AVM patients. The significance of this rare event in pediatric patients with AVMs warrants further investigation, but may be related to the persistence of blood vessel growth factors in the growing child.

The Experience with Arteriovenous Malformations at the University of Virginia

Patient Population

A total of 1,400 AVM patients who underwent Gamma Knife surgery (GKS) at the University of Virginia between 1989 and 2009 have been reviewed. The large patient number and relatively long-term follow-up allowed us to investigate the postradiosurgical hemorrhage rate and retrospectively the hemorrhage rate of AVMs before GKS. Our follow-up protocol was magnetic resonance images every 6 months for 2 years then yearly thereafter. When MRI showed that there was no flow void visible, cerebral angiography was recommended to confirm obliteration of the nidus. CT or MRI was performed if patients developed new or worsened symptoms such as headaches, seizures or neurological deficits. Hemorrhagic events in this study were defined as clinically symptomatic events with signs of hemorrhage on either CT or MRI. Additionally, asymptomatic hemorrhages which were only identified on follow-up images were also included. The clinical information was obtained from examining the patients or from patients' referring physicians or families.

Because the purpose of the present report is also to investigate the effect of GKS on the hemorrhage rate, 105 patients with large AVMs which were only partially treated were excluded from analysis. Additionally, 91 patients lost to follow-up were excluded leaving 1,204 AVM patients in the present study for analysis.

Patient Demographics and AVM Characteristics

There were 637 males and 567 females with a mean age of 35.3 years (range 3–82 years). The initial presentations leading to the diagnosis of AVMs were hemorrhage in 605 (50.2%), seizures in 271 (22.5%), headache in 163 (13.5%), neurological deficits in 89 (7.4%) and other symptoms (e.g. vertigo, bruits, tinnitus) in 33 (2.7%). In 43 (3.6%) patients, the AVMs were incidental findings. Additionally, 50 patients who initially presented with symptoms other than a hemorrhage experienced at least 1 episode of bleeding between the diagnosis of their AVMs and GKS. One hundred and thirty-eight patients had a partial resection of the nidus and 298 underwent a partial embolization of the nidus before undergoing GKS.

The locations of the AVMs were in the cerebral hemispheres in 742 (61.6%), basal ganglia in 92 (7.6%), thalamus in 104 (8.6%), corpus callosum in 47 (3.9%), brainstem in 99 (8.2%), cerebellum in 90 (7.5%) and insula/sylvian fissure in 30 (2.5%) patients. The Spetzler-Martin grading of the AVMs were grade I in 204 (16.9%) patients, grade II in 455 (37.8%) patients, grade III in 452 (37.5%) patients, grade IV in 91 (7.6%) patients and grade V in 2 (0.2%) patients. The nidus volume ranged from 0.1 to 33 cm^3 (mean 3.4 cm^3). The venous drainage was superficial only in 600 AVMs, deep only in 475 and both deep and superficial in 129. Five hundred and thirty-five AVMs had multiple draining veins, and 669 had only a single dominant draining vein.

Gamma Knife Radiosurgery Technique

The Gamma Knife model U was used from 1989 until July 2001 when the C model replaced it. The Perfexion model was used after September 2009. The Kula system was used for treatment planning from 1989 to 1994 and then was replaced with Gamma Plan software. Stereotactic angiography was the only imaging modality available in the beginning for dose planning, and, in the early 1990s, MRI was added for target definition and dose planning.

The dose selection is based on the size and location of the nidus. The mean prescription dose was 21.2 Gy (range 5–36 Gy), and the mean maximum dose was 39.4 Gy (range 10–60 Gy). The mean isodose configuration was 55% (range 30–95%), and the mean number of isocenters was 2.8 (range 1–22).

Statistical Analysis

The annual hemorrhage rate was calculated as the number of hemorrhages divided by the patient-years at risk. The pre-radiosurgical hemorrhage rates were calculated in two ways. First, we assumed that patients were at risk for hemorrhage since their birth and the risk years were calculated from their birth dates to the dates of GKS. The pre-radiosurgical hemorrhage rates were calculated as total hemorrhagic events divided by the sum of patients' ages at the time of GKS. Alternatively, we calculated the risk of hemorrhage starting from the dates that the AVMs were diagnosed until the dates of GKS.

We have not observed any patients having a hemorrhage after the nidus had been declared obliterated based on angiography; therefore the rate of postradiosurgical annual hemorrhage was calculated by dividing the hemorrhagic events by the patient risk years for which the end points were the dates of nidus obliteration or the dates of last follow-up if the nidi remained patent. As the nidus should have become obliterated before the final image study concluding obliteration of the nidus, we assumed that the AVMs became obliterated at the midpoint between the dates of the last images showing the AVMs were still patent and the dates of the first images showing that the AVMs were obliterated. We chose the dates when the AVMs were concluded obliterated on MRI instead of angiograms because some patients refused to have follow-up angiography to confirm the nidus obliteration and angiography was usually performed after the MRI had suggested that the nidi had become obliterated. If errors were to be introduced by incorrectly judging that the nidus had become obliterated based on MRI, we actually avoided overestimating the patient-years at risk and therefore underestimating the hemorrhage rate.

Univariate and multivariate logistic regressions were used to test for an association with patient demographics (age, gender) and AVM characteristics (size, lobar vs. deep locations, superficial only vs. deep venous drainage, single vs. multiple draining veins) with hemorrhagic AVM presentation. Univariate and multivariate proportional hazard models were used to test the risk factors predisposing patients to hemorrhage in the period from the diagnosis of AVM to the date of GKS and the follow-up period after GKS. Patients were censored from the postradiosurgery bleeding risk group when the AVM was obliterated. In addition, they were censored if patients underwent repeat GKS, surgical resection or embolization after GKS, were lost to follow-up or died. Additional factors evaluated for hemorrhages from diagnosis to GKS included hemorrhagic or nonhemorrhagic presentation. Radiosurgical treatment parameters (i.e. prescription dose, maximum dose, isodose configuration, number of isocenters) were further added to evaluate the postradiosurgical risk of hemorrhage.

Outcome of GKS

The mean imaging follow-up was 71 months following GKS. GKS yielded a total angiographic obliteration in 584 (48.5%) and subtotal obliteration [41] (residual draining vein without visible nidus on angiography) in 43 (3.6%) patients. In 429 (35.6%) patients, the AVMs remained patent. In 148 patients (12.3%) no flow void was observed on MRI, but patients either had not reached the time point when the angiography should be performed or they refused to have follow-up angiography to confirm the obliteration of the nidus. If we exclude 151 patients with follow-up less than the 2 years of latency period, angiographic obliteration occurred in 55.5%, subtotal obliteration in 4.1%, no flow void on MRI in 14.1%, and the nidi remained patent in 26.4%.

Preradiosurgical Hemorrhage Rate and Rebleeding Rate

A total of 657 patients suffered 803 hemorrhagic events over 42,495 risk years before GKS assuming patients were at risk for hemorrhage since their birth. Five hundred and fifty-six patients had one, 74 had two, 20 had three, and 7 had four or more episodes of hemorrhages. The crude annual hemorrhage rate was 2.0%. If we calculate the hemorrhage rate after the diagnosis of the AVMs, there were 68 hemorrhages in 52 patients who initially presented with symptoms other than hemorrhage and 130 rebleeds in 90 patients who experienced hemorrhages leading to the diagnosis of AVMs. The hemorrhage rate calculated after the diagnosis of the AVMs is 6.6% (198 bleeds in 2,984 risk years).

We also calculated separately the hemorrhage rate in patients who initially presented with hemorrhage or other symptoms before diagnosis of the AVMs. The hemorrhage rate in the subgroup of 605 patients who initially presented with hemorrhage was 735 events divided by 19,712 risk years yielding a 3.7% annual hemorrhage rate assuming patients were at risk for hemorrhage since their birth. The hemorrhage rate would be 10.4% if we calculated the 130 hemorrhagic events in 1,243 risk years from the diagnosis of AVMs to the dates of GKS. In the subgroup of 599 patients who initially presented with symptoms other than hemorrhage, 52 patients experienced 68 episodes of hemorrhages between the diagnosis of AVMs and the time of GKS. The hemorrhage rate was 3.9% (68 events divided by 1,741 risk years) from the diagnosis of AVMs to the date of GKS (fig. 1).

In patients with prior hemorrhages, the annual rebleeding rate was 8.6% (146 hemorrhages in 1,581 risk years from the dates of initial hemorrhage to the dates of GKS). The rebleeding rate was 10.2% in the first year after the initial hemorrhage, 10.8% in the second year, 6.5% between the second and fifth years, 6.7% between the fifth and tenth years, and 8.8% after 10 years. The rebleeding rate was approximately 10% in

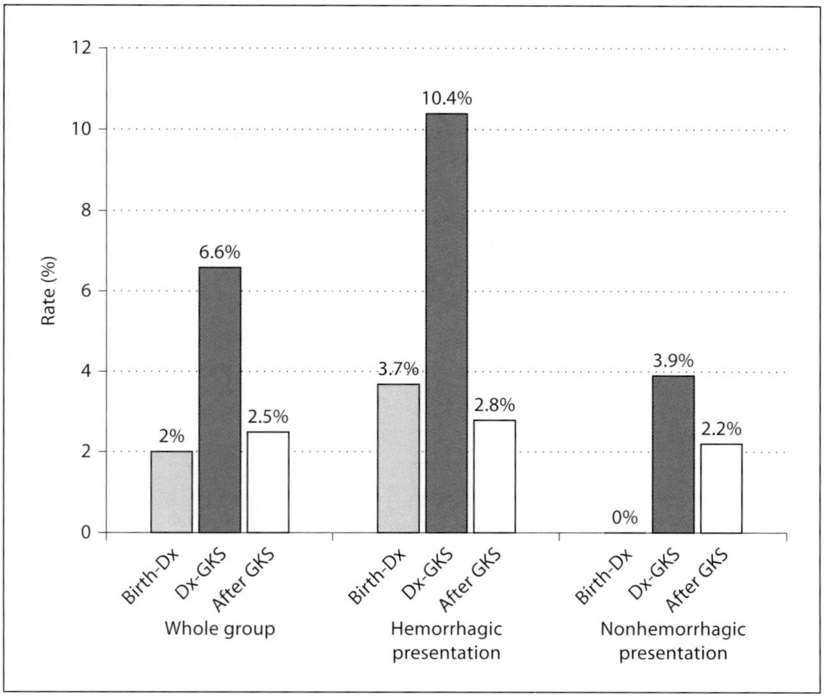

Fig. 1. Hemorrhage rates before and after GKS in patients who experienced at least 1 hemorrhage before GKS. Dx = Diagnosis.

the first and second years; it decreased but remained elevated in the first 5 years after an initial hemorrhage.

Patient Demographics and AVM Characteristics in Hemorrhagic or Nonhemorrhagic Presentation

Patients tending to present with hemorrhage were those of younger age, smaller volume AVMs in deep locations, and those with deep venous drainage or only a single draining vein (table 4). The same risk factors were checked for the period between the diagnosis of the AVMs and GKS. After the initial diagnosis, small and deep AVMs were no longer associated with an increased risk of hemorrhage, thereby suggesting that small and deep AVMs were more likely to be diagnosed after a hemorrhage, but that the small size or deep location were truly independent risk factors predisposing AVMs to rupture (table 5). A single draining vein was a risk factor for hemorrhage prior to and after the initial diagnosis. Patients with a prior hemorrhage are more likely to have a subsequent hemorrhage. Of 605 patients who had a hemorrhage leading to the diagnosis of the AVM, 90 developed a subsequent hemorrhage before GKS. Of the 599 patients who did not present with hemorrhage at the time of the diagnosis of the AVMs, 50 subsequently developed a hemorrhage ($p < 0.001$).

Table 4. Patient demographics and AVM characteristics in patients with hemorrhagic or non-hemorrhagic presentation

	Nonhemorrhagic presentation (n = 599)	Hemorrhagic presentation (n = 605)	p value (univariate)	p value (multivariate)
Patient demographics				
Male/female	316/283	321/284	0.916	
Age, years	35.2±15.7	30.6±16.7	<0.001	<0.001
AVM characteristics				
Location				
Lobar/deep	481/118	351/254	<0.001	<0.001
Venous drainage				
Superficial only/deep venous drainage	376/223	224/381	<0.001	<0.001
Single/multiple draining veins	278/321	391/214	<0.001	<0.001
Volume of the nidus, cm^3	4.0±3.3	2.8±3.0	<0.001	<0.001

Table 5. Risk factors of hemorrhages between the diagnosis of AVM and time of GKS

	No hemorrhage after diagnosis (n=1064)	Hemorrhage after diagnosis (n=140)	p value (univariate)	p value (multivariate)
Patient characteristics				
Male/female	564/498	73/69	0.693	–
Age of hemorrhage, years	33.5±16.2	28.5±15.9	0.858	–
AVM characteristics				
Location				
Lobar/deep	754/308	78/64	<0.001*	0.119
Venous drainage				
Superficial only/deep venous drainage	545/517	55/87	0.006*	0.774
Single/multiple draining veins	579/483	90/52	<0.001*	0.016*
Volume of the nidus, cm^3	3.4±3.3	3.6±2.8	0.060	–
Prior hemorrhage (no/yes)	547/515	52/90	<0.001*	<0.001*

Asterisks indicate statistically significant p values.

Postradiosurgical Hemorrhage Rate and Risk Factors of Hemorrhage

Following GKS, 94 patients had a hemorrhage, and 18 patients had 2. The postradiosurgical hemorrhage rate is 2.5% (130 hemorrhagic events in 5,239 risk years). The hemorrhage rate was 2.3% within 2 years following GKS, 2.2% between the second and fifth years, 2.5% between the fifth and tenth years, and 4.0% between the tenth and twentieth years (fig. 2). The postradiosurgical hemorrhage rate is fairly comparable to the reported natural hemorrhage rate of 2–4%.

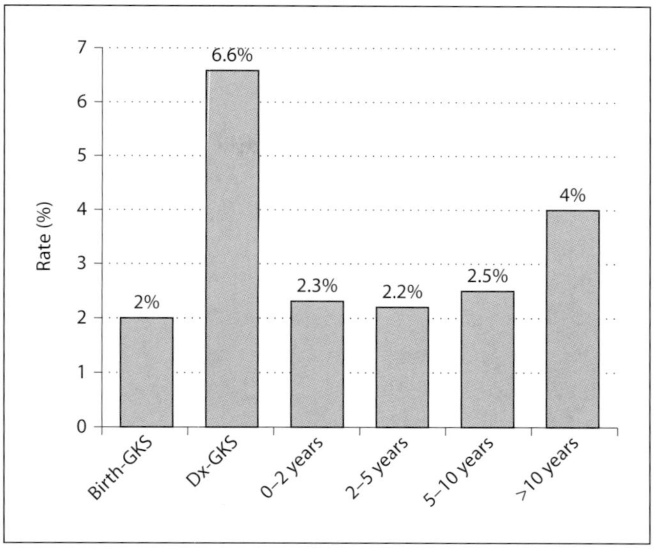

Fig. 2. Annual hemorrhage rates before and after GKS in our institutional experience for those with nonobliterated AVMs. Dx = Diagnosis.

In the subgroup of patients with preradiosurgical hemorrhage, 55 patients had 1 and 12 patients had 2 hemorrhages following GKS. The postradiosurgical hemorrhage rate in this subgroup was 2.8% (79 hemorrhagic events in 2,868 risk years) which seems to be lower than the preradiosurgical hemorrhage rates (3.7% calculated since birth or 10.4% calculated after diagnosis of the AVMs; fig. 1). The reduction of the hemorrhage rate from 10.4 to 2.8% seems to be quite significant. However, as we mentioned earlier, these data should be interpreted with caution since most believe that there is a temporarily increased risk for a subsequent hemorrhagic risk in the immediate period following a prior hemorrhage. Therefore, the reduction of the hemorrhage rate following GKS might represent the natural history of sporadic and temporal clustering of hemorrhages from AVMs.

Risk Factors Predicting Hemorrhage after GKS

Risk factors for at least 1 postradiosurgical hemorrhage were deep location, large nidus size and low prescription dose in univariate analysis. In multivariate analysis, only a low prescription dose remained to be associated with a high risk of hemorrhage (table 3). Of 657 patients who had a hemorrhage before GKS, 67 (10.2%) had hemorrhage during the follow-up. Of the 547 patients who did not have hemorrhage before GKS, 45 (8.2%) developed a hemorrhage during the follow-up ($p = 0.142$). Our institutional experience seems to be in keeping with the study from Karlsson et al. [42] showing that a low radiation dose is related to a continued risk for post-treatment hemorrhage. Higher doses of radiation trigger radiobiological pathways that lead to endothelial and perhaps intimal proliferation, decreased vessel diameter,

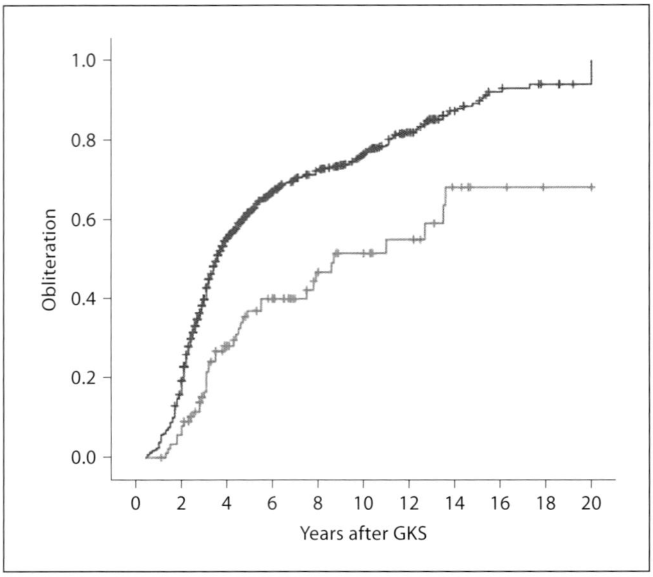

Fig. 3. Kaplan-Meier curves showing a higher obliteration rate in patients who did not have postradiosurgical hemorrhages (upper curve) compared to those with postradiosurgical hemorrhages (lower curve).

Table 6. Risk factors for a hemorrhage following Gamma Knife surgery

	No hemorrhage after GKS (n=1092)	Hemorrhage after GKS (n=112)	p value (univariate)	p value (multivariate)
Patient characteristics				
Male/female	581/511	56/56	0.928	–
Age of hemorrhage, years	35.4±16.1	34.4±17.0	0.826	–
AVM characteristics				
Location				
Lobar/deep	766/326	66/46	0.015*	0.271
Venous drainage				
Superficial only/deep venous drainage	546/546	54/58	0.982	–
Single/multiple draining veins	614/478	55/57	0.787	–
Prior hemorrhage (no/yes)	502/590	45/67	0.156	
Initial treatment parameters				
Volume of the nidus, cm^3	3.3±3.1	4.7±4.0	0.035*	0.214
Prescription dose, Gy	21.4±3.3	19.5±3.7	0.006*	0.046*
Maximum dose, Gy	39.6±7.3	37.4±6.9	0.231	–
Isodose line, %	55.2±11.4	52.6±8.4	0.081	–
Isocenters, n	2.8±2.2	2.9±1.7	0.480	–

Asterisks indicate statistically significant p values.

and eventual AVM obliteration [43]. A low dose of radiation delivered to an AVM is generally an ineffective dose as a peripheral dose of less than 16 Gy seldom achieves AVM obliteration.

Hemorrhage and AVM Obliteration

Among 1,054 patients with a follow-up of at least 2 years, the AVM obliteration rate (based on MRI or angiography) is lower in patients with postradiosurgical hemorrhage (fig. 3). In 92 patients with postradiosurgical hemorrhage, 51 (55.4%) AVMs remained patent at the last follow-up (mean follow-up 106.8 months, range 24–240 months). In 962 patients without hemorrhage, 271 (28.2%) AVMs remained patent ($p < 0.001$). None of our patients had sustained a hemorrhage following angiographic confirmation of AVM obliteration.

Conclusions

The natural hemorrhage rate in AVMs ranges from 2 to 4%, and the rate seems to be somewhat elevated in the immediate period following a prior hemorrhage. Although small AVMs are more likely to present with hemorrhage, smaller AVMs do not seem to be associated with a high hemorrhage rate once the AVMs have been diagnosed. Deeply located AVMs are more consistently associated with a hemorrhagic presentation as well as a higher rate of hemorrhage following their diagnosis. Other angioarchitectural features such as deep draining veins, venous stenosis or unsecured aneurysms are also associated with a higher hemorrhage rate.

Our experience and a review of the literature provide further evidence that patients remain at risk for hemorrhage as long as the nidus remains patent after radiosurgery. Although we have not observed a recurrent hemorrhage as long as the nidus was found to be obliterated based upon angiography, sporadic case reports of postobliteration hemorrhage call for continuous follow-up of the AVM patients even after radiographic confirmation of nidus obliteration.

References

1 Olivecrona H, Riives J: Arteriovenous aneurysms of the brain, their diagnosis and treatment. Arch Neurol Psychiatry 1948;59:567–602.

2 Brown RD Jr, Wiebers DO, Forbes G, O'Fallon WM, Piepgras DG, Marsh WR, et al: The natural history of unruptured intracranial arteriovenous malformations. J Neurosurg 1988;68:352–357.

3 Graf CJ, Perret GE, Torner JC: Bleeding from cerebral arteriovenous malformations as part of their natural history. J Neurosurg 1983;58:331–337.

4 Ondra SL, Troupp H, George ED, Schwab K: The natural history of symptomatic arteriovenous malformations of the brain: a 24-year follow-up assessment. J Neurosurg 1990;73:387–391.

5 Troupp H, Marttila I, Halonen V: Arteriovenous malformations of the brain. Prognosis without operation. Acta Neurochir (Wien) 1970;22:125–128.

6 Steiner L, Leksell L, Greitz T, Forster DM, Backlund EO: Stereotaxic radiosurgery for cerebral arteriovenous malformations. Report of a case. Acta Chir Scand 1972;138:459–464.

7 Steiner L, Lindquist C, Adler JR, Torner JC, Alves W, Steiner M: Clinical outcome of radiosurgery for cerebral arteriovenous malformations. J Neurosurg 1992;77:1–8.
8 Lunsford LD, Kondziolka D, Flickinger JC, Bissonette DJ, Jungreis CA, Maitz AH, et al: Stereotactic radiosurgery for arteriovenous malformations of the brain. J Neurosurg 1991;75:512–524.
9 Flickinger JC, Pollock BE, Kondziolka D, Lunsford LD: A dose-response analysis of arteriovenous malformation obliteration after radiosurgery. Int J Radiat Oncol Biol Phys 1996;36:873–879.
10 Kondziolka D, McLaughlin MR, Kestle JR: Simple risk predictions for arteriovenous malformation hemorrhage. Neurosurgery 1995;37:851–855.
11 Crawford PM, West CR, Chadwick DW, Shaw MD: Arteriovenous malformations of the brain: natural history in unoperated patients. J Neurol Neurosurg Psychiatry 1986;49:1–10.
12 Itoyama Y, Uemura S, Ushio Y, Kuratsu J, Nonaka N, Wada H, et al: Natural course of unoperated intracranial arteriovenous malformations: study of 50 cases. J Neurosurg 1989;71:805–809.
13 Yamane F, Takeshita M, Izawa M, Kagawa M, Sato K, Takakura K: Natural history of arteriovenous malformations: analysis of non-radically treated patients. J Clin Neurosci 1998;5(suppl):26–29.
14 Stefani MA, Porter PJ, ter Brugge KG, Montanera W, Willinsky RA, Wallace MC: Angioarchitectural factors present in brain arteriovenous malformations associated with hemorrhagic presentation. Stroke 2002;33:920–924.
15 Pollock BE, Flickinger JC, Lunsford LD, Bissonette DJ, Kondziolka D: Hemorrhage risk after stereotactic radiosurgery of cerebral arteriovenous malformations. Neurosurgery 1996;38:652–659, discussion 659–661.
16 Maruyama K, Kawahara N, Shin M, Tago M, Kishimoto J, Kurita H, et al: The risk of hemorrhage after radiosurgery for cerebral arteriovenous malformations. N Engl J Med 2005;352:146–153.
17 Maruyama K, Shin M, Tago M, Kishimoto J, Morita A, Kawahara N: Radiosurgery to reduce the risk of first hemorrhage from brain arteriovenous malformations. Neurosurgery 2007;60:453–458, discussion 458–459.
18 Mast H, Young WL, Koennecke HC, Sciacca RR, Osipov A, Pile-Spellman J, et al: Risk of spontaneous haemorrhage after diagnosis of cerebral arteriovenous malformation. Lancet 1997;350:1065–1068.
19 Stefani MA, Porter PJ, ter Brugge KG, Montanera W, Willinsky RA, Wallace MC: Large and deep brain arteriovenous malformations are associated with risk of future hemorrhage. Stroke 2002;33:1220–1224.
20 Halim AX, Johnston SC, Singh V, McCulloch CE, Bennett JP, Achrol AS, et al: Longitudinal risk of intracranial hemorrhage in patients with arteriovenous malformation of the brain within a defined population. Stroke 2004;35:1697–1702.
21 Stapf C, Mast H, Sciacca RR, Choi JH, Khaw AV, Connolly ES, et al: Predictors of hemorrhage in patients with untreated brain arteriovenous malformation. Neurology 2006;66:1350–1355.
22 Yamada S, Takagi Y, Nozaki K, Kikuta K, Hashimoto N: Risk factors for subsequent hemorrhage in patients with cerebral arteriovenous malformations. J Neurosurg 2007;107:965–972.
23 Hernesniemi JA, Dashti R, Juvela S, Vaart K, Niemela M, Laakso A: Natural history of brain arteriovenous malformations: a long-term follow-up study of risk of hemorrhage in 238 patients. Neurosurgery 2008;63:823–829, discussion 829–831.
24 Da Costa L, Wallace MC, ter Brugge KG, O'Kelly C, Willinsky RA, Tymianski M: The natural history and predictive features of hemorrhage from brain arteriovenous malformations. Stroke 2009;40:100–105.
25 Marks MP, Lane B, Steinberg GK, Chang PJ: Hemorrhage in intracerebral arteriovenous malformations: angiographic determinants. Radiology 1990;176:807–813.
26 Kader A, Young WL, Pile-Spellman J, Mast H, Sciacca RR, Mohr JP, et al: The influence of hemodynamic and anatomic factors on hemorrhage from cerebral arteriovenous malformations. Neurosurgery 1994;34:801–807, discussion 807–808.
27 Turjman F, Massoud TF, Vinuela F, Sayre JW, Guglielmi G, Duckwiler G: Correlation of the angioarchitectural features of cerebral arteriovenous malformations with clinical presentation of hemorrhage. Neurosurgery 1995;37:856–860, discussion 860–862.
28 Duong DH, Young WL, Vang MC, Sciacca RR, Mast H, Koennecke HC, et al: Feeding artery pressure and venous drainage pattern are primary determinants of hemorrhage from cerebral arteriovenous malformations. Stroke 1998;29:1167–1176.
29 Steinberg GK, Fabrikant JI, Marks MP, Levy RP, Frankel KA, Phillips MH, et al: Stereotactic heavy-charged-particle Bragg-peak radiation for intracranial arteriovenous malformations. N Engl J Med 1990;323:96–101.
30 Karlsson B, Lindquist C, Steiner L: Effect of Gamma Knife surgery on the risk of rupture prior to AVM obliteration. Minim Invasive Neurosurg 1996;39:21–27.

31 Colombo F, Pozza F, Chierego G, Casentini L, De Luca G, Francescon P: Linear accelerator radiosurgery of cerebral arteriovenous malformations: an update. Neurosurgery 1994;34:14–20, discussion 21.
32 Friedman WA, Blatt DL, Bova FJ, Buatti JM, Mendenhall WM, Kubilis PS: The risk of hemorrhage after radiosurgery for arteriovenous malformations. J Neurosurg 1996;84:912–919.
33 Kjellberg RN, Hanamura T, Davis KR, Lyons SL, Adams RD: Bragg-peak proton-beam therapy for arteriovenous malformations of the brain. N Engl J Med 1983;309:269–274.
34 Kasliwal MK, Kale SS, Gupta A, Kiran NA, Sharma MS, Agrawal D, et al: Does hemorrhagic presentation in cerebral arteriovenous malformations affect obliteration rate after gamma knife radiosurgery? Clin Neurol Neurosurg 2008;110:804–809.
35 Nataf F, Ghossoub M, Schlienger M, Moussa R, Meder JF, Roux FX: Bleeding after radiosurgery for cerebral arteriovenous malformations. Neurosurgery 2004;55:298–305, discussion 306.
36 Karlsson B, Lax I, Soderman M: Risk for hemorrhage during the 2-year latency period following gamma knife radiosurgery for arteriovenous malformations. Int J Radiat Oncol Biol Phys 2001;49: 1045–1051.
37 Liscak R, Vladyka V, Simonova G, Urgosik D, Novotny J Jr, Janouskova L, et al: Arteriovenous malformations after Leksell gamma knife radiosurgery: rate of obliteration and complications. Neurosurgery 2007;60:1005–1014, discussion 1015–1016.
38 Lindquist C, Steiner L: Stereotactic radiosurgical treatment of arteriovenous malformations; in Lunsford LD (ed): Modern Stereotactic Neurosurgery. Boston, Nijhoff, 1988, pp 491–505.
39 Lindqvist M, Karlsson B, Guo WY, Kihlstrom L, Lippitz B, Yamamoto M: Angiographic long-term follow-up data for arteriovenous malformations previously proven to be obliterated after gamma knife radiosurgery. Neurosurgery 2000;46:803–808, discussion 809–810.
40 Kader A, Goodrich JT, Sonstein WJ, Stein BM, Carmel PW, Michelsen WJ: Recurrent cerebral arteriovenous malformations after negative postoperative angiograms. J Neurosurg 1996;85:14–18.
41 Yen CP, Varady P, Sheehan J, Steiner M, Steiner L: Subtotal obliteration of cerebral arteriovenous malformations after gamma knife surgery. J Neurosurg 2007;106:361–369.
42 Karlsson B, Lindquist C, Steiner L: Prediction of obliteration after gamma knife surgery for cerebral arteriovenous malformations. Neurosurgery 1997; 40:425–430, discussion 430–431.
43 Schneider BF, Eberhard DA, Steiner LE: Histopathology of arteriovenous malformations after gamma knife radiosurgery. J Neurosurg 1997;87: 352–357.

Jason P. Sheehan, MD, PhD
Department of Neuroscience, University of Virginia
PO Box 801392
Charlottesville, VA 22908 (USA)
Tel. +1 434 924 2203, E-Mail jps2f@Virginia.edu

Niranjan A, Kano H, Lunsford LD (eds): Gamma Knife Radiosurgery for Brain Vascular Malformations.
Prog Neurol Surg. Basel, Karger, 2013, vol 27, pp 22–34 (DOI: 10.1159/000341625)

The Technical Evolution of Gamma Knife Radiosurgery for Arteriovenous Malformations

L. Dade Lunsford · Ajay Niranjan · Hideyuki Kano · Douglas Kondziolka

Department of Neurological Surgery and Center for Image-Guided Neurosurgery, University of Pittsburgh Medical Center, Pittsburgh, Pa., USA

Abstract

Gamma Knife stereotactic radiosurgery was first applied for the treatment of an intracranial arteriovenous malformation (AVM) in 1968. Using biplane angiography to target a small-volume, deep-seated lesion, photons were cross-fired on the pathological shunt. The AVM was obliterated within 3 years. This began a cautious introduction of Gamma Knife radiosurgery in the 1970s. As the Gamma Knife technology spread to sites in Europe, South America and the USA in the 1980s, AVM radiosurgery became a primary indication. During the early years the usual standard was to deliver a single radiosurgical isocenter to the target defined by 2-dimensional angiography. Most patients had small-volume AVMs unsuitable for surgical excision. Over time the technique of Gamma Knife AVM surgery evolved to include: careful patient selection, discussion of appropriate treatment strategies, anticonvulsant administration for lobar locations and intraoperative targeting using both high-resolution axial plane imaging – usually magnetic resonance imaging – coupled with biplane digital subtraction angiography. High-speed computer dose planning integrated with more detailed imaging strategies facilitated conformal radiation delivery in a single treatment session coupled with high selectivity of the dose delivered. Multiple isocenters became routine. Long-term follow-up care included serial imaging evaluations to assess the response and to detect complications. Imaging was critical to confirm the desired radiobiological response – complete obliteration. Long-term follow-up after obliteration confirmed that AVM radiosurgery had a high success rate for properly selected patients and a risk-benefit profile that substantiated patient safety. Twenty-year results after Gamma Knife radiosurgery for AVMs are currently available. Established roles have been found for pediatric cases and for larger-volume AVMs unsuitable for surgical removal. The role and technique of embolization prior to radiosurgery continue to be evaluated. Current dose response data based on volume and predictions of adverse radiation effects guide current care.

The First Applications of Radiosurgery for Arteriovenous Malformations

The relative rarity of brain arteriovenous malformations (AVMs) – with perhaps only 10,000 new patients identified in the USA each year – has led to considerable debate as to which management strategies are best for individual patients. Patients with symptomatic hemorrhages, recurrent seizures or increasing neurological deficits are often selected for surgical removal by craniotomy. Increasingly, endovascular procedures designed for reduction of the AVM flow or even obliteration were added into the overall management algorithm. Despite advances in surgical, endovascular and critical care of patients with AVMs, not all patients had satisfactory outcomes, and some had no management options at all. Deep-seated AVMs in critical locations were considered unsuitable for surgery because of the excessive risks.

Lars Leksell first coined the term and described the field of stereotactic radiosurgery (SRS) in 1951. He initially coupled an orthovoltage X-ray tube with an early-generation brain stereotactic guiding device in order to precisely irradiate the gasserian ganglion in patients with intractable, medically unresponsive trigeminal neuralgia. Leksell envisioned a cautious growth of this field and during the next 35 years explored a variety of radiosurgical technologies as he sought to offer potentially safer, minimally invasive, more precise brain surgery. Discouraged by the often poor outcomes of patients subjected to conventional management in the era between 1930 and 1970, he believed that a less invasive methodology might improve patient outcomes in a wide variety of functional disorders as well as various brain tumors. This brilliant surgeon and neurophysiologist collaborated extensively with radiobiologist and physicist Borje Larsson at both the Karolinska Hospital in Stockholm and the Gustaf Werner Institute in Uppsala, Sweden. Larsson directed the proton beam project in Uppsala. Leksell had developed a specially designed, human stereotactic guiding device that could treat patients with selective movement disorders and severe neurotic behavior disorders in an era when there were few medical alternatives. Their work was carefully based on ongoing radiobiological research in animals. The goat was the chosen investigational animal. After proton beam radiosurgery (using cross-fired proton beams rather than the Bragg peak effect), Larsson cared for the goats on his farm in Sweden. At the time of the goat's natural death, the brains were studied to assess the pathological response.

Leksell was not happy with the logistical difficulties of transporting patients from the hospital environment in Stockholm to Uppsala in order to undergo proton radiosurgery. Leksell and Larsson decided that a dedicated hospital unit that generated similar energy photons (6 MeV) was a better solution. The first *strålkniven* – Gamma Knife – contained 179 cobalt sources arrayed in a hemisphere. Photon beams emitted by the cobalt sources were focused via a secondary collimator helmet to an intracranial target defined by imaging after a stereotactic head frame had been attached to the head for target recognition using various imaging modalities. The first Gamma Knife was placed in the Sophiahemmet in Stockholm in 1968. However, the first patient (with a craniopharyngioma) was treated by Leksell and Backlund in 1968 at the site of the Gamma Knife manufacturing site in Linkoping. Leksell and selected members of his faculty at the Karolinska Hospital thereafter collaborated on the introduction of the Gamma Knife for a variety of emerging clinical indications. Although Leksell's primary interest was in functional disorders such as chronic pain, movement disorders and refractory neuroses, he was persuaded by his colleagues to cautiously introduce focused irradiation for other potential vascular and neoplastic lesions. Working with George Norén, they treated the first acoustic neuroma in 1971.

Ladislau Steiner persuaded Leksell to allow him to treat a single AVM patient. Leksell was a cautious individual, and he desired evidence that applications of the Gamma Knife were both safe and effective in the context of each clinical disorder. He authorized Steiner to treat the first patient in 1968, and their initial publication that described the results of the first patient was published in 1972 [1]. This initial patient had a deep-seated AVM identified by biplane angiography. A maximum dose of 50 Gy was administered to the small-volume AVM using the prototype Gamma Knife unit. The appropriate therapeutic dose was unknown, and the early dose planning systems were rudimentary compared to today's technologies. Within a matter of several years, Steiner demonstrated that follow-up angiography showed complete obliteration of the AVM.

This first successful case opened the door for an increasing application of radiosurgery in the management of small-volume AVMs. The Karolinska Hospital became a worldwide referral site for AVM treatment. By the time the senior author studied in Stockholm between 1980 and 1981, a large volume of patients were being treated on an annual basis. Characteristically, these AVMs had small volumes, were deeply located and received a relatively high dose in a single session, that being the paradigm of radiosurgery established by Leksell. The technology required biplane angiography for targeting and then calculation of the appropriate dose by the resident medical physicist, most commonly Jurgen Arndt, who was himself a pioneer in radiosurgery. By 1975, the potential value of Gamma Knife radiosurgery had been realized by Leksell and his team. Leksell and Larsson arranged for construction of a second Gamma Knife, modified to have more spherical collimator openings that facilitated more volumetric shaping of 3-dimensional morphological targets within the brain.

Disciples of Leksell, specifically David Forster in Sheffield, UK, and Hernan Bunge in Buenos Aires, Argentina, persuaded Leksell to allow construction of two additional Gamma units. Built in Switzerland in the early 1980s, units III and IV initially envisioned a technology that in practice would take more than 20 years to eventually reach introduction as the Perfexion® model. The patient was to be fixed to the bed which would move robotically to place the brain target at the center of the 179 converging photon beams. Unfortunately, the vision was premature compared to the engineering technologies then available, and eventually both units were reconfigured to have the operating surgeon manually place the patient's head frame in the focus of the beams.

In 1987, Gamma unit V – the first to have 201 cobalt sources and the larger 18-mm diameter collimator helmet – was installed at the University of Pittsburgh. The most common indication in the first years was, in fact, AVM. During the course of the first 4 years, more than 220 patients underwent Gamma Knife radiosurgery for their AVM [2]. Replicating the initial work of Leksell and Steiner, single isocenters were used in 52% of patients and multiple isocenters in 48%. In most patients, targeting was performed using biplane angiography. Within 4 years, it became obvious that additional imaging in the axial plane would enhance additional 3-dimensional analysis of complex AVMs. Axial plane imaging help facilitated better 3-dimensional planning by showing not only the AVM nidus, but also the surrounding brain outside of the target. Using the earliest 0.5-tesla generation of magnetic resonance imaging (MRI), we soon replaced computed tomography with MRI, since better contrast resolution of the target and the brain was immediately obvious. Graphic recognition of the AVM volume in 3 dimensions began.

Over the next 10 years, increasing attention was paid to improve targeting, improve dose planning to obtain high-definition imaging in multiple planes under stereotactic conditions, and to eventually move from conventional magnification subtraction angiography to digital subtraction angiography.

By 2011 more than 11, 000 patients had undergone radiosurgery at the University of Pittsburgh, and more than 1,300 had AVMs. Tracking data provided by the manufacturer of the Gamma Knife, AB Elekta, indicated that more than 60,000 patients worldwide had undergone radiosurgery for AVMs by 2011.

Particle Beam Radiosurgery

Leksell was well aware of contemporaneous efforts of Raymond Kjellberg, who used the proton beam generated by the cyclotron donated to Harvard University by the US Department of the Navy in recognition of efforts done during World War II. Leksell also corresponded with the teams working with protons at the Lawrence Livermore Laboratory in Berkeley, Calif. Although the initial investigators used protons as early as 1954 for pituitary ablation, the synchrocyclotron was eventually modified to generate helium ion beams. Both the Boston and Berkeley sites used the Bragg peak delivery concept of particle radiation energy. At Berkeley Jack Fabrikant and Gary Steinberg treated a large volume of intracranial AVM patients, usually using a staged approach of three fractions [3]. Kjellberg in Boston preferred the single treatment technique, which he called stereotactic Bragg peak irradiation. Although it fit the paradigm of radiosurgery, i.e. a single treatment session done under stereotactic conditions, Kjellberg himself was averse to the term radiosurgery. He irradiated more than 1,000 patients using the proton beam prior to his death [4].

Kjellberg hypothesized that the biological effect of the single treatment session radiation would lead to intravascular luminal changes and eventually reduce the risk of bleeding events by stabilization of the blood vessel walls. Approximately 19% of his patients achieved angiographically confirmed complete obliteration of the AVM [5]. Kjellberg maintained that the treatment reduced death rates from bleeding compared to a life table insurance survival analysis that he used as a comparison group. In part because of the high expense and poor access to proton facilities, the Gamma Knife became an increasingly valuable alternative at major medical centers. The field of SRS for AVMs blossomed.

Current Technique for Gamma Knife Radiosurgery

Initial Evaluation

As in all neurosurgical procedures, optimal patient selection is necessary in order to maximize benefits and to reduce risks. Most AVM patients suitable for radiosurgery have relatively small AVMs located in critical structures of the brain and have high risks for alternative managements including surgery and endovascular embolization. Many patients have already suffered a bleeding event. Recent data suggests that such a bleeding event significantly increases subsequent risks of additional episodes, especially in the first 6 months after the bleed [6]. Additional patients may present with a seizure disorder or on rare occasions stepwise neurological deterioration. AVMs located within or adjacent to the motor cortex or the corticospinal tract itself often lead to earlier recognition because of their effect on motor movement. AVMs are easily confirmed now using computed tomography or MRI. When all therapeutic options including primary surgery are to be considered, patients need to have high-definition, high-resolution digital subtraction angiography. Relatively few patients are selected for radiosurgery based on MRI alone. In rare cases, patients with relatively small AVMs in deep, critical locations (for which neither surgery nor embolization are good alternatives) may have the angiogram performed during the time of the Gamma Knife procedure itself.

Patient Selection

The patient's diagnostic imaging studies, including MRI and angiography, are reviewed by a multidisciplinary team who can best advise the patient and family relative to therapeutic options. Many patients obtain opinions from various centers. Patients who wish to undergo Gamma Knife management are seen in advance of the scheduled procedure, and their physical findings and medical history are reviewed. It is important to eliminate antiplatelet agents in preparation for angiography. Unless patients need such agents because of other medical conditions such as stents or coronary artery disease, we prefer that all AVM patients remain off antiplatelet agents until their AVM is confirmed as obliterated. Patients with subcortical lobar AVMs with seizure disorders are maintained on their current medications, and anticonvulsant levels are checked for appropriate therapeutic doses when feasible. For patients with subcortical lobar AVMs without a history of prior seizures, we begin anticonvulsants several days before the procedure. At the present time, we prefer to use levetiracetam in doses starting at 1,000 mg/day. We have found this agent to be effective and to have a lower side effect profile compared to the usage of phenytoin. In the past we found that phenytoin was associated with significant side effects, including drug reactions, in up to 10% of patients.

Informed consent is obtained from the patient and family. Pediatric patients less than the age of 12 or 13 years, are seen by a member of the anesthesia department, who prepares the patient and family for anesthesia administration during the procedure the following day. Older children and adults also watch a teaching video of the procedure. This video demonstrates the nature of stereotactic head frame application and the role of intraoperative sedation as needed.

The Day of the Procedure

On the day of the procedure, patients and families arrive by 6 o'clock in the morning. Patients are prepared by the nursing team with an intravenous line and are given lorazepam 1 mg sublingually. After this, additional conscious sedation is administered using titrated dosages of midazolam and fentanyl in order to achieve satisfactory pain management. We balance the sedation in order to still have an awake and cooperative patient with normal vital signs and adequate respiration during the subsequent transport to the imaging sites. Blood pressure, electrocardiographic and pulse oxygenation measurements are made continually during the time of stereotactic head frame application. The Leksell model G stereotactic head frame is attached to the head using quick fixation titanium pins after regional infiltration of a combination of half-strength Marcaine and half-strength xylocaine. Some colleagues prefer to add small amounts of sodium bicarbonate to the local anesthetic in order to reduce burning from the injection. Others have abandoned the bicarbonate because of the occasional development of edema surrounding the pin site after frame removal. After the stereotactic head frame has been secured to the patient's head, coordinate measurements are made of the frame, and a bubble chamber is used to make radius measurements of the skull geometry (fig. 1). This data is introduced into the dose planning computer system. We began our Gamma Knife experience using the Kula system, and then supplemented it with an in-house image integrated planning system that ran on a Silicone Graphics computer. As the manufacturer began to introduce successive generations of the image integrated planning system known as Gamma Plan®, we switched to the use of a company-marketed planning system (AB Elekta, Stockholm, Sweden).

Next, the patient is transported to MRI and undergoes a full head, 2-mm contrast-enhanced volume acquisition followed by whole-head 3-mm nonskipping T_2-weighted images. In selected small-volume tumors or AVMs we use 1- to 1.5-mm slices to image the area of interest. The images are transferred electronically through the hospital Ethernet to the dose planning computer system. Dose planning is begun immediately using the MRI data, while the patient is transported to the angiographic suite. Under the direction of a trained endovascular specialist, digital subtraction biplane angiography is performed to identify the AVM target, to recognize proximal or intranidal aneurysms, and to assess venous outflow restrictions.

Preradiosurgery embolization has been used in between 15 and 18% of our patients, usually based on the nature of the referral pattern. We usually wait a minimum of 1 month after the last embolization procedure before considering radiosurgery. We

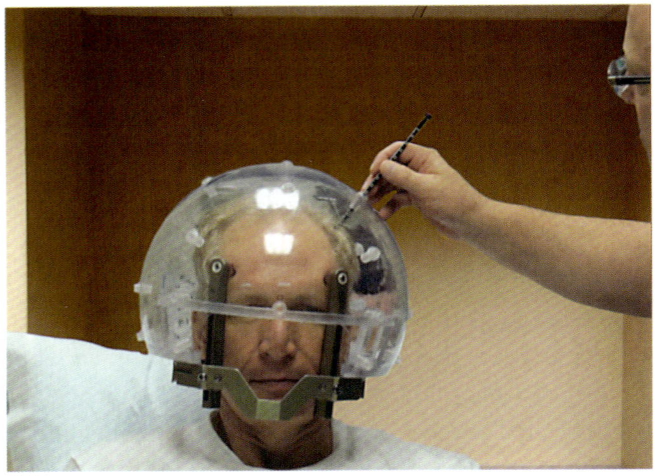

Fig. 1. After stereotactic head frame application, skull radius measurements are made and entered into the Gamma Plan dose planning system. These measurements are used for dose calculations and possible collision during the treatment. These measurements also confirm the correct patient when the subsequent stereotactic volumetric MRI images are downloaded into the dose planning computer.

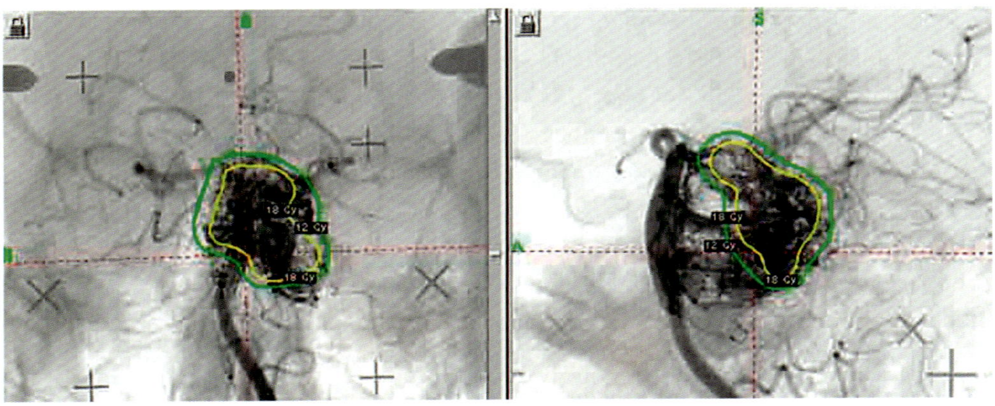

Fig. 2. Anterior and lateral vertebral artery angiograms documenting an AVM in the pons. The yellow line defines the radiosurgical target which will receive a minimal dose of 18 Gy. The maximal and marginal doses are selected based on the probability of obliteration and estimated risk of AREs, as suggested by the volume that receives ≥12 Gy in the single SRS procedure.

believe that this delay reduces the risk of delayed brain reactive changes or adverse radiation effects (AREs) after SRS.

Dose planning is completed after the digital subtraction angiograms have been chosen and scanned into the planning system (Leksell version 9.0–10.0). We review the necessary vascular injections needed to visualize the AVM with the angiographer in advance, and we select appropriate angiographic films to digitize into the dose planning computer. In general, anteroposterior and lateral images are selected (fig. 2). The views must define the nidus (the vascular shunt that lies between afferent feeding arteries and draining veins). We also select at least one view that demonstrates any early draining veins.

Dose planning is completed under the direction of the responsible neurosurgeon, a radiation oncologist and the medical physicist (fig. 3). After conformal planning, usually using the 50% isodose at the edge of the AVM, the dose volume histogram is reviewed. The edge dose is optimized, and the volume enclosed with the edge dose is chosen. For volumes less than 10 cm^3, we normally treat the AVM in a single session. For AVMs greater than 15 cm^3 in volume, we recommend staging of selected anatomical components of the AVM separated by at least 3 months. For AVMs in the 10- to 15-cm^3 range, we weigh staging versus a single session based on a number of other factors. These factors include the AVM volume, its location, the need to safely deliver ≥17 Gy to the margin of the AVM, and the age of the patient (for example children may require general anesthesia).

Currently, we use either the Leksell 4C or the Leksell Perfexion Gamma Knife. For deep-seated, more centrally located AVMs, the 4C is an excellent and reliable tool. For more eccentrically placed AVMs that are far lateral, or far anterior or posterior in the brain, the Perfexion unit, which is fully robotic at all times, has proven valuable (fig. 4).

Dose volume selections are based on our experience in more than 11,000 patients, a variety of publications from other centers, and estimation of the ARE related to the volume treated. Dose selection is modified based on the anatomical location of the AVM. AREs are much more likely to be detected in AVMs located in areas of critical brain function. The dose is selected after discussion between the physicist, the surgeon and the radiation oncologist. The dose plan specifies the location and the maximum and marginal dose. The plan is exported to the Gamma Knife itself, after which the patient is positioned on the bed. The final prescription is signed by the responsible neurosurgeon, radiation oncologist and medical physicist.

Postoperative Care

At the conclusion of the procedure, the patient's stereotactic head frame is removed, and the patient receives a single intravenous dose of 40 mg of methylprednisolone adjusted somewhat for age and weight. Headache after frame removal responds to acetaminophen or oxycodone. An additional anticonvulsant dose is delivered orally for patients with subcortical lobar AVMs. Currently, patients having angiography may be able to have their angiographic puncture closed using a quick-close technique, thereby allowing them to be up at 3 h. Previously, bed rest for 8 h after angiography was routine, and such patients routinely spent the night prior to discharge the next day. Most patients now go home on the same day, and the entire procedure is performed as an outpatient.

Long-Term Follow-Up

The response of the AVM to Gamma Knife SRS is assessed at selected intervals using clinical examinations and follow-up MRI. Our normal protocol is to obtain evaluations and imaging at 6 months, 1, 2 and 3 years. The response of the AVM is serially

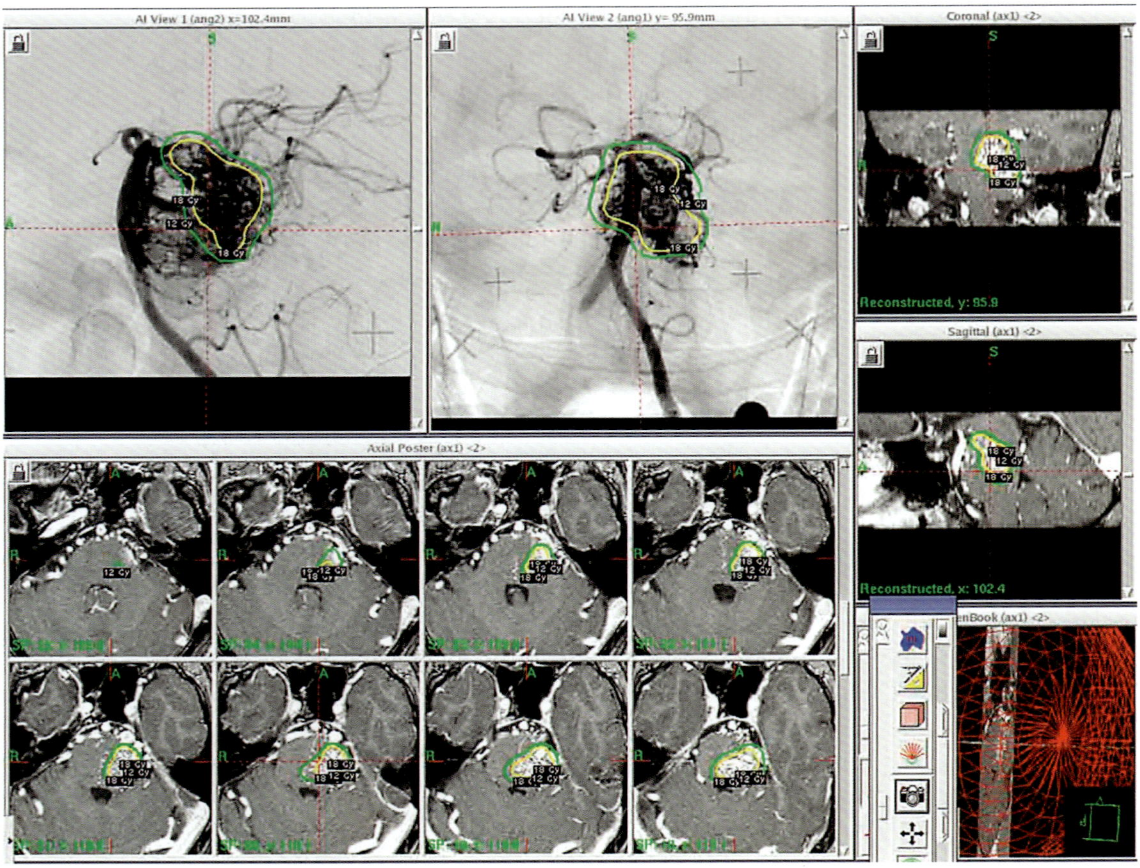

Fig. 3. Gamma Knife planning for a pontocerebellar AVM includes digital subtraction angiographic anteroposterior and lateral images, which are coupled with axial plane contrast-enhanced 1- to 2-mm images as well as T_2-weighted images.

Fig. 4. The patient is in position for SRS using the Leksell Perfexion Gamma Knife. After initiation of treatment, the patient is advanced into the Gamma Knife so that the 192 photon beams intersect at the initial isocenter. The bed robotically moves the patient to each successive isocenter as needed until the entire dose is delivered.

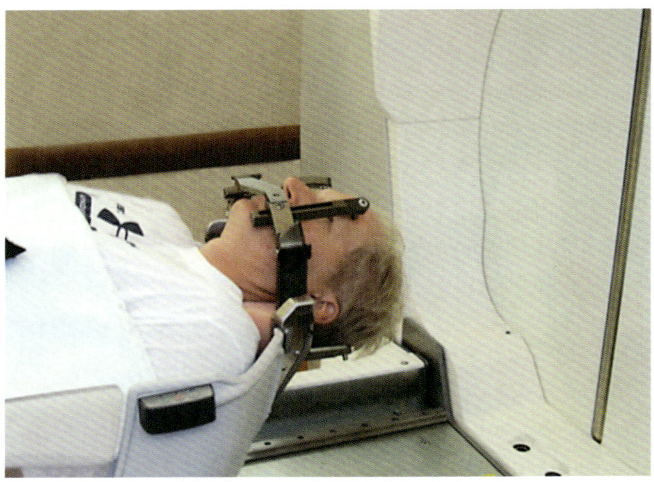

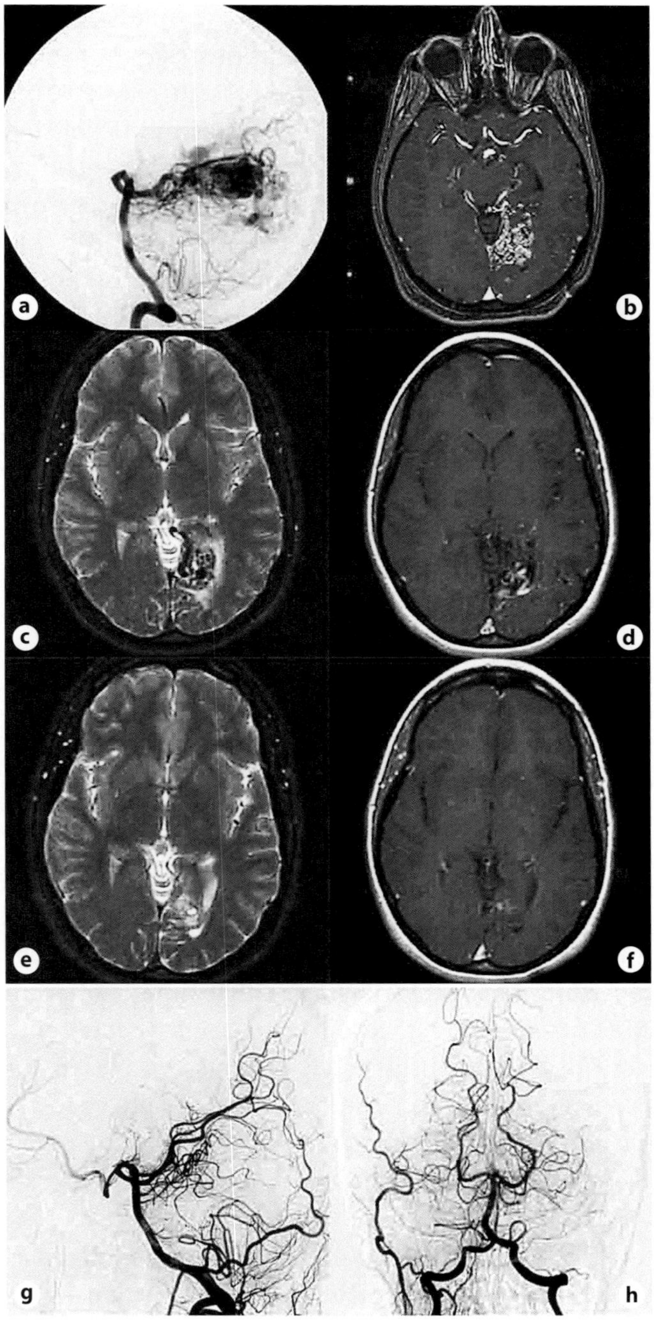

Fig. 5. **a** Lateral vertebral artery angiogram documenting an AVM in the left occipital lobe. **b** Axial T_1-weighted contrast-enhanced MR image showing a left occipital AVM. **c**, **d** Axial T_2- and T_1-weighted contrast-enhanced MR images obtained 1 year after radiosurgery showing a reduction of AVM nidus. **e**, **f** Axial T_2- and T_1-weighted contrast-enhanced MR images obtained 2 years after SRS showing the absence of a nidus. **g**, **h** Lateral and anteroposterior vertebral artery angiograms obtained 2 years after SRS showing the absence of a nidus and early venous drainage.

assessed with the expectation to see a gradual reduction in the MRI-defined flow voids over the course of several years (fig. 5). Patients are counseled that between 40 and 50% of optimally treated patients may have obliteration within the first year and 70–80% within the next 2 years. If an MRI including T_2-weighted imaging suggests complete obliteration of the AVM at the end of 3 years, then angiography is recommended at that time. If the angiogram confirms obliteration, the patients are recommended to get follow-up MRI at 2, 4 and 8 years after the procedure in order to monitor the long-term response and to assess for any potential long-term side effects.

Late cyst development has been seen in 1–2% of patients undergoing radiosurgery at our center. It appears to be more common in patients who originally had an intracerebral hemorrhage at the time of AVM presentation. We suspect that residual hemosiderin pigment acts as a radiation sensitizer which increases the risk of late brain cavitation at the target site.

Management of Adverse Radiation Effects

Although increasing data related to the risks of radiation injury is available, the development of AREs is not always predictable. Perhaps 4% of the world's population are hypersensitive to radiation, and even for small-volume AVMs treated with appropriate guideline doses, late radiation-related side effects can develop. AREs are usually related to the dose, volume and location.

In certain patients, nidus obliteration leads to a gradual reduction in flow through the shunt followed by an ictal thrombosis of the venous outflow. Such patients often have a sudden, severe headache, and a few may even have a seizure. Emergent imaging at that time is often thought to reveal a bleed, but MRI often shows that this represents venous outflow thrombosis rather than an AVM hemorrhage. Such patients are placed for approximately 2 weeks on corticosteroids, and such symptoms usually abate. At any time when a new ictal event occurs during the follow-up interval (including a seizure or suspected AVM bleed), we order a computed tomogram or preferably MRI to assess the patient status.

Patients with suspected AREs (defined as significant contrast uptake at the target site usually surrounded by a disproportionate high T_2-weighted signal change compatible with increased brain water content or cerebral edema) are first treated with corticosteroids. If admission is required, intravenous corticosteroids are used and then converted to oral corticosteroids. The senior author prefers methylprednisolone, since in his experience methylprednisolone has a lower risk profile, less potential for exacerbating glucose abnormalities and a reduced risk of steroid myopathy in comparison to dexamethasone. After 2 weeks, still symptomatic patients are usually switched to a combination of vitamin E 400 IU twice per day and Trental 400 mg twice per day [7]. These agents are used for a period of 3 months and have been shown to be associated with an increasing reduction of edema in the serial imaging studies [7].

The Roles of Gamma Knife Radiosurgery

Over the last 24 years, a steady growth in scientific publications has established the role of Gamma Knife radiosurgery in the management of small-volume AVMs, pediatric AVMs, brainstem, basal ganglia, thalamic and larger-volume AVMs unsuitable for surgical management. The role of embolization before or after radiosurgery continues to be evaluated. Increasing success with embolization has been reported by a variety of centers worldwide. Some centers report success rates (complete AVM closure) in the range of 40–70% [8–11]. Newer agents such as Onyx, a slower-polymerizing agent, has also been evaluated. Embolization per se may have a more important role in preparation for surgical removal of an AVM, since flow reduction may significantly improve surgical outcomes during craniotomy. Flow reduction alone has little value in the preparation for radiosurgery. Embolization must instead significantly and permanently exclude a component of the AVM, thereby reducing the volume of the target that needs to undergo radiosurgery. In our experience permanent volume reduction of a component of the AVM has proven to be a more elusive outcome after embolization. Embolization in the absence of volume reduction appears to have little benefit in the preparation for radiosurgery. In the future, embolization technologies that allow us to deliver AVM endothelial sensitizers or brain protectors may be an innovative method to improve the therapeutic index of embolization in combination with radiosurgery.

Conclusions

Since the first brilliant insight of Lars Leksell, radiosurgery has gradually matured and become a mainstream strategy for AVM management. Using highly refined imaging performed under stereotactic guidance, targeting of the pathological AVM shunt has become possible. Modern dose planning systems are very efficient. Using a multidisciplinary team to select, to target and to treat AVM patients has resulted in steadily improving results.

References

1 Steiner L, Leksell L, Greitz T, Forster DM, Backlund EO: Stereotaxic radiosurgery for cerebral arteriovenous malformations. Report of a case. Acta Chir Scand 1972;138:459–464.

2 Lunsford LD, Kondziolka D, Flickinger JC, Bissonette DJ, Jungreis CA, Maitz AH, Horton JA, Coffey RJ: Stereotactic radiosurgery for arteriovenous malformations of the brain. J Neurosurg 1991;75:512–524.

3 Fabrikant JI, Levy RP, Steinberg GK, Silverberg GD, Frankel KA, Phillips MH, Lyman JT: Heavy-charged-particle radiosurgery for intracranial arteriovenous malformations. Stereotact Funct Neurosurg 1991;57:50–63.

4 Kjellberg RN, Hanamura T, Davis KR, Lyons SL, Adams RD: Bragg-peak proton-beam therapy for arteriovenous malformations of the brain. N Engl J Med 1983;309:269–274.

5 Kjellberg RN: Stereotactic Bragg peak proton beam radiosurgery for cerebral arteriovenous malformations. Ann Clin Res 1986;18(suppl 47):17–19.

6 Pollock BE, Flickinger JC, Lunsford LD, Bissonette DJ, Kondziolka D: Factors that predict the bleeding risk of cerebral arteriovenous malformations. Stroke 1996;27:1–6.

7 Williamson R, Kondziolka D, Kanaan H, Lunsford LD, Flickinger JC: Adverse radiation effects after radiosurgery may benefit from oral vitamin E and pentoxifylline therapy: a pilot study. Stereotact Funct Neurosurg 2008;86:359–366.

8 Andrade-Souza YM, Ramani M, Scora D, Tsao MN, ter Brugge K, Schwartz ML: Embolization before radiosurgery reduces the obliteration rate of arteriovenous malformations. Neurosurgery 2007;60:443–451, discussion 451–452.

9 Gobin YP, Laurent A, Merienne L, Schlienger M, Aymard A, Houdart E, Casasco A, Lefkopoulos D, George B, Merland JJ: Treatment of brain arteriovenous malformations by embolization and radiosurgery. J Neurosurg 1996;85:19–28.

10 Henkes H, Nahser HC, Berg-Dammer E, Weber W, Lange S, Kuhne D: Endovascular therapy of brain AVMs prior to radiosurgery. Neurol Res 1998;20:479–492.

11 Miyachi S, Negoro M, Okamoto T, Kobayashi T, Kida Y, Tanaka T, Yoshida J: Embolisation of cerebral arteriovenous malformations to assure successful subsequent radiosurgery. J Clin Neurosci 2000;7(suppl 1):82–85.

L. Dade Lunsford, MD, FACS
Lars Leksell Distinguished Professor of Neurological Surgery
University of Pittsburgh, Suite B-400, UPMC Presbyterian
200 Lothrop Street
Pittsburgh, PA 15213 (USA)
Tel. +1 412 647 6781, E-Mail lunsfordld@upmc.edu

Niranjan A, Kano H, Lunsford LD (eds): Gamma Knife Radiosurgery for Brain Vascular Malformations.
Prog Neurol Surg. Basel, Karger, 2013, vol 27, pp 35–48 (DOI: 10.1159/000341628)

Targeting and Conformality in Arteriovenous Malformation Radiosurgery

Ian Paddick[a–e] · Enrico Motti[f,g]

[a]Cromwell Gamma Knife Centre and [b]London Gamma Knife Centre at Barts, London, and [c]Thornbury Radiosurgery Centre, Sheffield, [d]National Centre for Neurology and Neurosurgery, Queen Square, London, UK; [e]St. Elisabeth Hospital, Tilburg, The Netherlands; [f]Department of Neurological Sciences, Neurosurgery, Università di Milano, Milano, and [g]Neurosurgery, Maria Cecilia Hospital, Ravenna, Italy

Abstract

The struggle to achieve a high degree of conformity around targets of complex morphology has been one of the driving forces in the development of ever more sophisticated radiosurgical devices and intricate treatment delivery. Rarely are radiosurgical targets more complex in shape than those associated with arteriovenous malformations (AVMs). In this report we examine theoretical and practical issues of target delineation and creation of conformal AVM treatment plans, and comment on the concepts of gradient and homogeneity.

Arteriovenous malformations (AVMs) are widely considered as technically tricky radiosurgical indications to treat, in terms of targeting, due to additional imaging procedures and an apparent 'subjectivity' of target delineation, as demonstrated in papers showing significant interobserver variation [1, 2]. Conformity, the principle of maximizing coverage of the target and minimizing dose to normal tissues, should in theory increase nidal obliteration rates and reduce complications. Certainly, the fact that radiosurgery of a brain lesion is at all possible is due to the high conformity of the dose. However, as yet, there is little evidence in the literature that conformity to the nidal target is related to successful treatment. This is possibly due to many other clinical and dose plan-related variables that confound the data.

Paradoxically, the world's first successful radiosurgery treatment of an AVM by Steiner in 1970 was far from conformal [3]. Only a small fraction of the nidus was covered by the prescription dose of 25 Gy. Instead of aiming for conformity, a single isocentre was used to target the main feeding artery. While this planning technique could be considered suboptimal when compared with modern techniques, the remarkable efficacy of this early treatment suggests that some AVMs require very little therapy to precipitate closure. Therefore, conformity indices are not the only method that should be used to evaluate the suitability of AVM treatment plans. Indeed, the current planning philosophy of delineating the margin of the vascular lesion then working on conformal coverage may need to be re-evaluated.

Most planning techniques described in this report are those applied with Gamma Knife radiosurgery (GKRS), being the most widely used device in the treatment of AVMs, with over 66,000 having been treated with this technique up to December 2010. However, general aspects of target definition and planning techniques covered here can be applied to all radiosurgical devices.

Imaging Methods

Magnetic resonance imaging has now become standard for targeting in GKRS. Other digital imaging modalities serving special radiosurgery niches – computed tomography (CT), positron emission tomography, magneto-encephalography – are supplementary. For AVMs the valuable information provided by magnetic resonance imaging must be integrated with the dynamic information provided by digital subtraction angiography [4]. Angio-CT has been employed [5], but appealing as it is to obtain angio-architectural information by a non-invasive method, the technique is currently inadequate on a number of levels and will likely be entirely superseded by 3-dimensional rotational angiography as soon as the tools that allow its registration in stereotactic space become more widely available [6].

Target Definition

The outlining of a solid tumour on a gadolinium-enhanced T_1-weighted image sequence is often as simple as segmenting between high and low signal strengths. However, an AVM nidus rarely allows us the luxury of such simple delineation. The notion of defining an AVM anatomically is simplistic. AVMs vary greatly in their shape, size and complexity [7]. Whilst some malformations are inherently well defined, with an easily perceived margin, others may be much more diffuse. Additionally, there may be associated vascular changes, so-called neovascularization, angiogenesis or recruitment meaning the pressing into exceptional service (and consequent dilation/hypertrophy) of normal vessels, which are otherwise invisible on normal angiograms due to their small diameter. This produces regions adjacent to an AVM in which the blood vessels appear abnormal, but are not part of the shunting malformation. As a consequence, exactly what constitutes the AVM nidus is open to a degree of interpretation, and the extent of this will vary depending on the AVM morphology (compact or diffuse). For this reason, a much higher level of clinical input and review is required for AVM planning, often including a radiologist, neurosurgeon and physicist

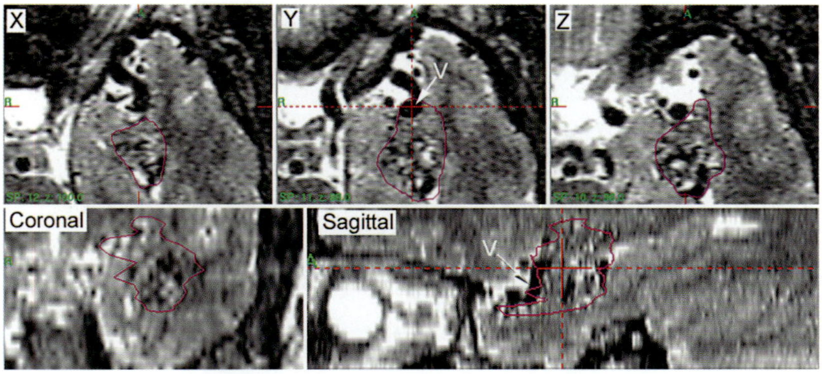

Fig. 1. A target outlined (in magenta) by a radiologist on 2-mm-thick T_2-weighted magnetic resonance images. While slice Y covers the vessel labelled 'v', the outlines on the slices on either side, X and Z, omit this vessel. It will be impossible for the treatment planner to avoid spilling dose outside the target on slices X and Z if they are to cover the target on slice Y. Unless corrected, the dose planner pays a penalty in terms of conformity for this inconsistency. Note the telltale zigzag appearance of the target on the coronal and sagittal images.

amongst others: we take exception with the view that in AVMs radiosurgical success is not as reliant on the expertise of practitioners as the dexterity of the neurosurgeon is for microsurgery [8].

A consistent and smooth outlining of the nidus is essential if the treatment planner is to have a possibility of achieving a conformal plan. This does not mean that the shape of the nidal target needs to be simplified, but it is essential that the outline remains consistent from slice to slice and structures that are outlined on one slice are not unintentionally excluded on neighbouring slices. For Gamma Knife users, the 'display volume templates' function in Leksell Gamma Plan allows an outline to be projected onto its neighbouring slice. Equivalent features exist in other radiosurgery planning systems. This ensures that the clinician outlining the target is aware of which adjacent structures have already been defined as target, aiding consistency. A simple test to confirm consistency is to view the target outline on planes orthogonal to the images used for delineation (e.g. sagittal and coronal images if axial images were used for outlining). These reconstructed outlines should be no more meandering than the original outlines used to construct them. Reconstructed outlines with a tell-tale zigzag betray targeting inconsistencies (fig. 1).

Conformity Indices

Delineation of nidal volumes is susceptible to interobserver variability [1, 2]. However, without outlining, conformity is merely a subjective notion. A degree of objectivity may need to be applied, via an index. There are many definitions of conformity, with their respective indices. The two most commonly used are the Prescription Isodose to Target Volume Ratio (PITV) as defined by Shaw et al. [9] and the New Conformity Index by Paddick [10]. These are defined respectively as:

$$\mathrm{PITV} = \frac{\mathrm{PIV}}{\mathrm{TV}} \qquad (1)$$

where PIV is the prescription isodose volume and TV is the target volume, and

$$\text{New Conformity Index (Paddick)} = \frac{\mathrm{TV}_{\mathrm{PIV}}}{\mathrm{TV}} \times \frac{\mathrm{TV}_{\mathrm{PIV}}}{\mathrm{PIV}} = \frac{\mathrm{TV}_{\mathrm{PIV}}^{2}}{\mathrm{TV} \times \mathrm{PIV}} \qquad (2)$$

where $\mathrm{TV}_{\mathrm{PIV}}$ is the volume of target encompassed by the prescription isodose.

While the former index is simple to calculate, it does not take into account either the proportion of the target treated or the amount of normal tissue covered by the prescription isodose. As a result, false 'perfect' scores can be obtained when scoring far-from-conformal plans. The Paddick index takes into account the amount of over- and undertreatment, ensuring no false perfect scores. An ideal score with Shaw's index is 1.00, or slightly higher (experienced users know that a perfect score of 1.00 is usually a false one). A score of less than unity suggests a lack of target coverage, and a score over unity suggests excessive treatment of normal tissues. Paddick's index is between 0 and 1, with the highest score representing the most conformal plan.

Every treatment plan is a compromise between conformity and practicability (treatment time, number of beams). The art of the treatment planner is knowing when this balance is achieved and further refinement of the plan will merely increase treatment time, with negligible increases in conformity or clinical efficacy.

To maintain this balance, the radiosurgeon may sometimes have to prioritize which parts of the nidal border are 'conformal' and which ones are 'suboptimal'. Neighbouring structures often include cerebrospinal fluid of the ventricles/cisterns, haemorrhage traces, gliotic tissue and embolus. These structures appear to present a negligible risk from extraneous radiation. On the other hand, neighbouring healthy brain should be protected, and priority can be given to functional areas while keeping the number of isocentres/beams and the resulting treatment time to an acceptable level (fig. 2, 3). In this respect, the singular task of obtaining the best possible conformity index for a treatment plan is not the clinical goal.

While spilling dose into non-eloquent areas is likely to have a negligible effect on treatment complications, it must be remembered that for every unit (millijoule) of energy 'spilled' inside the primary beam, approximately 50 units are delivered to the rest of the head in the form of lower doses to a large volume (dependent on beam energy, size of patient and target). This may increase the overall radiation burden on the patient and increase the small chance of inducing future malignancies [11].

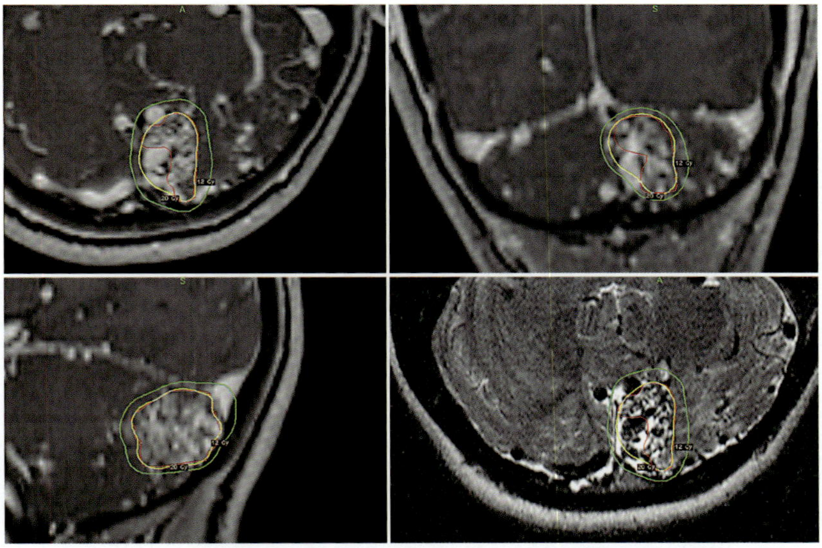

Fig. 2. Axial, coronal and sagittal images of a cerebellar AVM treatment plan. The 20- and 12-Gy isodoses are displayed in yellow and green, respectively, the target in red. While clearly not conformal in the traditional sense, it is extremely conformal on the lateral edges of the nidus which border normal brain tissue, with dose 'spilled' only onto the medial dura/sinus/draining vein.

However, this risk is extremely small compared with other risks of complications/bleeding. A simple rule of thumb is to ensure that all beams are directed onto and through the target and isocentres are not placed on the edge of the volume. Placing isocentres on the periphery of the target is a great temptation for the treatment planner; it creates a more homogeneous dose distribution, but at the expense of increasing the dose to normal tissues outside the target [15]. Here the clinician also has the option of treating younger people with a lower dose (reducing the dose to normal tissues and therefore the risk of future malignancies in this group of likely longer survivors). In doing so, he can maintain the equivalent 'adult' efficacy since younger patients have been shown to have earlier/higher rates of successful obliteration [12].

Dose Gradient

While the matching of the prescription isodose to the target is normally considered the definition of conformity, in AVM radiosurgery other dose planning parameters could be considered to be of equal importance, such as selectivity, which is a quality describing the dose fall-off outside the target. Flickinger et al. [13] and Voges et al. [14] have demonstrated a relationship between treatment complications and the volume of the 12- and 10-Gy isodoses, respectively. These values are typically about

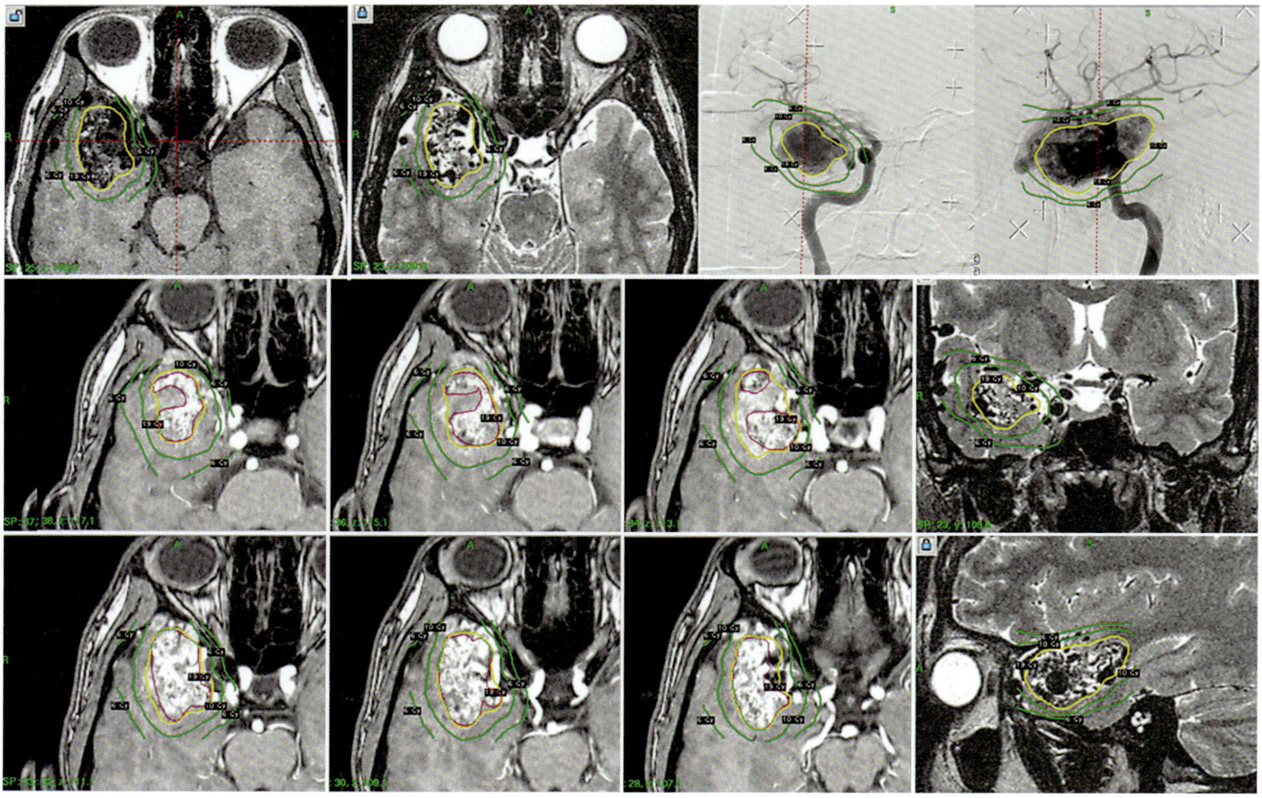

Fig. 3. Example of 'crowding' of isodoses to ensure a steep decrease in irradiation at the lateral margin of the right optic nerve, with widely spaced gradients toward the relatively indifferent cranial base in the middle fossa. Note the highly conformal lateral edge on two slices bottom right, where the target immediately neighbours normal brain, while on other slices, there is a general spill of dose outside the target into ischaemic brain and draining veins.

half of the prescription dose required for AVM obliteration. The Gradient Index proposed by Paddick and Lippitz [15] allows the dose planner to quantify this important parameter, and to use it as a quality check or to compare potential treatment plans.

Homogeneity

The homogeneity/inhomogeneity argument has historically presented inhomogeneity in tumour radiosurgery as basically negative (by itself perceived as an unhealthy word and concept), but later recognized as a possible factor leading to superior GKRS efficacy when compared to linear accelerator-based radiosurgery [16]. When applied to AVMs, the argument remains controversial as it is often voiced that inhomogeneity is intrinsically dangerous if applied to tangles of vessels by potentially causing hazardous localized stop flows and selectively weakening vessel walls inside the nidus. However, homogeneous treatments delivered by linear accelerator instrumentation have proved less efficient [17] and none of the dire consequences of eminently inhomogeneous volume-staged treatments have materialized. On the contrary, they have proved safe and effective [18]. The argument against inhomogeneity has become less frequent after the adoption by the radiotherapeutical community of dedicated linear accelerator instrumentation (Cyberknife), which often favours conformity over homogeneity.

Steering the Internal Dose Gradient

The large internal dose gradient of Gamma Knife treatment plans, seen by some as a disadvantage, can be used to the radiosurgeon's advantage when covering heterogeneous targets. A typical nidal target can be subdivided into its constituent parts: true nidus (microscopic shunting vessels), larger vessels suspected of containing shunts, draining veins enclosed by nidus and gliotic tissue. By steering 'hot spots' onto areas considered 'true nidus', higher doses can be concentrated where they are likely to be more efficacious. This can be performed by either increasing the weighting of isocentres in these areas or by adding additional shots or beams on top of a completed conformal plan to make 'colder spots' hotter.

When treatment planning larger AVMs of complex shape, the radiosurgeon is faced with compromise between planning time, beam on time, conformity and dose gradient, amongst others. However, this is especially pertinent for the planning of AVMs of complex morphology. These are sometimes referred to as 'woolly balls': a target which on a macroscopic level is simple but, due to smaller uneven 'snaking' deviations from its macroscopic shape, is very complex, requiring many smaller shots or beams to enable conformal coverage. In this example, the most efficient course of action is to cover the macroscopic shape with larger shots or beams, but use many lower weighted smaller beams to cover the many microscopic undulations that constitute the edge of the target. This method is certainly more efficient in terms of 'beam on time' than covering the whole target with smaller beams (fig. 4).

Embolization

As complete embolization of an AVM nidus is rarely attained, referral to radiosurgery of partially embolized cases has become increasingly common. This is not being perceived as failure of the endovascular technique but as a facilitating preliminary procedure that is supposed to reduce the volume for subsequent radiosurgery or protect the patient from a bleeding event [19]. Conspicuous literature exists that proves that both aims are seldom if ever reached and on the contrary the risks of both procedures cumulate with lower efficacy and consistently larger morbidity/mortality [20–23].

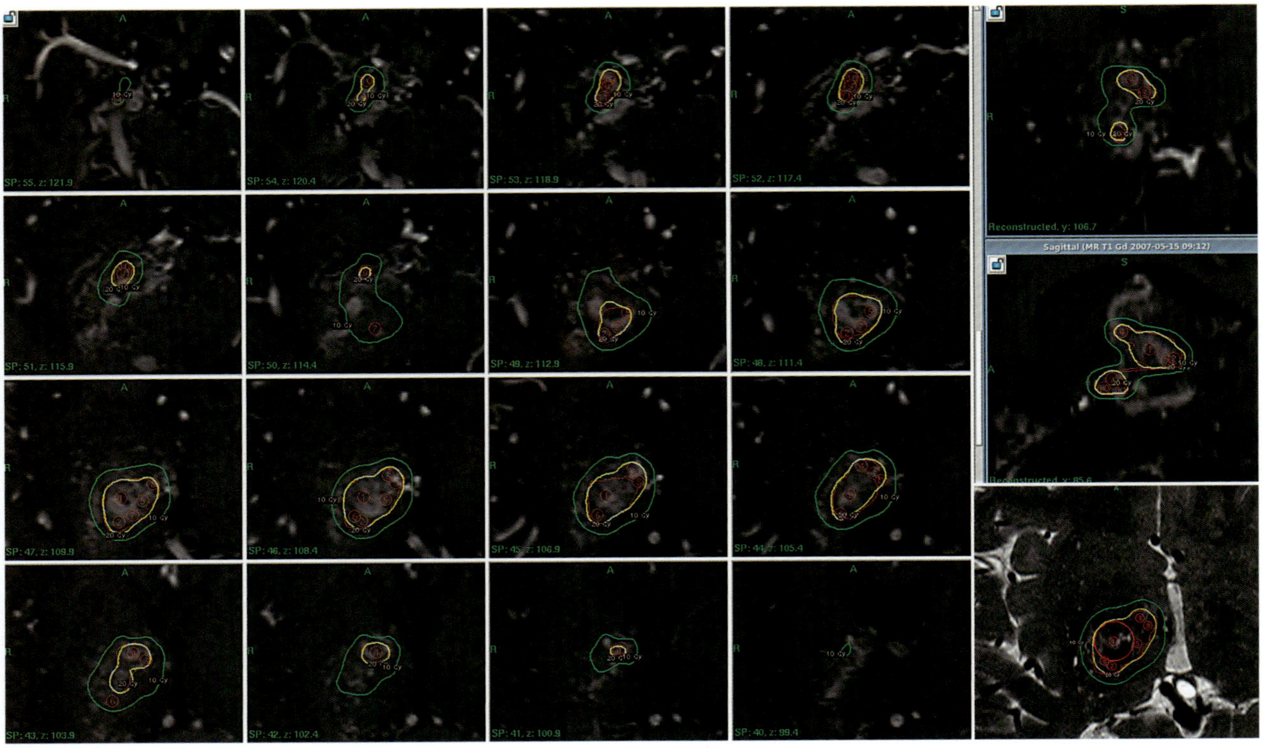

Fig. 4. A complex right thalamic AVM. 20 Gy was prescribed to the 45% isodose. The 20- and 10-Gy isodoses are displayed in yellow and green, respectively, the target in red. Despite the complex shape, good conformity was achieved using 11 isocentres and a beam on time of less than 1 h. This was aided by a single, heavily weighted 8-mm isocentre in the centre of the target (shown as a circle in the bottom right axial image). All other isocentres were lower weighted 4-mm shots. PITV = 1.12, New Paddick Conformity Index = 0.79, Gradient Index = 2.89.

Notwithstanding rote statements in the literature that treatment decisions in AVMs belong to multidisciplinary teams competent in vascular neurosurgery, interventional techniques and radiosurgery, most patient's primary treatments are decided upon by the physician of first referral, more often than not the neuroradiologist.

Conformality becomes a theoretical subject in the course of radiosurgical planning for the large partially embolized AVM nidus that after a series of interventional sessions has become a 'patchwork' lesion (fig. 5).

The problem is represented by the twin facts of an effectively unchanged volume and the necessity of sparing as much as possible surrounding healthy tissue from further damage [24], often in a patient that has become neurologically symptomatic. The obvious strategy, to cover as little volume as possible, must be balanced against the possibility that low-flow scarcely visible areas of pathological circulation may become revascularized in the course of time following radiosurgery. Radiosurgery appears less effective in reaching complete obliteration of an AVM after previous interventional

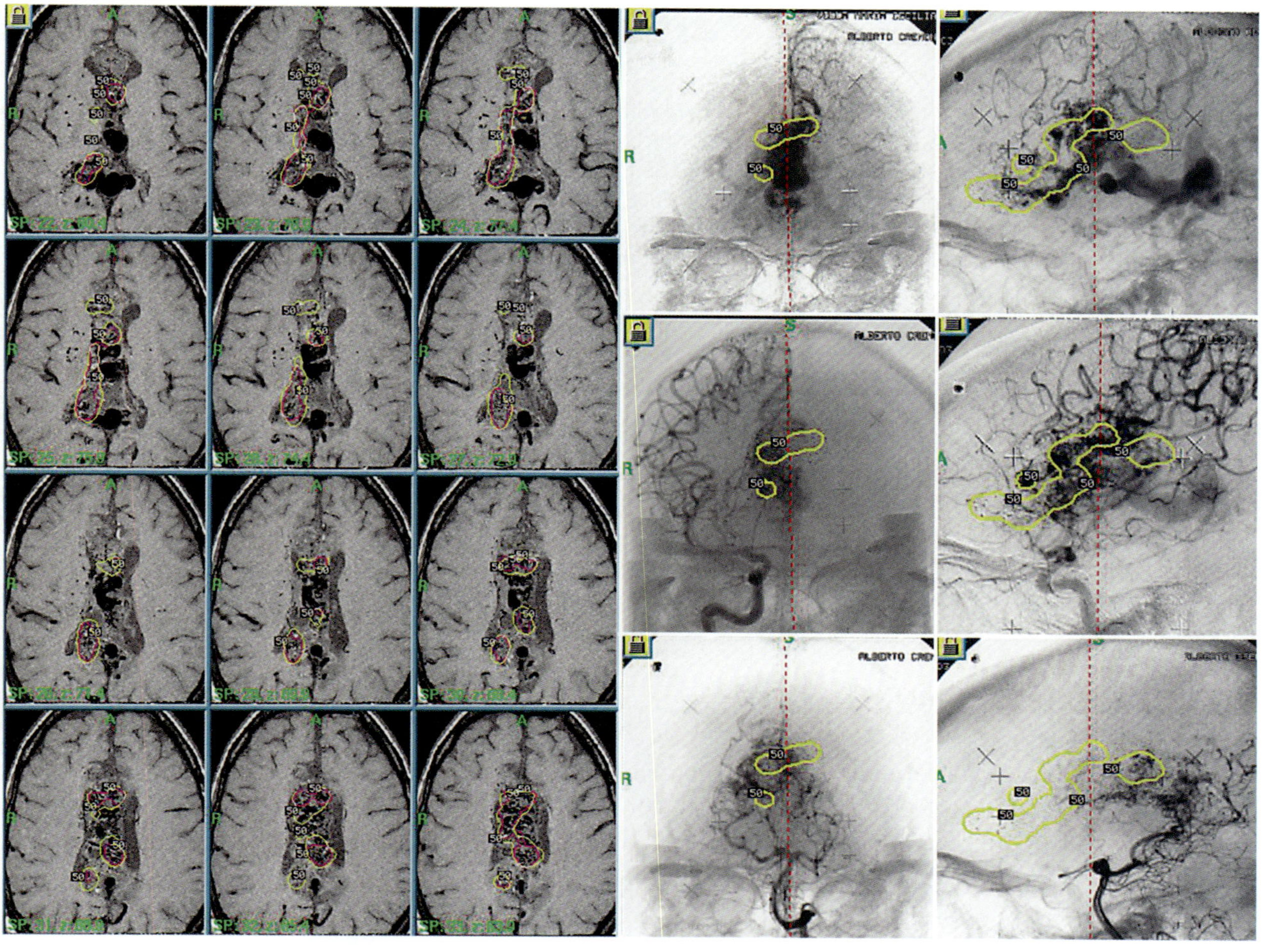

Fig. 5. Female patient aged 34 years – large AVM diagnosed following haemorrhage in 1994 (at the age of 18 years) – who underwent 10 embolization sessions in a 3-year period (June 1994 to June 1997) by a very experienced team. Starting 1 year after the last embolization session, a high number of bleeds (9 CT verified) and transitory neurological deficits occurred over a period of 5 years. After another unsuccessful interventional procedure, she was referred (aged 26) to radiosurgery and underwent GKRS treatment twice: in March 2003 and, after a further single intervening bleed, in February 2008. In both procedures the target was represented by a 'patchwork' of strictly collimated selective subtargets within a very complex angio-architecture made up by residual and by revascularized portions, the latter partly misjudged as occluded at the time of the first GK procedure.

attempts [25] thus further raising the challenge, against poor odds, to not add injury and to maximize efficacy. While obvious following embolization by metallic materials in AVMs (relatively rare, fig. 6), Shtraus et al. [26] noted the dosimetric effects of Onyx due to its high electron density. In radiosurgery systems where CT electron density corrections are made, dose errors are likely due to the excessive distortion of CT, from which the electron density of tissues is calculated. Although Onyx is

Fig. 6. Haemorrhagic right capsular AVM with 2 compartments, the anterior portion of which underwent successful occlusion by Onyx and retrograde venous coiling in September 2008. GKRS on residual nidus fed by the right posterior choroidal artery in January 2010. The significant artefacts on CT, which extend many centimetres from the lesion, cause unreliable dose density corrections.

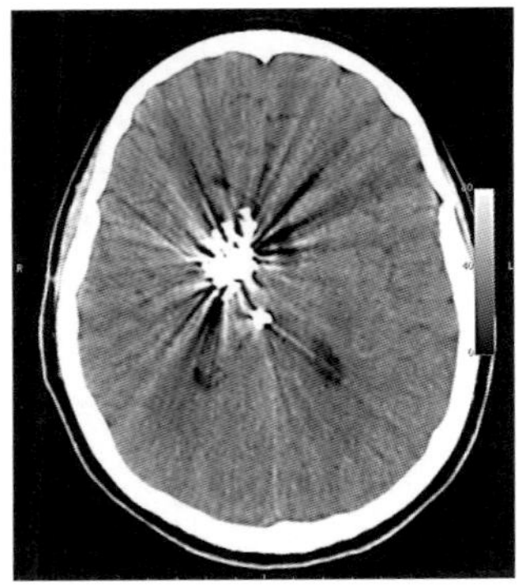

more attenuating than water, overestimation of this effect can result in an overdose of the target. In systems where no compensation is made for tissue heterogeneity, the presence of Onyx will slightly reduce the dose from the beams that pass through the embolus.

General Considerations

In another defining aspect, compared to radiotherapy, radiosurgery is not limited to tumoral targets. On the contrary, historically, it was first used in neurosurgical functional interventions. Adoption of radiosurgery for the treatment of cerebral AVMs, a non-functional and non-tumoral target, was a later development and the object of controversy amongst pioneers.

Although there has been occasional discussion about the alpha/beta ratio of brain tissue and cerebral vessel walls [27], the matter is highly speculative and serves at present no useful purpose. In AVMs radiosurgery does not aim to kill malignant cells or reverse the growth tendency of the target tissue, but rather it aims to induce those changes in the vessel wall (foremost hypertrophy and myofibroblast proliferation [28]) that will eventually obliterate the lumen via an inflammatory process [29]. Apparently, the inflammation induced by radiosurgery prods the vessel wall toward the desired degeneration/hypertrophy only if a measure of modification already exists: tunica media changes and intimal proliferation are the histological markers of vessels belonging to the arteriovenous malformative tract [30, 31].

The wealth of anatomical, metabolical and ultrastructural investigations may obscure the simple fact that vessel walls sustaining the cerebral circulation are not just the obvious hollow scaffold to healthy and deranged tissue (all but similar to the plumbing distribution in a building), but rather possibly the closest interface the brain has with the external environment after sensory organs. Not unlike the skin, the endothelial lining is subjected to tear and stress and develops bourses, creases, fatty deposits etc. and in the process continually sheds its worn component cells. These dynamic processes are exaggerated in AVMs with a range of mechanical stresses and pathological changes that in time make them the complex vascular anomalies we recognize at diagnosis. A high rate of proliferation and a reduced apoptotic response to inflammatory mediators has been described in human brain endothelial cells [32]. The angiogenic factors, i.e. vascular endothelial growth factor and endothelin-1, which are not normally produced by 'quiescent' brain vasculature, have been found in endothelial cells of brain AVMs [32]. These appear to be the most radiosensitive layer of the vessel wall, which separate and become disrupted in response to radiation [32]. However, no evidence of occlusion in normal cerebral arteries following GKRS has accrued in the tens of thousands of treated AVMs and even the occasional recognition of focal wall changes in a normal vessel warrants a case report [17]. Histopathological changes following radiosurgery are most prominent in the abnormal vessels within the AVM, whereas normal arteries within the field are relatively unaffected [33]. Veins have also been found to be insensitive to radiation but still undergo vessel wall fibrosis [34].

There is indication that the exaggerated dynamic processes in the vessel wall of key arteries and veins in an AVM have a possible end point which is not only haemorrhage and angio-architectural and neural distortion/derangement, but also spontaneous occlusion [1]: rarely described, but undetectable in clinically silent, undiagnosed AVMs. Radiosurgery appears then only to take advantage of the underlying self-obliterating mechanism, prodding it to completion. One could say that radiosurgery in AVMs is a 'physiological therapy' that extends nature's work.

The insight gained by spontaneous occlusion, where, among other factors, the presence of a single draining vein seems to play a determinant role, may guide us in treatment planning: radiosurgery may obliterate a relatively small nidus with a single efferent vein in a time scale too precipitous to be safe (fig. 7).

This occurrence, relatively rare in our series (3 in 500 AVM cases – unreported) is currently an object of analysis awaiting final outcome with at least 3 years of follow-up in all cases. The observation of precocious venous occlusion, with its attending dramatic side effects, represents indication that conformal treatment planning in AVMs should not only aim to attain complete coverage of the malformed vascular tissue, carefully sparing normal brain tissue, but that sometimes careful conformation and 'steering' of hot spots ought to be employed also for avoidance of the origin of efferent veins. One possible interpretation of undesired precocious venous occlusion would be to attribute single large draining veins a much higher sensitivity to radiation than currently thought: this would confer a susceptibility for occlusion greater than that of nidal arteries and multiple venous efferents. Obliteration of the whole AVM with no side effects (and possibly no intervening haemorrhage) is the aim of a properly conformal treatment. Closure of the draining vessels is part of the goal, but the time course of the obliteration process as it affects the different component vessels (afferents, fistulous tracts, efferents) is likely to be central to an uneventful curative process, and treatment planning will have to take into account these features, once they become fully understood.

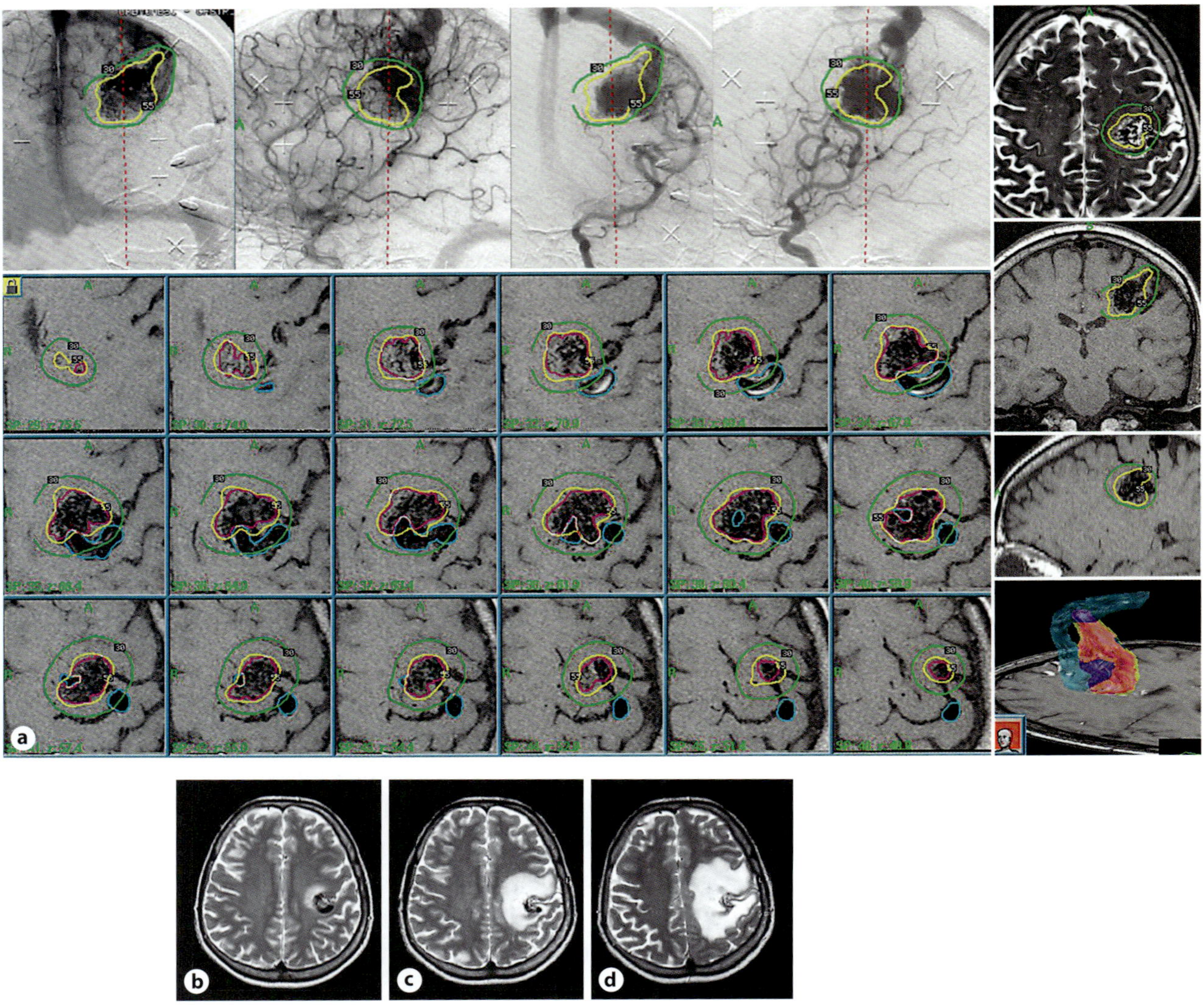

Fig. 7. Female patient aged 40 years, non-haemorrhagic left motor AVM. The treatment plan (**a**) shows careful avoidance of the draining vein (outlined in blue) as soon as it emerges from the nidus volume (5 cm^3, 19 Gy at 55% isodose). **b–d** The course of rapid obliteration and drastic reduction of efferent vein diameter at 9, 14 and 17 months following GKRS, respectively, is shown along with concomitant excessive signal modification in satellite tissue. Sudden worsening of right hand paresis (which, originally minor, had led to recognition of the AVM) took place about 15 months following radiosurgery.

Conclusion

Unlike in oncological radiosurgery the complete aim of treatment is not just reversal of a growing lesion, but also the elimination of functional changes (in a way akin to pituitary adenoma radiosurgery) represented in AVM patients by derangement of function (seizures, steal, neuropsychological function, headache) and life-threatening haemorrhage risk. Full conformal coverage of the lesion must therefore require preliminary analysis that includes not only the requirements of oncological treatment planning, i.e. confine radiation to the target and spare healthy tissue, but also takes into account special needs different from other common conditions treated by radiosurgery. Patient characteristics (age, symptoms, history) play a role just as relevantly as the required identification of feeders, fistulous nidal areas, efferents, reactive modifications already present in the normal circulation and nearby eloquent areas.

Interpretation of the above factors and details of treatment in these mostly young, otherwise healthy individuals is even more important than in oncological radiosurgery; the first major historical advances in the treatment of AVMs came following the recognition that they were not just tumorous angiomas, but consisted of relatively few crucial blood vessels that must be occluded to attain cure. Contrary to common belief [8], in radiosurgery of AVMs as in microsurgery, success may as well be contingent on the expertise of the skilled practitioner in modalities of visualization [35] and target identification [36], who by careful delineation and anatomical conformity strives to maximize the gradient around the target in order to maximize obliteration rates and lower associated complications.

References

1 Buis DR, Lagerwaard FJ, Barkhof F, Dirven CM, Lycklama GJ, Meijer OW, et al: Stereotactic radiosurgery for brain AVMs: role of interobserver variation in target definition on digital subtraction angiography. Int J Radiat Oncol Biol Phys 2005;62:246–252.

2 St George EJ, Butler P, Plowman PN: Can magnetic resonance imaging alone accurately define the arteriovenous nidus for gamma knife radiosurgery? J Neurosurg 2002;97:464–470.

3 Steiner L, Leksell L, Greitz T, Forster DM, Backlund EO: Stereotaxic radiosurgery for cerebral arteriovenous malformations. Report of a case. Acta Chir Scand 1972;138:459–464.

4 Yu C, Petrovich Z, Apuzzo ML, Zelman V, Giannotta SL: Study of magnetic resonance imaging-based arteriovenous malformation delineation without conventional angiography. Neurosurgery 2004;54: 1104–1107, discussion 1108–1010.

5 Sanelli PC, Mifsud MJ, Stieg PE: Role of CT angiography in guiding management decisions of newly diagnosed and residual arteriovenous malformations. AJR Am J Roentgenol 2004;183:1123–1126.

6 Colombo F, Cavedon C, Francescon P, Casentini L, Fornezza U, Castellan L, et al: Three-dimensional angiography for radiosurgical treatment planning for arteriovenous malformations. J Neurosurg 2003; 98:536–543.

7 Zipfel GJ, Bradshaw P, Bova FJ, Friedman WA: Do the morphological characteristics of arteriovenous malformations affect the results of radiosurgery? J Neurosurg 2004;101:393–401.

8 Andisheh B, Brahme A, Bitaraf MA, Mavroidis P, Lind BK: Clinical and radiobiological advantages of single-dose stereotactic light-ion radiation therapy for large intracranial arteriovenous malformations. Technical note. J Neurosurg 2009;111:919–926.

9 Shaw E, Kline R, Gillin M, Souhami L, Hirschfeld A, Dinapoli R, et al, Radiation Therapy Oncology Group: Radiosurgery quality assurance guidelines. Int J Radiat Oncol Biol Phys 1993;27:1231–1239.

10 Paddick I: A simple scoring ratio to index the conformity of radiosurgical treatment plans. Technical note. J Neurosurg 2000;93(suppl 3):219–222.

11 Ganz JC: Gamma knife radiosurgery and its possible relationship to malignancy: a review. J Neurosurg 2002;97:644–652.

12 Pollock BE, Flickinger JC, Lunsford LD, Maitz A, Kondziolka D: Factors associated with successful arteriovenous malformation radiosurgery. Neurosurgery 1998;42:1239–1244, discussion 1244–1247.

13 Flickinger JC, Kondziolka D, Lunsford LD, Kassam A, Phuong LK, Liscak R, et al: Development of a model to predict permanent symptomatic postradiosurgery injury for arteriovenous malformation patients. Arteriovenous Malformation Radiosurgery Study Group. Int J Radiat Oncol Biol Phys 2000;46:1143–1148.
14 Voges J, Treuer H, Sturm V, Buchner C, Lehrke R, Kocher M, et al: Risk analysis of linear accelerator radiosurgery. Int J Radiat Oncol Biol Phys 1996;36:1055–1063.
15 Paddick I, Lippitz B: A simple dose gradient measurement tool to complement the conformity index. J Neurosurg 2006;105(suppl):194–201.
16 Shaw E, Scott C, Souhami L, Dinapoli R, Kline R, Loeffler J, et al: Single dose radiosurgical treatment of recurrent previously irradiated primary brain tumors and brain metastases: final report of RTOG protocol 90-05. Int J Radiat Oncol Biol Phys 2000;47:291–298.
17 Pedroso AG, De Salles AA, Tajik K, Golish R, Smith Z, Frighetto L, et al: Novalis shaped beam radiosurgery of arteriovenous malformations. J Neurosurg 2004;101(suppl 3):425–434.
18 Sirin S, Kondziolka D, Niranjan A, Flickinger JC, Maitz AH, Lunsford LD: Prospective staged volume radiosurgery for large arteriovenous malformations: indications and outcomes in otherwise untreatable patients. Neurosurgery 2008;62(suppl 2):744–754.
19 Cockroft KM, Rosenwasser RH: Cerebrovascular-endovascular. Prog Neurol Surg 2006;19:107–122.
20 Han PP, Ponce FA, Spetzler RF: Intention-to-treat analysis of Spetzler-Martin grades IV and V arteriovenous malformations: natural history and treatment paradigm. J Neurosurg 2003;98:3–7.
21 Jayaraman M, Cloft HJ: Embolization of brain arteriovenous malformations for cure: because we could or because we should? AJNR Am J Neuroradiol 2009;30:107–108.
22 Pollock BE, Flickinger JC, Lunsford LD, Bissonette DJ, Kondziolka D: Hemorrhage risk after stereotactic radiosurgery of cerebral arteriovenous malformations. Neurosurgery 1996;38:652–659, discussion 659–661.
23 Wikholm G, Lundqvist C, Svendsen P: The Goteborg cohort of embolized cerebral arteriovenous malformations: a 6-year follow-up. Neurosurgery 2001;49:799–805, discussion 806.
24 Lekovic GP, Kim LJ, Gonzalez LF, Bice A, Albuquerque FC, McDougall CG: Radiation exposure during endovascular procedures. Neurosurgery 2008;63:ONS81–85, discussion ONS85–86.
25 Andrade-Souza YM, Ramani M, Scora D, Tsao MN, ter Brugge K, Schwartz ML: Embolization before radiosurgery reduces the obliteration rate of arteriovenous malformations. Neurosurgery 2007;60:443–451, discussion 451–452.
26 Shtraus N, Schifter D, Corn BW, Maimon S, Alani S, Frolov V, et al: Radiosurgical treatment planning of AVM following embolization with Onyx: possible dosage error in treatment planning can be averted. Journal of Neurooncol 2010;98:271–276.
27 Qi XS, Schultz CJ, Li XA: Possible fractionated regimens for image-guided intensity-modulated radiation therapy of large arteriovenous malformations. Phys Med Biol 2007;52:5667–5682.
28 Szeifert GT, Timperley WR, Forster DM, Kemeny AA: Histopathological changes in cerebral arteriovenous malformations following Gamma Knife radiosurgery. Prog Neurol Surg 2007;20:212–219.
29 Chen Y, Zhu W, Bollen AW, Lawton MT, Barbaro NM, Dowd CF, et al: Evidence of inflammatory cell involvement in brain arteriovenous malformations. Neurosurgery 2008;62:1340–1349, discussion 1349–1350.
30 Isoda K, Fukuda H, Takamura N, Hamamoto Y: Arteriovenous malformation of the brain – histological study and micrometric measurement of abnormal vessels. Acta Pathol Jpn 1981;31:883–893.
31 Wong JH, Awad IA, Kim JH: Ultrastructural pathological features of cerebrovascular malformations: a preliminary report. Neurosurgery 2000;46:1454–1459.
32 Sammons V, Davidson A, Tu J, Stoodley MA: Endothelial cells in the context of brain arteriovenous malformations. J Clin Neurosci 2011;18:165–170.
33 O'Connor MM, Mayberg MR: Effects of radiation on cerebral vasculature: a review. Neurosurgery 2000;46:138–149, discussion 150–151.
34 Fajardo LF: Morphologic patterns of radiation injury. Front Radiat Ther Oncol 1989;23:75–84.
35 Maitz AH, Niranjan A, Jungreis CA, Kondziolka D, Flickinger JC, Lunsford LD: Tube angulation improves angiographic targeting of arteriovenous malformations during stereotactic radiosurgery. Comput Aided Surg 2001;6:225–229.
36 Ellis TL, Friedman WA, Bova FJ, Kubilis PS, Buatti JM: Analysis of treatment failure after radiosurgery for arteriovenous malformations. J Neurosurg 1998;89:104–110.

Ian Paddick
Medical Physics Limited, Lilley Farm
Pond Lane
Mapledurham, Oxfordshire RG4 7TY (UK)
Tel. +44 7956 295 390, E-Mail ian@physicsconsulting.co.uk

Niranjan A, Kano H, Lunsford LD (eds): Gamma Knife Radiosurgery for Brain Vascular Malformations.
Prog Neurol Surg. Basel, Karger, 2013, vol 27, pp 49–57 (DOI: 10.1159/000341623)

Dose Selection in Stereotactic Radiosurgery

John C. Flickinger[a,b] · Hideyuki Kano[b] · Ajay Niranjan[b] ·
Douglas Kondziolka[a,b] · L. Dade Lunsford[a–c]

Departments of [a]Radiation Oncology, [b]Neurological Surgery and [c]Radiology, University of Pittsburgh School of Medicine, Pittsburgh, Pa., USA

Abstract

Selection of the prescription dose for arteriovenous malformation (AVM) radiosurgery is the final step in treatment planning. Physicians need to choose a prescription dose that provides an optimal middle ground between optimizing AVM obliteration with high radiation doses and limiting complication risks with the lowest doses. Accurately predicting complication risks for individual patients is a complex process that is highly dependent on the radiosurgery treatment volume, the target location and the nature of the target tissue. This article reviews the principles and data guiding dose selection for AVM radiosurgery.

Basic Principles

Creating a radiosurgical treatment plan is a multiple step process. After defining the target volume on stereotactic images, we create a treatment plan with a treatment volume (volume receiving the prescription dose) that closely matches the target volume. At some point, we must decide what radiation dose will be prescribed to the treatment volume. It is helpful to use radiobiological principles to understand and interpret the limited outcome data from past radiosurgery experience to select optimal doses for individual patients.

Dose-Volume Effects

With most conventional fractionated radiotherapy treatment plans, treatment volumes are huge in comparison to radiosurgery in part because large margins are added to the treatment volume to account for setup errors and patient motion. Within the range of large conventional radiotherapy treatment volumes, most differences in treatment volume between one patient and the next have only minor effects on radiation tolerance. With large-field conventional fractionated radiotherapy, it may be necessary to decrease the dose by 5% or less to keep the same complication risk when the treatment volume is doubled. Because of this, volume effects can be safely ignored in many conventional, fractionated radiotherapy dose prescriptions. Radiosurgery treatment volumes, on the other hand, commonly vary by a factor of 300 (0.1–30 cm^3) for most of the indications treated. The change in radiation tolerance across this range of treatment volumes used in radiosurgery is tremendous compared with those seen over the volumes treated in conventional fractionated radiotherapy. Because of these steep dose-volume effects, we can safely give a radiosurgery treatment volume of 1 cm^3 or less to a dose of 25 Gy in a single fraction, while the same single-fraction dose administered to a conventional radiotherapy field enclosing half the brain would be lethal.

Early Dose-Volume Guidelines

There was little laboratory or clinical investigation to define dose-volume effects in the early years of radiosurgery, even though Leksell published the concept of high-dose small-volume stereotactic brain irradiation and coined the term 'radiosurgery' as far back as 1951 [1]. Kjellberg et al. [2] plotted 1 and 99% dose-volume isoeffect lines for brain necrosis on log-log axes from data from animal experiments and human clinical experience with photon and proton beams. They included data from one of the best studies of volume effects at the time: the 1963 study by Berg and Lindgren [3] of the variation in radiation tolerance for fields encompassing between 25 and 100% of rabbit brains. Kjellberg used the resulting 1% dose-volume isoeffect line for radiation necrosis as his guideline for most of his subsequent dose prescriptions for proton beam radiosurgery. These plots were used as initial guidelines for linear accelerator radiosurgery dose prescriptions [4]. Leksell's group in Stockholm varied their dose prescriptions for the Gamma Knife that they developed according to their slowly accumulating clinical and laboratory experience. By the mid-1980s they felt that marginal doses of 25 Gy seemed optimal for treating arteriovenous malformations (AVMs), acoustic neuromas and meningiomas with their 4-, 8- and 14-mm diameter collimators.

When the University of Pittsburgh Gamma Unit became operational in August of 1987, there was little else to guide dose prescriptions. This new unit was equipped with 18-mm diameter collimators (in addition to the 4-, 8- and 14-mm collimators with prior models) and better treatment planning software, making it easier to treat larger volumes than Stockholm had treated in the past. We could not rely on Stockholm's dose prescription policies to be safe for larger volumes and questioned whether Kjellberg's guidelines were appropriate. The integrated logistic formula developed to address these issues with brain necrosis risk predictions estimated over radiosurgery dose-volume histograms [5]. The formula parameters were fitted to the scant clinical and laboratory data available at the time, and resulted in dose-volume prescription guidelines almost identical to Kjellberg's.

Table 1 compares these two guidelines for spherical targets of different diameters. Both the integrated logistic formula and Kjellberg's 1% isoeffect line were intended

Table 1. A comparison of dose-volume prescription guidelines for different mean tumor diameters from Kjellberg's 1% radionecrosis isoeffect line, 3% necrosis risk predictions from the integrated logistic formula, and the risk levels in the RTOG phase I study for malignant brain tumors with prior irradiation [2, 4–6]

Mean diameter	Volume, cm^3	1% isoeffect, Gy	3% int. log., Gy	RTOG, Gy
12.5 mm	1.02	27.5	34.0	24 (10%)
15.0 mm	1.77	25.0	29.0	24 (10%)
17.5 mm	2.81	22.5	23.0	24 (10%)
20.0 mm	4.19	20.0	18.0	18 (20%)
22.5 mm	5.96	18.7	16.5	18 (20%)
25.0 mm	8.18	17.5	14.5	18 (20%)
27.5 mm	10.9	16.5	13.5	18 (20%)
30.0 mm	14.1	15.0	13.0	15 (14%)
32.5 mm	18.0	14.0	12.5	15 (14%)

for predicting only necrosis of brain parenchyma. They were never intended to predict injury to cranial nerves that were known to be more sensitive. These guidelines were not intended to predict asymptomatic or temporary postradiosurgery sequelae, which were not described by then.

Dose-Volume Effect Studies in Radiosurgery

The RTOG 90-05 Phase I Study Guidelines

The RTOG 90-05 phase 1 dose escalation study for radiosurgery included adults with previously irradiated cerebral or cerebellar solitary nonbrainstem tumors ≤40 mm in maximum diameter [6]. Brainstem tumors were excluded. The final report included 156 analyzable patients entered between 1990 and 1994: 36% with recurrent primary brain tumors (median prior dose 60 Gy) and 64% with recurrent brain metastases (median prior dose 30 Gy). Doses were prescribed within 3 maximum tumor diameter groupings: <20, 21–30 and 31–40 mm. Starting doses for this dose-escalation study were 18 Gy for tumors ≤20 mm, 15 Gy for 21–30 mm and 12 Gy for 31–40 mm. Doses were escalated in 3-Gy increments as long as the incidence of acute (within 3 months of radiosurgery) unacceptable toxicity remained <20% for each dose level. They defined unacceptable toxicity as irreversible grade 3 (severe) or any grade 4–5 (life-threatening or fatal) central nervous system (CNS) toxicity. In total, 22% (35/156) of the subjects developed unacceptable acute and chronic toxicities. Out of this total, 15 were irreversible grade 3 (severe; 10% of all patients, 42% of unacceptable toxicity group), 16 were grade 4 (life-threatening; 10% of all patients, 46% of unacceptable toxicity group), and 4 were grade 5 (fatal; 3% of all patients, 11% of unacceptable toxicity group). The 15 grade 3 toxicities were cases of irreversible edema requiring inpatient intravenous steroids. Grade 3 toxicities developed at a median time of 4.5 months following radiosurgery (range 0.5–36 months). The 16 grade 4 toxicities included 15 cases of radionecrosis requiring operation and 1 case of clinically and radiographically suspected radionecrosis that was subsequently confirmed at autopsy. Grade 4 toxicities occurred at a median interval of 5.0 months following protocol radiosurgery (range 4.0–27 months). The actuarial incidence of radionecrosis was 5, 8, 9 and 11% at 6, 12, 18 and 24 months following radiosurgery, respectively. The 4 grade 5 (fatal) toxicities were initially acute or chronic grade 3 or 4 CNS toxicities that ultimately proved fatal. They occurred with a median time of 2.5 months following radiosurgery (range 1.0–65 months).

Maximum Diameter <20 mm

For tumors ≤20 mm, radiosurgical doses were escalated from 18 to 21 Gy and then to 24 Gy in 12, 18 and 10 subjects, respectively without reaching an unacceptable incidence of acute CNS toxicity. For the ≤20 mm maximum diameter cohort, the dose was not escalated beyond 24 Gy because of investigators' reluctance to give a single radiosurgical dose of 27 Gy. No irreversible grade 3 toxicity developed in <3 months but late toxicity developed in 8, 11 and 10% of 12, 18 and 10 subjects at 18, 21 and 24 Gy, respectively. A maximum tolerable dose was assigned to be 24 Gy, but it is unclear whether unacceptable toxicity would have been reached at 27 Gy.

Maximum Diameter 21–30 mm

Within the cohort with 21- to 30-mm tumors, dose was escalated from 15 Gy (where 7% acute and 7% late toxicity developed in 15 subjects) to 18, 21 and finally 24 Gy. The 24-Gy dose level quickly proved unacceptable in 12 subjects with acute, chronic and total CNS toxicities of 23, 35 and 58%. Although 21 Gy initially appeared tolerable in 13 subjects based on acute toxicity (8%), unacceptable late CNS toxicity (31%) developed at 21 Gy. The maximum tolerable dose for 21–30 mm was therefore lowered to 18 Gy where 0% acute and 20% late toxicity developed in 15 subjects.

Maximum Diameter 31–40 mm

For the cohort with 31- to 40-mm tumors, radiosurgical doses were escalated from 12 Gy in 21 subjects (with 5% acute and 5% late toxicity) to 15 Gy and then to 18 Gy. The maximum tolerable dose was 15 Gy (where 0% acute and 14% late toxicity developed in 21 subjects), because both unacceptable acute (17%) plus chronic (33%) toxicity (total 50%) developed with 18 Gy.

Additional Tolerance Data with RTOG Maximum Tolerated Doses

RTOG 9508 randomized 167 subjects with 1–3 brain metastases to whole-brain radiotherapy followed by stereotactic radiosurgery (SRS) with the maximum tolerable doses of 24, 18 or 15 Gy and compared them to 164 randomized to whole-brain radiotherapy alone [7]. In this study grade 2 CNS toxicity was defined as any subjective weakness with no objective findings, mild paresthesias or loss of deep tendon reflexes. Grade 3 was mild or moderate objective weakness or objective sensory loss/paresthesias without impairment of function. Grade 4 was objective weakness or severe sensory loss/paresthesias that interfere with function. Out of the 167 subjects who underwent radiosurgery, 24, 5 and 4% developed acute or late grade 2, 3 and 4 acute toxicity. That compared to 33, 2 and 1% grade 2, 3 and 4 toxicities with whole-brain radiotherapy alone. Out of 33, 29 and 20 subjects undergoing radiosurgery after whole-brain radiotherapy for solitary brain metastases measuring <20, 21–30 and 31–40 mm, grade ≥2 toxicities developed in 6, 27 and 20% of subjects, respectively. All but 2 toxicities were grade 2, with 1 grade 3 (3%) for <20 mm and 1 grade 4 (3%) for 21–30 mm.

Radiation Injury Responses in AVM versus Tumors

Radiosurgery toxicity studies in patients with malignant tumors, and specifically brain metastases, are compromised by difficulty distinguishing radiation injury from tumor progression along with follow-up limitations as a result of patients dying from advancing metastatic and primary disease. Improvements in distinguishing radiation injury from progression of brain metastases on imaging studies have only been recent [8]. We compared the rate of developing postradiosurgery imaging changes (new increased T_2-weighted signal in surrounding brain) in 138 AVM patients and 139 benign tumor patients (84 vestibular schwannomas and 55 meningiomas) all with >2-year follow-up who were treated with similar doses in our early experience [9]. Thirty percent of the AVM versus 10% of the benign tumor patients developed postradiosurgery imaging changes. More recently we performed a multivariate logistic regression modeling comparison of postradiosurgery imaging changes (symptomatic or asymptomatic edema) in 307 AVM patients and 291 meningioma patients with 2 or more years of follow-up. With multivariate modeling controlling for effects of volume ($p = 0.007$) and dose with a linear-quadratic model ($p = 0.0143$ and 0.0148 for dose and dose squared), we found the rate of postradiosurgery imaging changes was significantly higher ($p < 0.0001$) in the AVM patients with an odds ratio of 7.5 (95% confidence interval 3.4–16.4). Thus, it is clear that a greater degree of postradiosurgery injury is expected in treating AVMs.

Early AVM Radiosurgery Tolerance Studies

Our initial analyses of AVM radiosurgery complications found that the integrated logistic model did not adequately predict imaging changes [10]. A comparison of various models with best-fitting exponents found a better fit of data for postradiosurgery sequelae in AVM patients for a logistic dose-volume threshold model compared to the integrated logistic model or a stem cell depletion model [9]. The logistic dose-volume threshold model is a function of the volume of tissue receiving above a specified threshold dose.

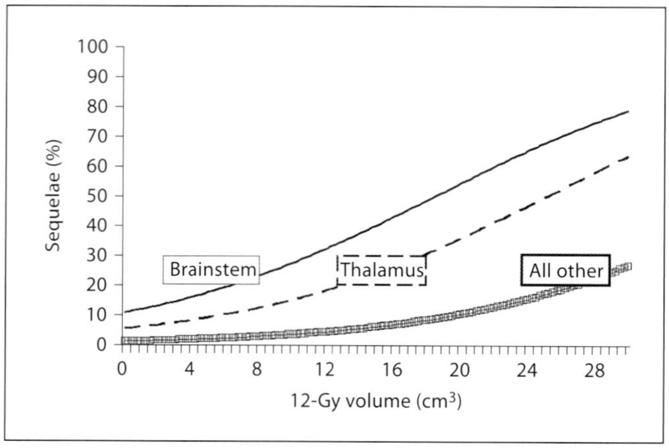

Fig. 1. Risk prediction curves correlating the probability of developing persistent symptomatic postradiosurgery sequelae for 815 AVM patients according to the volume of tissue receiving 12 Gy or more and location (brainstem, thalamus or other).

Our next study evaluated 307 AVM patients who received Gamma Knife radiosurgery at the University of Pittsburgh between 1987 and 1993 [11]. All patients had a regular clinical or imaging follow-up for a minimum of 2 years (range 24–96 months, median 44 months). The rate of developing any postradiosurgery imaging changes 2 (and 7) years after radiosurgery was 30.5%; for symptomatic changes it was 10.5%. Symptomatic postradiosurgery imaging changes resolved in 53% of patients within 3 years of onset which was significantly less ($p = 0.0274$) than the 95% resolution rate for asymptomatic postradiosurgery imaging changes. The actuarial rate for developing persistent symptomatic postradiosurgery imaging changes (radiation necrosis) was 5.05% at 7 years.

Multivariate analysis of various treatment parameters identified a significant correlation of any postradiosurgery imaging change only with the total volume of AVM plus surrounding tissue receiving a radiation dose greater than 12 Gy, termed the 12-Gy volume. None of the other factors tested including target dose inhomogeneity, dose rate, number of isocenters, maximum or minimum AVM nidus dose, treatment volume, 8- or 10-Gy volumes, or 8- to 12-Gy marginal volumes (in surrounding tissue excluding the target volume) were independently correlated with postradiosurgery imaging changes in any significant way. The 12-Gy volume reflects both the treatment volume and the minimum dose to the AVM nidus used in the radiosurgical treatment but correlates more closely with the risk of radiation sequelae than dose or treatment volume alone.

Recent AVM Radiation Tolerance Studies

We recently analyzed radiation tolerance in 815 AVM patients with >3 years of follow-up who underwent radiosurgery at the University of Pittsburgh between 1987 and 2007. Figure 1 shows the risk of persistent postradiosurgery neurological sequelae according to a 12-Gy volume and by location (brainstem, thalamic or all others). The odds ratios for developing permanent neurological sequelae following AVM radiosurgery were significantly higher for thalamic ($p = 0.004$, odds ratio 7.47) and brainstem (pons, medulla, midbrain, pineal) locations ($p = 0.000001$, odds ratio 34.8).

Dose Response for AVM Obliteration

Successful AVM obliteration depends on accurate stereotactic definition of the nidus and the radiosurgical dose administered. Our 1996 analysis of 197 AVM patients with 3-year angiographic follow-up showed an overall complete obliteration rate of 72% after a single Gamma Knife radiosurgery procedure [12]. In 20 of 197 patients (10%), the targeted nidus failed to become obliterated. The other 35 patients (18% of those treated) who failed to obliterate the nidus had only a residual AVM nidus outside the treatment volume. Thus, problems with target definition were the single greatest reason for failure to achieve obliteration in our early experience. Our next follow-up analysis included 351 AVM patients with a >2-year follow-up after radiosurgery. We found 18% of 48 patients embolized with the older techniques used at the time (polyvinyl chloride particles as opposed to glue or Onyx used now) had a persistent nidus outside the radiosurgery treatment volume compared to 5% out-of-field nidus in the 303 nonembolized patients. Older embolization techniques were associated with higher recanalization rates leading to greater risks of persistent out-of-field nidus (marginal target miss) since embolized nidus with no evidence of flow is not normally targeted within radiosurgery treatment volumes. Multimodality imaging, including magnetic resonance imaging, magnetic resonance angiography and angiography, is crucial to obtain the best result [12, 13]. In these studies obliteration correlated with prescription dose but no significant volume effects on obliteration were identified.

The true radiobiological dose response for AVM obliteration can be elucidated from in-field AVM obliteration data [12, 13] and also mathematical models that can account for marginal misses [13].

We recently analyzed the dose response in 515 AVM patients who underwent radiosurgery at the University of Pittsburgh and had a minimum of 5 years of follow-up after radiosurgery. When both dose and dose squared were included in the dose response model to make it a linear-quadratic model, the small negative coefficient for the dose-squared factor leads to an α/β ratio of –45.9. The dose response is shown in figure 2. The maximum obliteration rates in this model were 95.7% with no embolization and 91.8% with prior embolization. The dose response is relatively steep between 12 and 17 Gy, leveling out at around 20 Gy with 50% obliteration occurring at approximately 14 Gy.

Repeat Radiosurgery

Since radiation is used to target AVMs composed of nonneoplastic tissue with normal individual cells, AVM radiosurgery shares many characteristics with normal tissue injury responses seen with other radiation treatments. Because radiation injury

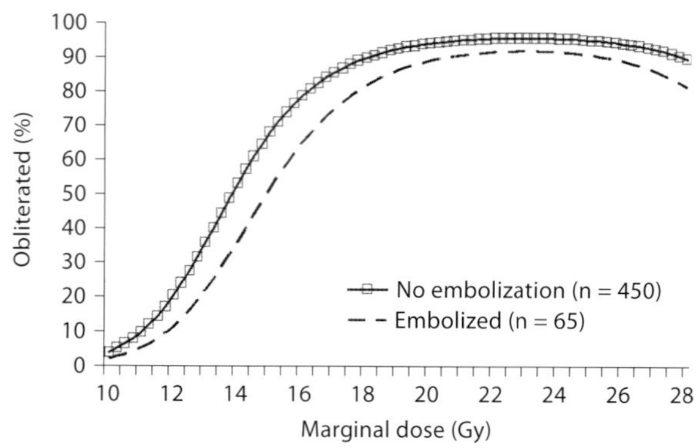

Fig. 2. Dose response curves for AVM obliteration according to prescription dose and history of prior embolization from 515 patients with >5 years of follow-up. Logistic model, $\alpha/\beta = -45.9$; maximum obliteration at 23 Gy; 95.7% with no embolization, 91.8% with prior embolization.

reactions occur more commonly when there has been prior radiation, it would be reasonable to expect that repeat previously irradiated AVMs could be obliterated using lower radiation doses at the time of retreatment than previously untreated AVM. Our dose response analysis for repeat radiosurgery in 2000 disproved this expectation [14]. Similar or more likely higher doses were needed to achieve the same obliteration rates as with the initial treatment.

We recently reviewed our experience with repeat AVM radiosurgery. Between 1989 and 2006, we repeated AVM radiosurgery in 105 patients with incompletely obliterated AVMs at a median of 40.9 months after initial SRS (range 27.5–139 months). The median AVM target volume at initial SRS was 6.4 cm^3 (range 0.2–26.3 cm^3) and was reduced to 2.3 cm^3 (range 0.1–18.2 cm^3) at the time of repeat radiosurgery. The median margin dose at both initial SRS and repeat SRS was 18 Gy. The actuarial total obliteration rates after repeat SRS were 35, 68, 77 and 80% at 3, 4, 5 and 10 years, respectively. Factors associated with a higher rate of AVM obliteration were smaller residual AVM target volume ($p = 0.038$) and ≥50% of volume reduction after the initial procedure ($p = 0.014$). Seven patients (7%) had a hemorrhage in the interval between initial SRS and repeat SRS. Seventeen patients (16%) had hemorrhage after repeat SRS and 6 patients died. The cumulative actuarial rates of new AVM hemorrhage after repeat SRS were 1.9, 8.1, 10.1 and 22.4% at 1, 2, 3–5 and 10 years, respectively, This translates into annual hemorrhage rates of 4.05% for years 0–2 and 1.79% for years 2–10 following repeat radiosurgery. Factors associated with higher hemorrhage risks after repeat SRS were a larger number of prior hemorrhages ($p = 0.008$), larger AVM target volume ($p = 0.002$), initial AVM volume reduction <50% ($p = 0.034$), and a higher Pollock-Flickinger score ($p = 0.010$). Symptomatic adverse radiation effects developed in 5 patients (4.7%) after initial SRS in these patients (lower than the 10% expected from unselected initial treatment series) and 10 patients (9.5%) after repeat SRS. Prior embolization ($p = 0.022$) and higher Spetzler-Martin grade ($p = 0.004$) were significantly associated with higher rates of adverse radiation effects. Five patients (4.8%) developed delayed cyst formation at a median of 108 months after repeat SRS (range 47–184 months). The lower rates of adverse symptomatic postradiosurgery sequelae after unsuccessful initial radiosurgery and relatively low complication rates with retreatment in these patients suggest that some of these patients may possess at least a slight radioresistance within the target cells in their AVM and in their surrounding normal tissue. It also suggests that the AVM obliteration response may be contributing to the normal tissue injury response.

References

1 Leksell L: The stereotaxic method and radiosurgery of the brain. Acta Chir Scand 1951;102:316–319.
2 Kjellberg R, Hanamura T, Davis K, Lyons S, Butler W, Adams R: Bragg-peak proton-beam therapy for arteriovenous malformations of the brain. N Engl J Med 1983;309:269–274.
3 Berg NO, Lindgren M: Relation between field size and tolerance of rabbit's brain to roentgen irradiation (200 kV) via a split-shaped field. Acta Radiol 1963;1:147–150.
4 Loeffler JS, Alexander E, Siddon R, Saunders W, Coleman N, Winston K: Stereotactic radiosurgery for intracranial arteriovenous malformations using a standard linear accelerator. Int J Radiat Oncol Biol Phys 1989;17:673.
5 Flickinger JC: The integrated logistic formula and prediction of complications from radiosurgery. Int J Radiat Oncol Biol Phys 1989;17:879–885.
6 Shaw E, Scott C, Souhami L, Dinapoli R, Kline R, Loeffler J, Farnan N: Single dose radiosurgical treatment of recurrent previously irradiated primary brain tumors and brain metastases: final report of RTOG protocol 90-05. Int J Radiat Oncol Biol Phys 2000;47:291–298.
7 Andrews DW, Scott CB, Sperduto PW, Flanders AE, Gaspar LE, Schell MC, Werner-Wasik M, Demas W, Ryu J, Bahary JP, Souhami L, Rotman M, Mehta MP, Curran WJ Jr: Whole brain radiation therapy with or without stereotactic radiosurgery boost for patients with one to three brain metastases: phase III results of the RTOG 9508 randomised trial. Lancet 2004;363:1665–1672.
8 Kano H, Kondziolka D, Lobato-Polo J, Zorro O, Flickinger JC, Lunsford LD: T_1/T_2 matching to differentiate tumor growth from radiation effects after stereotactic radiosurgery. Neurosurgery 2010;66:486–491.
9 Flickinger JC, Lunsford LD, Kondziolka D: Radiosurgical dosimetry: principles and clinical implications; in De Salles AF, Goetsch S (eds): Stereotactic Surgery and Radiosurgery. Madison, Medical Physics Publishing, 1993, pp 293–306.
10 Flickinger JC, Lunsford LD, Kondziolka D, Maitz AM, Epstein A, Simons S, Wu A: Radiosurgery and brain tolerance: an analysis of neurodiagnostic imaging changes following gamma knife radiosurgery for arteriovenous malformations. Int J Radiat Oncol Biol Phys 1992;23:19–25.
11 Flickinger JC, Kondziolka D, Pollock BE, Maitz AH, Lunsford LD: Complications from arteriovenous malformation radiosurgery: multivariate analysis and risk modeling. Int J Radiat Oncol Biol Phys 1997;38:485–490.
12 Flickinger JC, Pollock BE, Kondziolka D, Lunsford LD: A dose-response analysis of arteriovenous malformation obliteration after radiosurgery. Int J Radiat Oncol Biol Phys 1996;36:873–879.
13 Flickinger JC, Kondziolka D, Maitz AH, Lunsford LD: An analysis of the dose-response for arteriovenous malformation radiosurgery and other factors affecting obliteration. Radiother Oncol 2002;63:347–354.
14 Maesawa S, Flickinger JC, Kondziolka D, Lunsford LD: Repeated radiosurgery for incompletely obliterated arteriovenous malformations. J Neurosurg 2000;92:961–970.

John C. Flickinger, MD
Joint Radiation Oncology Center
5230 Centre Avenue
Pittsburgh, PA 15232 (USA)
E-Mail flickingerjc@upmc.edu

Niranjan A, Kano H, Lunsford LD (eds): Gamma Knife Radiosurgery for Brain Vascular Malformations.
Prog Neurol Surg. Basel, Karger, 2013, vol 27, pp 58–66 (DOI: 10.1159/000341620)

Development and Testing of a Radiosurgery-Based Arteriovenous Malformation Grading System

Bruce E. Pollock

Departments of Neurological Surgery and Radiation Oncology, Mayo Clinic College of Medicine, Rochester, Minn., USA

Abstract

Stereotactic radiosurgery is an accepted management option for many patients with intracranial arteriovenous malformations (AVMs). The Spetzler-Martin grading scale is the most widely accepted and utilized method to predict outcomes after surgical resection of intracranial AVMs but is not sensitive to factors that correlate with successful AVM radiosurgery. The need for a system that accurately predicts patient outcomes after AVM radiosurgery led to the development of the radiosurgery-based AVM score (RBAS). The RBAS has evolved and has been modified over the years to reflect changes in AVM radiosurgical technique and has been validated by numerous centers using the Gamma Knife®, modified LINAC and the CyberKnife®. Use of the RBAS permits an accurate prediction of outcomes from radiosurgery to guide choices between observation, surgical resection or radiosurgery for individual AVM patients, and should be used in future studies on AVM radiosurgery to stratify patients for more precise comparative analyses.

More than 40 years have passed since Dr. Ladislau Steiner and colleagues reported that single-fraction, high-dose irradiation could be used to manage patients with intracranial arteriovenous malformations (AVMs) [1]. Notably, 204 of the first 762 patients (27%) undergoing Gamma Knife® radiosurgery at the Karolinska Institute had AVMs partly because these lesions could be visualized by cerebral angiography before the advent of axial neuroimaging [2]. At the same time, Kjellberg et al. [3] and Steinberg et al. [4] were using heavy charged particles instead of photons to irradiate AVMs, and later papers showed that AVM radiosurgery could be performed successfully using modified linear accelerators (LINACs) [5–7]. These pioneering studies showed that nidus irradiation caused progressive obliteration of AVMs and provided patients with protection against later hemorrhage. Stereotactic radiosurgery has become an accepted option for patients with intracranial AVMs, and numerous improvements to this technique have been documented over the past decades. Despite its acknowledged role in the treatment of patients with intracranial AVMs, the indications for this technique continue to be debated and refined. To that end, a method that reliably predicts patient outcomes after AVM radiosurgery is needed to allow direct comparison with the natural history of untreated lesions and the risk associated with surgical resection or endovascular therapies. In this report, the author describes the development and testing of a grading system for AVM radiosurgery.

Defining End Points after Arteriovenous Malformation Radiosurgery

The results of AVM radiosurgery have traditionally been defined based on 3 factors: obliteration rate, the risk of radiation-related complications and the chance of a postradiosurgical hemorrhage. Each of these variables has been independently analyzed and can be summarized quite simply. First, the chance of AVM obliteration directly correlates with the radiation dose delivered to the margin of the malformation [8, 9]. Provided that the radiation delivery is well targeted, the chance of AVM obliteration is approximately 70, 80 and 90% for radiation doses of 16, 18 and 20 Gy, respectively. Second, radiation-related complications after AVM radiosurgery relate to the radiation exposure to the surrounding tissue and the location of the AVM [10–12]. Patients with deeply located AVMs (thalamus, basal ganglia or brainstem) are more likely to develop neurological deficits secondary to imaging changes noted on magnetic resonance imaging (MRI). Third, radiosurgery does not increase the bleeding rate of AVMs [13–17], and some degree of protection against hemorrhage may be conferred even in the absence of AVM obliteration. It has also been recognized that late complications can occur many years after AVM radiosurgery including bleeding from previously obliterated lesions [18], delayed cyst formation [19, 20] and radiation-induced tumors [21]. Fortunately, the incidence of these late complications is very low and should not be overemphasized when deciding whether radiosurgery is an appropriate treatment strategy for individual AVM patients.

Reporting the results of AVM radiosurgery based on the individual factors of obliteration status, radiation-related deficits or postradiosurgical hemorrhage is not sufficient. For example, a patient could have complete AVM obliteration demonstrated on angiography but suffer a significant decline in functional status from radiation necrosis. If the end point is obliteration status alone, then this patient would be considered to have a good outcome. Conversely, a patient may continue to demonstrate some residual nidus after radiosurgery but has no new deficits from either radiation-related complications or bleeding. This patient would be considered a treatment failure despite having suffered no adverse events from either the procedure or the AVM itself. If one is to fully describe the desired outcome of AVM radiosurgery, the defined outcome should be the number of patients that achieve obliteration without new neurological deficits, regardless of whether the morbidity was from radiation-related complications or AVM bleeding after the procedure [22, 23]. However, some cerebrovascular neurologists now feel that neurosurgeons have been overly aggressive in the management of AVM patients, especially for patients with unruptured AVMs [24]. They argue that the morbidity associated with AVM bleeding is less than previously thought [25], and the chance of neurological deficits after treatment of unruptured AVMs may be greater than previously described [26]. Consequently, future AVM studies on observation, surgical resection, embolization and radiosurgery should document not only the obliteration status and treatment-related morbidity, but also use standardized measures such as the modified Rankin Score (MRS) to assess patient outcomes and permit accurate comparisons for the different treatment techniques.

The Radiosurgery-Based Arteriovenous Malformation Grading System

The Spetzler-Martin grading system is the most widely utilized grading system for intracranial AVMs [27]. Based on the AVM size, location and pattern of venous drainage, this grading scale has been validated prospectively [28], and by numerous neurosurgeons to predict patient outcomes after AVM resection [29, 30]. However, the factors related to successful surgical removal of brain AVMs are not exactly the same as the factors associated with successful AVM radiosurgery (fig. 1). For example, the Spetzler-Martin grading scale ranks AVM size as less than 3 cm (1 point), 3–6 cm (2 points) and greater than 6 cm (3 points) in greatest linear dimension. Conversely, the vast majority of AVMs having single-session radiosurgery are less than 3 cm in greatest dimension with typical treatment volumes ranging from less than 1 cm^3 to approximately 14 cm^3. Thus, it is clear that the Spetzler-Martin grading scale is relatively insensitive to AVM volume which is a significant factor associated with successful AVM radiosurgery. In addition, the various cortical regions considered 'eloquent' in the Spetzler-Martin grading system are less susceptible to injury from radiosurgery, and so the risk of these areas should not be equated to the risk of radiosurgery for AVMs in the basal ganglia, thalamus or brainstem. Recognizing the shortcomings of this system in predicting outcomes from AVM radiosurgery, the Mayo Clinic in collaboration with the University of Pittsburgh have worked over the past 15 years to develop a radiosurgery-based AVM grading system to help guide the management for individual AVM patients (table 1).

Initially we performed a multivariate analysis on 220 patients having AVM radiosurgery at the University of Pittsburgh to determine factors that correlated with AVM obliteration without new neurological deficits after single-session AVM radiosurgery [22]. These results were used to calculate the Pittsburgh Arteriovenous Malformation Radiosurgery grading scale [31]. Unfortunately, this grading scale was

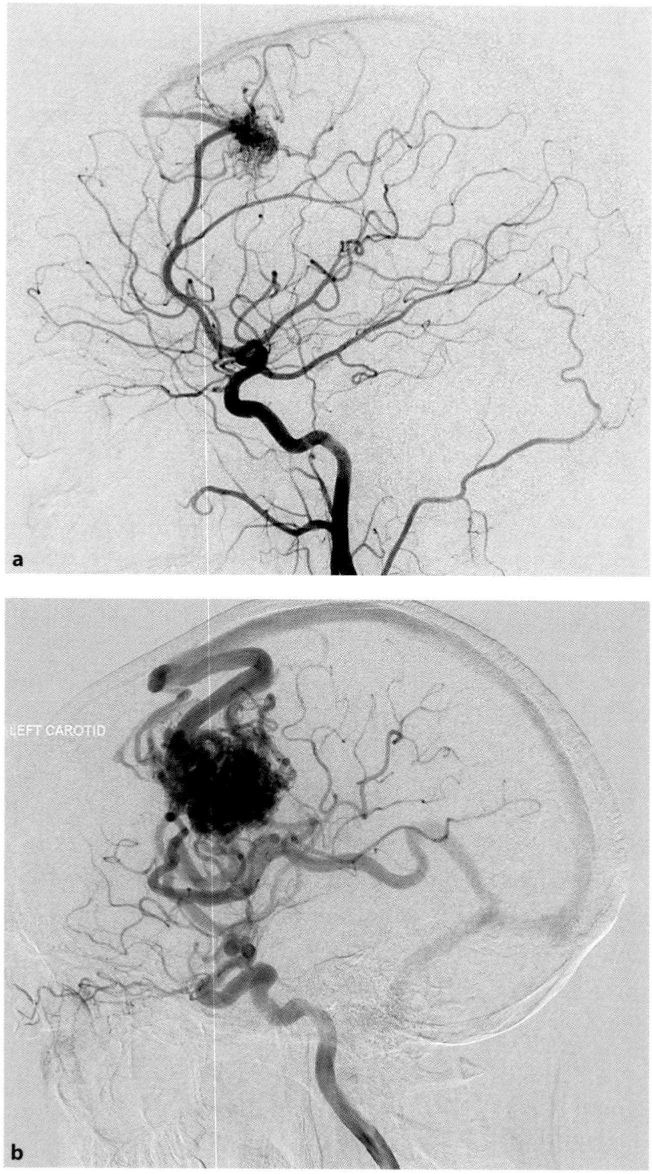

Fig. 1. Lateral cerebral angiograms of 2 patients with Spetzler-Martin grade I–II AVMs that have significantly different risks from radiosurgery. **a** Nineteen-year-old woman with headaches who was found to have a 1.2-cm right frontal AVM (Spetzler-Martin grade I). The patient underwent single-session radiosurgery (margin dose, 25 Gy); the modified RBAS was 0.48. **b** Sixteen-year-old boy who had tonic-clonic seizure and was found to have a 4-cm left frontal AVM (Spetzler-Martin grade II). The patient underwent staged-volume radiosurgery (margin dose, 15 Gy); the modified RBAS was 2.14.

too complicated for practical application requiring 5 separate variables (AVM volume, patient age, AVM location, prior embolization and number of draining veins) as well as a y-intercept value. Recognizing the difficulty in using the Pittsburgh Arteriovenous Malformation Radiosurgery grading scale, we used regression analysis modeling and removed 2 variables (prior embolization, number of draining veins) from the Pittsburgh Arteriovenous Malformation Radiosurgery grading scale to develop the radiosurgery-based AVM score (RBAS) [32]. The RBAS was then tested on 136 patients having AVM radiosurgery at the Mayo Clinic from 1990 to

Table 1. Evolution of the radiosurgery-based AVM grading system

Grading system	Scores
Pittsburgh AVM Radiosurgery Scale [31]	Score = 0.13 + (0.1) (AVM volume, cm^3) + (0.03) (patient age, years) + (0.64) (AVM location)[a] + (0.67) (embolization; 0 = no, 1 = yes) + (0.35) (number of draining veins)
Radiosurgery-based AVM score [32]	Score = (0.1) (AVM volume, cm^3) + (0.02) (patient age, years) + (0.3) (AVM location)[a]
Modified radiosurgery-based AVM score [33]	Score = (0.1) (AVM volume, cm^3) + (0.02) (patient age, years) + (0.5) (AVM location)[b]

[a] Location defined as: 0 = frontal/temporal; 1 = parietal/occipital/intraventricular/corpus callosum/cerebellum; 2 = basal ganglia/thalamus/brainstem.
[b] Location defined as: 0 = hemispheric/corpus callosum/intraventricular/cerebellum; 1 = basal ganglia/thalamus/brainstem.

1997 and was found to accurately predict outcomes after a single radiosurgical procedure. Of significance, the grading system does not include any treatment-related factors such as radiation dose, so it can be used to counsel individual patients on the chance of success with AVM radiosurgery at the time of consultation. Moreover, despite significant differences between the patients having AVM radiosurgery at the University of Pittsburgh and the Mayo Clinic with regard to age, presentation, prior embolization and size, the RBAS predicted outcomes well for both patient cohorts confirming that it is robust and sensitive to different radiation prescription guidelines.

A number of advances in AVM radiosurgery occurred over the time interval that the RBAS was developed, the most significant being the routine use of stereotactic MRI in conjunction with angiography for dose planning. Although multivariate analysis of patients treated using angiography alone for dose planning clearly showed that outcomes were best predicted using location as a 3-tiered variable [10, 22, 31, 32], it was unclear that segregation of hemispheric or cerebellar AVMs was needed when more contemporary dose planning techniques were employed. We recently tested whether simplification of the RBAS using location as a 2-tiered variable (basal ganglia, thalamus or brainstem vs. other) detracted from the accuracy of the scale [33]. Overall, there was no difference between the original or modified RBAS with regard to AVM obliteration without new neurological deficits or decline in MRS after radiosurgery (fig. 2).

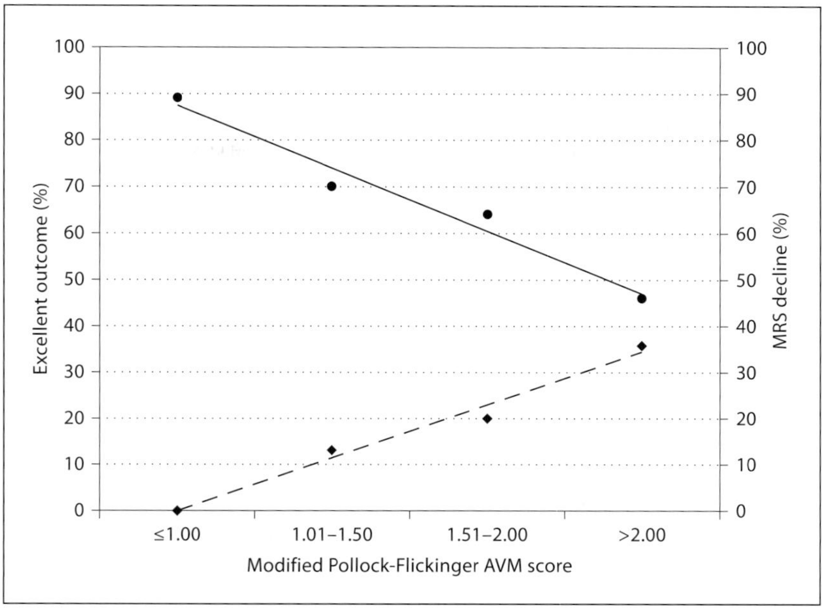

Fig. 2. Graph showing percentage of AVM patients that achieve an excellent outcome (nidus obliteration without new neurological deficits; solid line) or decline in the modified Rankin Score (MRS) (dashed line) based on the modified RBAS.

Validation of the Radiosurgery-Based Arteriovenous Malformation Score

Since 2002, a number of studies tested the RBAS as a method to predict outcomes after AVM radiosurgery (table 2) [23, 34–44]. Specifically, the RBAS has been validated for patients with deep AVMs [35, 39, 42], pediatric AVM patients [36], outcomes after one or more radiosurgical procedures [23], and the chance of neurological decline after AVM radiosurgery [39, 41]. In addition, although the RBAS was developed on AVM patients having Gamma Knife radiosurgery, it has been found to be equally effective for patients undergoing LINAC-based procedures [34, 35, 38, 43]. Raffa et al. [43] analyzed 403 patients undergoing LINAC-based AVM radiosurgery at the University of Florida from 1988 and 2008. Obliteration without new deficits was achieved for 74, 64, 50 and 11% of patients with AVM scores of <1.0, between 1.0 and 1.8, between 1.8 and 2.5, and ≥2.5, respectively. The RBAS has also been found to correlate with patient outcomes after CyberKnife® radiosurgery. Colombo et al. [37] reviewed 279 AVM patients having CyberKnife radiosurgery from 2003 and 2008. The median RBAS of 102 patients with follow-up >36 months was 1.41 (range, 0.46–10.1). No patient suffered a neurological deterioration. Univariate analysis showed a strong correlation between lower AVM scores and outcomes ($p < 0.01$).

Table 2. Validation of the RBAS

Series	Group tested	Technique	Conclusions
Pollock et al. [23], 2003	all locations	GK	RBAS predicted outcomes after 1 or more radiosurgical procedures
Pollock et al. [42], 2004	deep AVMs	GK	RBAS predicted outcomes for deep AVMs
Maruyama et al. [39], 2004	BS AVMs	GK	RBAS predicted complications for BS AVMs
Andrade-Souza et al. [34], 2005	deep AVMs	LINAC	RBAS predicted outcomes for deep AVMs
Andrade-Souza et al. [35], 2005	all locations	LINAC	RBAS predicted outcomes
Maruyama et al. [15], 2005	CC AVMs	GK	RBAS predicted outcomes for CC AVMs
Cohen-Gadol and Pollock [36], 2006	pediatric AVMs	GK	RBAS predicted outcomes for pediatric AVMs
Lee et al. [38], 2006	all locations	LINAC	RBAS predicted outcomes
Pollock and Brown [41], 2006	all locations	GK	RBAS predicted MRS decline
Raffa et al. [43], 2009	all locations	LINAC	RBAS predicted outcomes
Colombo et al. [37], 2009	all locations	CyberKnife	RBAS predicted outcomes
Wegner et al. [44], 2010	all locations	GK	modified RBAS predicted outcomes

BS = Brainstem; CC = corpus callosum; GK = Gamma Knife. Deep AVMs are defined as lesions located in the basal ganglia, thalamus or brainstem.

Conclusions

Routine use of the RBAS allows a more accurate prediction of outcomes from radiosurgery to guide choices between observation, surgical resection or radiosurgery for individual AVM patients. This system has been validated by numerous centers using the Gamma Knife, modified LINAC and CyberKnife, and should be used in future studies on AVM radiosurgery to stratify patients for more precise comparative analyses.

References

1 Steiner L, Leksell L, Grietz T, Forster DM, Backlund EO: Stereotaxic radiosurgery for cerebral arteriovenous malformations: report of a case. Acta Chir Scand 1972;138:459–464.

2 Leksell L: Stereotactic radiosurgery. J Neurol Neurosurg Psychiatry 1983;46:797–803.

3 Kjellberg RN, Hanamura T, Davis KR, Lyons SL, Adams RD: Bragg-peak proton-beam therapy for arteriovenous malformations. N Engl J Med 1983; 309:269–274.

4 Steinberg GK, Fabrikant JI, Marks MP, Levy RP, Frankel KA, Phillips MH, Shuer LM, Silverberg GD: Stereotactic heavy-charged-particle Bragg-peak radiation for intracranial arteriovenous malformations. N Engl J Med 1990;323:96–101.
5 Betti OO, Munari C, Rosler R: Stereotactic radiosurgery with the linear accelerator: treatment of arteriovenous malformations. Neurosurgery 1989; 24:311–321.
6 Columbo F, Pozza F, Chierego G, Casentini L, De Luca G, Francescon P: Linear accelerator radiosurgery of cerebral arteriovenous malformations: an update. Neurosurgery 1994;34:14–21.
7 Friedman WA, Bova FJ, Mendenhall WM: Linear accelerator radiosurgery for arteriovenous malformations: the relationship of size to outcome. J Neurosurg 1995;82:180–189.
8 Flickinger JC, Pollock BE, Kondziolka D, Lunsford LD: A dose-response analysis of arteriovenous malformation obliteration by radiosurgery. Int J Radiat Onc Biol Phys 1996;36:873–879.
9 Karlsson B, Lindquist C, Steiner L: Prediction of obliteration after gamma knife surgery for cerebral arteriovenous malformations. Neurosurgery 1997; 40:425–431.
10 Flickinger JC, Kondziolka D, Lunsford LD, Liscak R, Phuong LK, Pollock BE: Development of a model to predict permanent symptomatic post-radiosurgery injury for arteriovenous malformation patients. Int J Radiat Onc Biol Phys 2000;46:1143–1148.
11 Lax I, Karlsson B: Prediction of complications in gamma knife radiosurgery of arteriovenous malformations. Acta Oncol 1996;35:49–56.
12 Voges J, Treuer H, Lehrke R, Kocher M, Staar S, Muller RP, Sturm V: Risk analysis of linac radiosurgery in patients with arterio-venous malformations (AVM). Acta Neurochir 1997;68:118–123.
13 Friedman WA, Blatt DL, Bova FJ, Buatti JM, Mendenhall WM, Kubilis PS: The risk of hemorrhage after radiosurgery for arteriovenous malformations. J Neurosurg 1996;84:912–919.
14 Karlsson B, Lax I, Söderman M: Risk of hemorrhage during the 2-year latency period following gamma knife radiosurgery for arteriovenous malformations. Int J Radiat Oncol Biol Phys 2001;49:1045–1051.
15 Maruyama K, Kawahara N, Shin M, Tago M, Kishimoto J, Kurita H, Kawamoto S, Morita A, Kirino T: The risk of hemorrhage after radiosurgery for cerebral arteriovenous malformations. N Engl J Med 2005;352:146–153.
16 Nataf F, Ghossoub M, Schlienger M, Moussa R, Meder J, Roux F: Bleeding after radiosurgery for cerebral arteriovenous malformations. Neurosurgery 2004;55:298–305.
17 Pollock BE, Flickinger JC, Lunsford LD, Bissonette DJ, Kondziolka D: Hemorrhage risk after stereotactic radiosurgery of cerebral arteriovenous malformations. Neurosurgery 1996;38:652–661.
18 Shin M, Kawahara N, Maruyama K, Tago M, Ueki K, Kirino T: Risk of hemorrhage from an arteriovenous malformation confirmed to have been obliterated on angiography after stereotactic radiosurgery. J Neurosurg 2005;102:842–846.
19 Pollock BE, Brown RD Jr: Management of cysts arising after radiosurgery of intracranial arteriovenous malformations. Neurosurgery 2001;49:259–265.
20 Yamamoto M, Jimbo M, Hara M, Saito I, Mori K: Gamma knife radiosurgery for arteriovenous malformations: long-term follow-up results focusing on complications occurring more than 5 years after irradiation. Neurosurgery 1996;38:906–914.
21 Kaido T, Hoshida T, Uranishi R, Akita N, Kotani A, Nishi N, Sakaki T: Radiosurgery-induced brain tumor: case report. J Neurosurg 2001;95:710–713.
22 Pollock BE, Flickinger JC, Lunsford LD, Maitz AH, Kondziolka D: Factors associated with successful arteriovenous malformation radiosurgery. Neurosurgery 1998;42:1239–1247.
23 Pollock BE, Gorman DA, Coffey RJ: Patient outcomes after arteriovenous malformation radiosurgical management: results based on a 5- to 14-year follow-up study. Neurosurgery 2003;52:1291–1297.
24 Stapf C, Mohr JP, Choi JH, Hartmann A, Mast H: Invasive treatment of unruptured brain arteriovenous malformations is experimental therapy. Curr Opin Neurol 2006;19:63–68.
25 Hartmann A, Mast H, Mohr JP, Koennecke HC, Osipov A, Pile-Spellman J, Duong DH, Young WL: Morbidity of intracranial hemorrhage in patients with cerebral arteriovenous malformation. Stroke 1998;29:931–934.
26 Hartmann A, Stapf C, Hofmeister C, Mohr JP, Sciacca RR, Stein BM, Faulstich A, Mast H: Determinants of neurological outcome after surgery for brain arteriovenous malformations. Stroke 2000; 31:2361–2364.
27 Spetzler RF, Martin NA: A proposed grading system for arteriovenous malformations. J Neurosurg 1986: 65;476–483.
28 Hamilton MG, Spetzler RF: The prospective application of a grading system for arteriovenous malformations. Neurosurgery 1994;34:2–7.
29 Lawton MT, Du R, Tran MN, Achrol AS, McCulloch CE, Johnston SC, Quinnine NJ, Young WL: Effect of presenting hemorrhage on outcome after microsurgical resection of brain arteriovenous malformations. Neurosurgery 2005;56:485–493.

30 Davidson AS, Morgan MK: How safe is arteriovenous malformation surgery? A prospective, observational study of surgery as first-line treatment for brain arteriovenous malformations. Neurosurgery 2010;66:498–504.

31 Pollock BE, Flickinger JC, Lunsford LD, Maitz A, Kondziolka D: The Pittsburgh arteriovenous malformation radiosurgery (PAR) grading scale. Radiosurgery 1997;2:137–146.

32 Pollock BE, Flickinger JC: A proposed radiosurgery-based grading system for arteriovenous malformations. J Neurosurg 2002;96:79–85.

33 Pollock BE, Flickinger JC: Modification of the radiosurgery-based arteriovenous malformation grading system. Neurosurgery 2008;63:239–243.

34 Andrade-Souza YM, Zadeh G, Ramani M, Scora D, Tsao MN, Schwartz ML: Testing the radiosurgery-based arteriovenous malformation score and the modified Spetzler-Martin grading system to predict radiosurgical outcome. J Neurosurg 2005;103:642–648.

35 Andrade-Souza Y, Zadeh G, Scora D, Tsao MN, Schwartz ML: Radiosurgery for basal ganglia, internal capsule, and thalamus arteriovenous malformations: clinical outcomes. Neurosurgery 2005;56:56–64.

36 Cohen-Gadol AA, Pollock BE: Radiosurgery for pediatric arteriovenous malformations. J Neurosurg 2006;104(suppl):388–391.

37 Colombo F, Cavedon C, Casentini L, Francescon P, Causin F, Pinna V: Early results of CyberKnife radiosurgery for arteriovenous malformations. J Neurosurg 2009;111:807–819.

38 Lee JS, Girvigian MR, Miller MJ, Rahimian J, Chen JCT, Greathouse HE, Tome M: Validation of a radiosurgery-based grading system for arteriovenous malformations. Radiosurgery 2006;6:221–228.

39 Maruyama K, Kondziolka D, Niranjan A, Flickinger JC, Lunsford LD: Stereotactic radiosurgery for brainstem arteriovenous malformations: factors affecting outcome. J Neurosurg 2004;100:407–413.

40 Maruyama K, Shin M, Tago M, Kurita H, Kawamoto S, Morita A, Kirino T: Gamma knife surgery for arteriovenous malformations involving the corpus callosum. J Neurosurg 2005;102(suppl):49–52.

41 Pollock BE, Brown RD Jr: Use of the modified Rankin scale to assess outcome after arteriovenous malformation radiosurgery. Neurology 2006;67:1630–1634.

42 Pollock BE, Gorman DA, Brown PD: Radiosurgery for arteriovenous malformations of the basal ganglia, thalamus, and brainstem. J Neurosurg 2004;100:210–214.

43 Raffa SJ, Chi YY, Bova FJ, Friedman WA: Validation of the radiosurgery-based arteriovenous malformation score in a large linear accelerator radiosurgery experience. J Neurosurg 2009;111:832–839.

44 Wegner RE, Oysul K, Pollock BE, Sirin S, Kondziolka D, Niranjan A, Lunsford LD, Flickinger JC: A modified radiosurgery-based arteriovenous malformation grading scale and correlation with outcomes. Int J Radiat Oncol Biol Phys 2011;79:1147–1150.

Bruce E. Pollock, MD
Department of Neurological Surgery, Mayo Clinic
200 First Street SW
Rochester, MN 55905 (USA)
Tel. +1 507 284 5317, E-Mail pollock.bruce @mayo.edu

Niranjan A, Kano H, Lunsford LD (eds): Gamma Knife Radiosurgery for Brain Vascular Malformations.
Prog Neurol Surg. Basel, Karger, 2013, vol 27, pp 67–72 (DOI: 10.1159/000341639)

Radiosurgery for Brainstem Arteriovenous Malformation

Keisuke Maruyama[a] · Tomoyuki Koga[b] · Ajay Niranjan[c] · Douglas Kondziolka[c] · John C. Flickinger[c] · L. Dade Lunsford[c]

[a]Department of Neurosurgery, Kyorin University School of Medicine, and [b]University of Tokyo, Tokyo, Japan; [c]University of Pittsburgh Medical Center, Pittsburgh, Pa., USA

Abstract

The authors outlined the treatment result of arteriovenous malformations (AVMs) inside the brainstem by reviewing the 4 existing studies in detail. The majority of patients with brainstem AVMs had a history of hemorrhage, leading to neurological deficits at the time of treatment in 72–73% of patients. The most frequent location was the midbrain or the pons depending on studies, while the medulla oblongata was the least common location throughout the series. The obliteration rate after radiosurgery was 44–73%, which was generally lower than in other locations, while the complication rate was 5–14%, which was expectedly higher than in other locations. No objective evidence for size is known, and therefore, patient selection and treatment planning should be carefully performed after judicious assessment of treatment risks and benefits among limited treatment options.

Therapeutic options for arteriovenous malformations (AVMs) inside the brainstem are limited because of its dense concentration of critical neural structures [1–5]. Only a selected group of patients with brainstem AVMs is amenable to direct microsurgical resection [5]. For the remainder of lesions, stereotactic radiosurgery might be the only safe and effective treatment option. Also devastating morbidity and mortality by recurrent hemorrhages in the natural history after the first hemorrhage have to be taken into account when considering the treatment indication of these lesions. So far there are only 4 studies in the world literature that focus on radiosurgery for brainstem AVMs (table 1) [1–4]. Several other studies reported the treatment results combined with AVMs in deep locations including the basal ganglia, the thalamus and/or the corpus callosum [6–8], but the selected results of brainstem AVM were not demonstrated. Another study reported combined results of AVMs and angiographically occult vascular malformations, which was almost similar to cavernous malformations, in the brainstem [9].

Table 1. Previous reports on brainstem AVM radiosurgery

Authors	Year	Patient number	Follow-up period months	Obliteration rate	Complication rate	Institute
Kurita et al. [1]	2000	30	52	44	7	Tokyo
Massager et al. [2]	2000	87	38	73	5	Pittsburgh and Brussels
Maruyama et al. [3]	2004	50	72	66	14	Pittsburgh
Koga et al. [4]	2011	44	71	52	5	Tokyo

In this report, the authors outlined the treatment result of AVMs in the brainstem by reviewing all the 4 reported studies in detail.

Clinical Characteristics

The median patient age in the reported studies ranged from 35 to 39 years of age [2–4], which was almost similar to patients with AVMs in other locations. The majority of them (72–82%) had a history of hemorrhage [2–4], leading to new neurological deficits at the time of treatment in 72–73% of patients. The volume of treated AVMs ranged from 0.1 to 14 cm^3, where the median or mean volume was 1.3–1.5 cm^3 [2–4]. A majority of AVMs belonged to Spetzler-Martin grade VI (39–86%) [2, 3], which meant 'inoperable' [10]. The radiosurgery-based AVM score [11], which can estimate the risk of radiosurgery better than the Spetzler-Martin grade, was 1.5–1.6 at the median with a range of 0.75–2.89. This score was calculated according to the following equation: AVM score = (0.1)(AVM volume in cm^3) + (0.02)(patient age in years) + (0.3)(location of lesion: frontal or temporal = 0; parietal, occipital, intraventricular, corpus callosum, cerebellar = 1; basal ganglia, thalamic, brainstem = 2), which was later modified [11, 12]. The possible range of this score is from below 0.05 to above 6, and the score in brainstem AVMs tends to become larger because of its location, reflecting the higher treatment-related risk. The margin dose selected was similar to other locations (20–21 Gy) [2–4].

Arteriovenous Malformation Localization inside the Brainstem and Related Outcomes

The incidence of brainstem AVMs among all brain AVMs was less than 5% [2]. Localization inside the brainstem is shown in table 2. The most frequent location was the midbrain or the pons depending on studies (fig. 1), while the medulla oblongata was known to be the least common location throughout all the previous series [2–4].

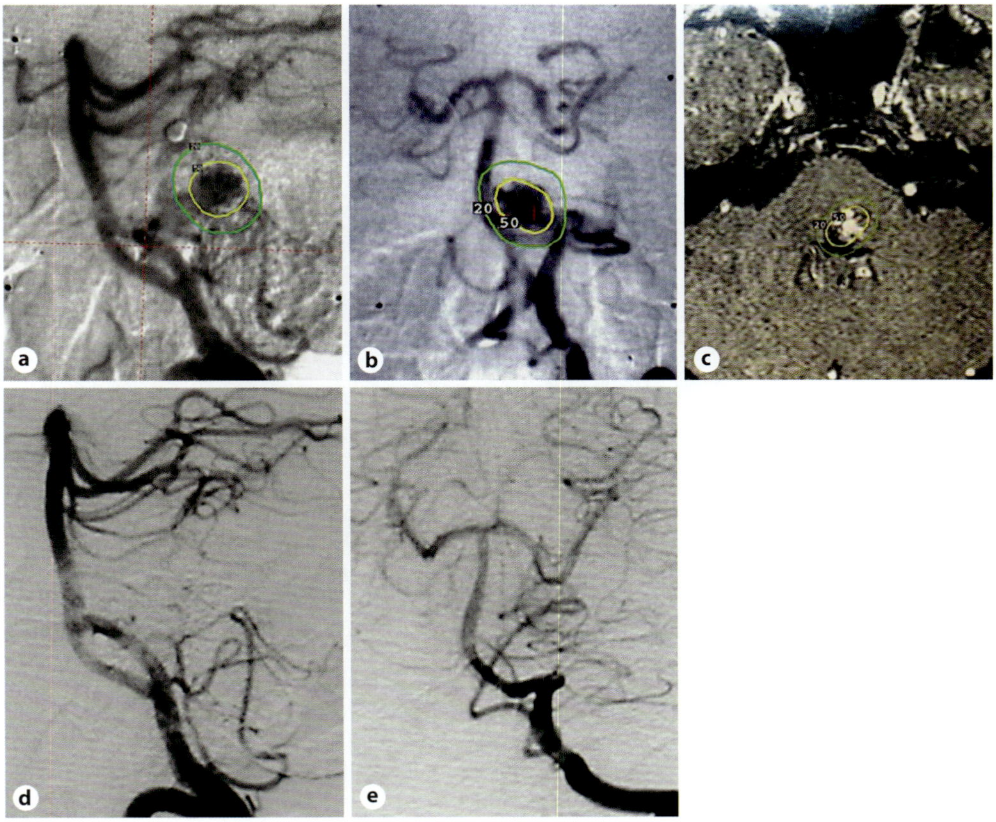

Fig. 1. Stereotactic vertebral arteriogram, lateral (**a**) and anteroposterior (**b**) views, and magnetic resonance imaging (**c**) of a 25-year-old patient showing a pontine AVM with superimposed 50% and 20% isodose lines. A follow-up angiogram 50 months after radiosurgery shows complete obliteration of AVM both in lateral (**d**) and anteroposterior (**e**) views.

Table 2. AVM localization (%) inside the brainstem

Authors	Midbrain	Pons	Medulla oblongata
Massager et al. [2]	78	33	7
Maruyama et al. [3][1]	78	40	6
Koga et al. [4]	36	48	14

[1] Multiple locations are included.

The tectal plate of the midbrain was the most vulnerable to adverse radiation effects probably because of dense confinement of multiple cranial nerve nuclei relating to eye movement or the medial longitudinal fasciculus, and also because of the possibility of aqueductal stenosis due to adverse radiation effects of the brainstem parenchyma (fig. 2) [3].

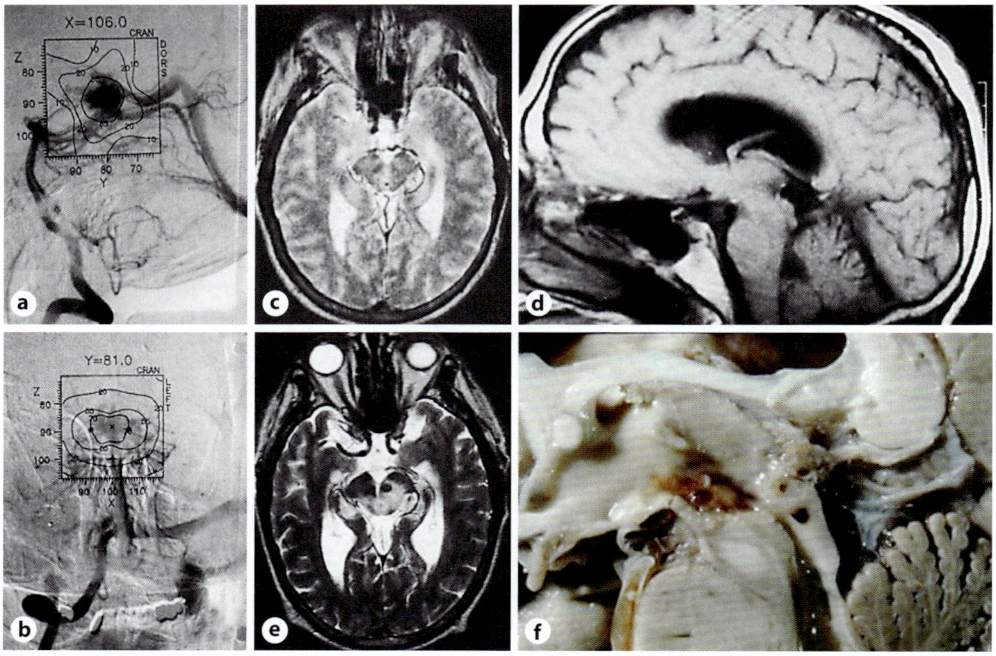

Fig. 2. Stereotactic vertebral arteriogram, lateral (**a**) and anteroposterior (**b**) views, and magnetic resonance imaging, axial (**c**) and sagittal (**d**) views, of a 63-year-old patient showing an AVM in the tectal plate. Twenty grays were administered to the AVM margin (**a**). (**e**) A T_2-weighted magnetic resonance image 28 months later shows an adverse radiation effect. This patient died of unrecognized hydrocephalus 35 months after radiosurgery. (**f**) A postmortem specimen shows minimal parenchymal damage or necrosis at the site of treatment.

Direct surgical approach to the medulla oblongata can cause damage to the respiratory center of the medulla. However, radiosurgery to this region can be applied safely according to the reported series. At the same time, one has to be aware that such treatment results might be the consequence of careful patient selection and judicious treatment planning by a specialized team of stereotactic radiosurgeons.

The Effect of Treatment in Terms of Obliteration Result

The rate of obliteration of brainstem AVMs several years after radiosurgery was 44–73%, which was generally lower than other locations [1–4]. The reason of this finding was a possible reduction of the applied dose in critical brain locations in order to minimize treatment-related morbidity [1, 3, 4]. However, the risk of hemorrhage was reduced after treatment in all reviewed studies [3, 4]. This might be the result of a protective effect of radiosurgery even before evidence of angiographic obliteration [13].

According to the statistical analyses, factors for higher obliteration were more spherical lesions necessitating fewer isocenters [3], history of hemorrhage [4] and higher margin dose [4].

Treatment-Related Morbidity

The rate of complication was 5–14% [1–4], which was higher than in other locations, a result anticipated based on the location of the AVM. AVM locations in the tectal plate, older patient age, and higher radiosurgery-based score were reported to be the factors that influenced the morbidity of radiosurgery [3]. However, radiosurgical complications were reduced after the integration of magnetic resonance imaging and treatment planning [3]. High-resolution magnetic resonance imaging supplemented by digital subtraction angiography remains the contemporary gold standard for the treatment of AVMs. Biplane angiography alone was utilized for treatment planning in the earlier radiosurgery era.

One concern for radiosurgeons might be the limit of the treatable size of AVMs. Exposure of the brainstem to more than 12 Gy at volumes as low as 0.1 cm^3 can produce adverse radiation imaging effects and new neurological deficits [14]. One guideline suggested inclusion of less than one third of the volume of brainstem parenchyma on axial neuroimaging studies [1]. As a general rule, patient selection and treatment planning should be carefully performed after judicious assessment of treatment risks and benefits in view of the limited treatment options.

Recently radiosurgery that incorporates diffusion tensor tractography has been reported [15, 16]. However, application of this technique to treat brainstem AVMs is not recommended because diffusion tensor imaging is sensitive to significant susceptibility artifacts around the brainstem. Successful conformal treatment planning should be made based on high-definition imaging, and anatomical understanding of the critical neural structure within which such AVMs are located.

References

1 Kurita H, Kawamoto S, Sasaki T, Shin M, Tago M, Terahara A, Ueki K, Kirino T: Results of radiosurgery for brain stem arteriovenous malformations. J Neurol Neurosurg Psychiatry 2000;68:563–570.

2 Massager N, Regis J, Kondziolka D, Njee T, Levivier M: Gamma knife radiosurgery for brainstem arteriovenous malformations: preliminary results. J Neurosurg 2000;93(suppl 3):102–103.

3 Maruyama K, Kondziolka D, Niranjan A, Flickinger JC, Lunsford LD: Stereotactic radiosurgery for brainstem arteriovenous malformations: factors affecting outcome. J Neurosurg 2004;100:407–413.

4 Koga T, Shin M, Terahara A, Saito N: Outcomes of radiosurgery for brain stem arteriovenous malformations. Neurosurgery 2011;69:45–51.

5 Nozaki K, Hashimoto N, Kikuta K, Takagi Y, Kikuchi H: Surgical applications to arteriovenous malformations involving the brainstem. Neurosurgery 2006;58(suppl 2):270–279.

6 Kiran NA, Kale SS, Kasliwal MK, Vaishya S, Gupta A, Singh Sharma M, Shankar Sharma B, Kumar Mahapatra A: Gamma knife radiosurgery for arteriovenous malformations of basal ganglia, thalamus, and brainstem – a retrospective study comparing the results with that for AVMs at other intracranial locations. Acta Neurochir (Wien) 2009;151:1575–1582.
7 Zabel-du Bois A, Milker-Zabel S, Huber P, Schlegel W, Debus J: Stereotactic linac-based radiosurgery in the treatment of cerebral arteriovenous malformations located deep, involving corpus callosum, motor cortex, of brainstem. Int J Radiat Oncol Biol Phys 2006;64:1044–1048.
8 Pollock BE, Gorman DA, Brown PD: Radiosurgery for arteriovenous malformations of the basal ganglia, thalamus, and brainstem. J Neurosurg 2004;100:210–214.
9 Duma CM, Lunsford LD, Kondziolka D, Bissonette DJ, Somaza S, Flickinger JC: Radiosurgery for vascular malformations of the brain stem. Acta Neurochir (Wien) 1993;58(suppl):92–97.
10 Spetzler RF, Martin NA: A proposed grading system for arteriovenous malformations. J Neurosurg 1986;65:476–483.
11 Pollock BE, Flickinger JC: A proposed radiosurgery-based grading system for arteriovenous malformations. J Neurosurg 2002;96:79–85.
12 Pollock BE, Flickinger JC: Modification of the radiosurgery-based arteriovenous malformation grading system. Neurosurgery 2008;63:239–243.
13 Maruyama K, Kawahara N, Shin M, Tago M, Kishimoto J, Kurita H, Kawamoto S, Morita A, Kirino T: The risk of hemorrhage after radiosurgery for cerebral arteriovenous malformations. N Engl J Med 2005;352:146–153.
14 Sharma MS, Kondziolka D, Khan A, Kano H, Niranjan A, Flickinger JC, Lunsford LD: Radiation tolerance limits of the brainstem. Neurosurgery 2008;63:728–733.
15 Maruyama K, Kamada K, Shin M, Itoh D, Aoki S, Masutani Y, Tago M, Kirino T: Integration of three-dimensional corticospinal tractography into treatment planning for gamma knife surgery. J Neurosurg 2005;102:673–677.
16 Maruyama K, Kamada K, Ota T, Koga T, Itoh D, Ino K, Aoki S, Tago M, Masutani Y, Shin M, Saito N: Tolerance of pyramidal tract to gamma knife radiosurgery based on diffusion-tensor tractography. Int J Radiat Oncol Biol Phys 2008;70:1330–1335.

Keisuke Maruyama, MD, PhD
Department of Neurosurgery, Kyorin University School of Medicine
6-20-2 Shinkawa
Mitaka City, Tokyo 181-8611 (Japan)
Tel. +81 422 47 5511, E-Mail kskmaru-tky@umin.ac.jp

Niranjan A, Kano H, Lunsford LD (eds): Gamma Knife Radiosurgery for Brain Vascular Malformations.
Prog Neurol Surg. Basel, Karger, 2013, vol 27, pp 73–80 (DOI: 10.1159/000341629)

Multistaged Volumetric Management of Large Arteriovenous Malformations

Hideyuki Kano[a,c] · Douglas Kondziolka[a,c] · John C. Flickinger[b,c] · Kyung-Jae Park[a,c] · Phillip V. Parry[a] · Huai-che Yang[a,c] · Sait Sirin[a,c] · Ajay Niranjan[a,c] · Josef Novotny Jr.[b,c] · L. Dade Lunsford[a,c]

Departments of [a]Neurological Surgery and [b]Radiation Oncology and [c]Center for Image-Guided Neurosurgery, University of Pittsburgh School of Medicine, Pittsburgh, Pa., USA

Abstract

We sought to define the long-term outcomes and risks of arteriovenous malformation (AVM) management using 2 or more stages of stereotactic radiosurgery (SRS) for symptomatic large-volume AVMs unsuitable for surgery. Two decades ago, we prospectively began to stage anatomical components in order to deliver higher single doses to AVMs >10 cm^3 in volume. Forty-seven patients with large AVMs underwent volume-staged SRS. The median interval between the two SRS procedures was 4.9 months (range, 3–14 months). The median nidus volume was 11.5 cm^3 (range, 4.0–26 cm^3) in the first stage of SRS and 9.5 cm^3 in the second. The median margin dose was 16 Gy (range, 13–18 Gy) for both SRS stages. The actuarial rates of total obliteration after 2-staged SRS were 7, 20, 28 and 36% at 3, 4, 5 and 10 years, respectively. Sixteen patients needed additional SRS at a median interval of 61 months (range, 33–113 months) after the 2-staged SRS. After repeat procedure(s), the eventual obliteration rate was 66% at 10 years. The cumulative rates of AVM hemorrhage after SRS were 4.3, 8.6, 13.5 and 36.0% at 1, 2, 5 and 10 years, respectively. Symptomatic adverse radiation effects were detected in 13% of patients. Successful prospective volume-staged SRS for large AVMs unsuitable for surgery requires 2 or more procedures to complete the obliteration process. Patients remain at risk for hemorrhage if the AVM persists.

Stereotactic radiosurgery (SRS) is an effective treatment option for patients with intracranial arteriovenous malformations (AVMs). SRS has become the first-line management for patients with small to medium-volume AVMs. The rate of total obliteration of such AVMs varies from 70 to 95% at 3–5 years after the procedure [1, 2]. However, the management of larger AVMs still poses a significant challenge. When larger AVMs are treated with SRS, the doses are lowered in order to maintain safety. The lower doses are however associated with significantly lower total obliteration rates after a single SRS procedure [3]. Single-stage radiosurgery of a large-volume

AVM either results in unacceptable radiation-related risks or low obliteration efficacy. Although selected centers have advocated staged radiosurgery for large AVMs, relatively few published reports establish outcomes after such an approach. The obliteration response of an AVM is dependent on dose and volume; for larger volumes, the dose must be reduced for safety. In 1992, we began to stage anatomical components of large-volume AVMs in order to improve the obliteration rate (using higher doses) and potentially to reduce the hemorrhage risk of AVMs that otherwise have no other effective therapeutic options.

Pittsburgh Experience

Forty-seven patients (26 males, 21 females; median age, 33 years; range, 6–57 years) underwent prospective volume-staged SRS. All patients had symptomatic AVMs >10 ml in volume. Symptoms included hemorrhage in 18 patients (38%), seizures in 9 (19%), headaches in 7 (15%) and neurological deficits in 9 (19%). Four patients had incidentally diagnosed AVMs. Three patients had undergone attempted surgical resection for their AVM and 21 patients (45%) had prior embolization. The AVM locations included cerebral hemispheres (n = 34), thalamus (n = 6), basal ganglia (n = 5) and cerebellum (n = 2). Patients were categorized according to Spetzler-Martin grades. There were 5 patients (11%) in Spetzler-Martin grade III, 28 (60%) in grade IV and 14 (30%) in grade V. Patients underwent high-resolution axial plane magnetic resonance imaging (MRI) followed by conventional or digital subtraction biplane stereotactic angiography at the time of the first procedure. Volumetric 3-dimensional dose planning was performed using Leksell Gamma Plan® software. After outlining the total volume of the AVM nidus on the MRI, the malformation was divided into approximately equal volumes using identified landmarks such as major vessels, the ventricles or brain anatomical structures. A dose plan was designed for the entire volume, after which isocenters were gradually subtracted until approximately 50% of the total volume remained. After 2006 computer dose planning was performed using coregistration of the initial MRI treatment plan and the second treatment plan. By the time of completion of the second procedure, the margin SRS dose included the entire AVM nidus volume. The median initial AVM volume was 22.0 cm^3 (range, 10.2–56.9 cm^3). The median target volume was 11.5 cm^3 (range, 4.0–26 cm^3) in the first stage of SRS and 9.5 cm^3 (range, 2.8–33.7 cm^3) in the second. The median total target volume was 22.0 cm^3 (range, 10.2–56.9 cm^3). The median margin dose was 16 Gy (range, 13–18 Gy) for both stages of SRS.

Complete AVM obliteration was defined using MRI as disappearance of the nidus in contrast-enhanced T_1- and T_2-weighted images and disappearance of flow voids in T_2-weighted images. Complete angiographic AVM obliteration was defined as disappearance of the nidus and absence of early venous drainage. At any time when a new neurological symptom or sign developed, the patient's new computed tomogram and/or MRI were obtained to rule out a hemorrhage or adverse radiation effects (AREs).

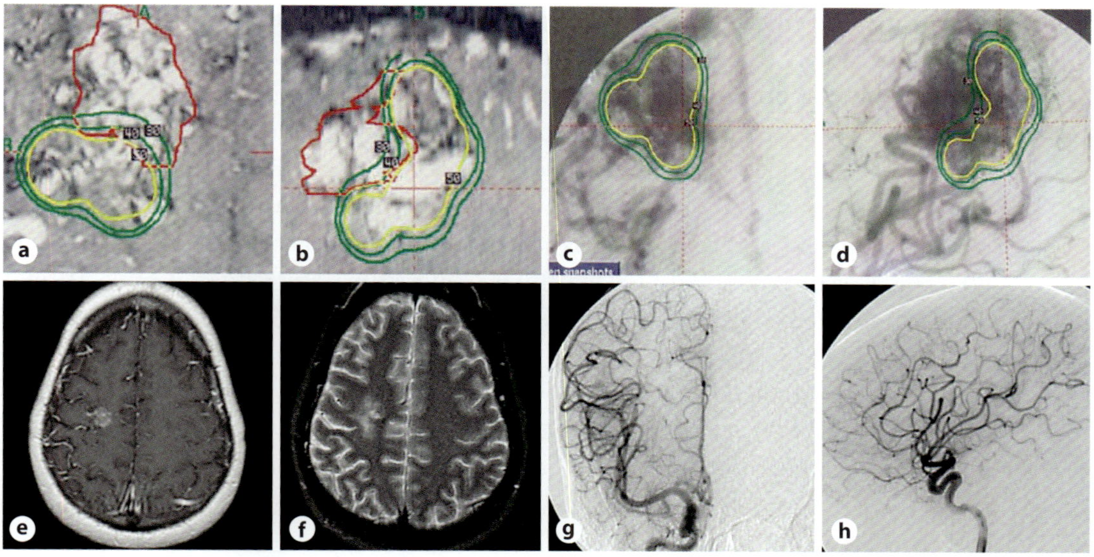

Fig. 1. A 33-year-old male who was diagnosed with a large right frontal AVM following a seizure event underwent staged SRS. Axial (**a**) and coronal (**b**) T1-weighted contrast-enhanced MR images at the time of 1st stage SRS show the anatomical components selected for the first (yellow and green lines) and the second (red line) volume staged SRS. The late arterial phase of the angiograms demonstrates multiple feeders from the right anterior and middle cerebral arteries. In anteroposterior (**c**) and lateral (**d**) views of the right internal carotid artery angiogram at the time of the initial volume-staged SRS, the total target volume was 16.7 cm^3 (stage 1: 10 cm^3, stage 2: 6.7 cm^3), and the margin dose was 17 Gy for both stages. Axial T_1-weighted contrast-enhanced (**e**) and T_2-weighted (**f**) MR images show total obliteration 38 months after the second volume-staged SRS. Anteroposterior (**g**) and lateral (**h**) views of the right internal carotid artery angiogram show total obliteration 38 months after the second volume-staged SRS.

At the time of final assessment, 9 patients had died from AVM hemorrhage. The median follow-up duration was 87 months (range, 0.4–206 months) after the second SRS. The obliteration rates after the initial 2-staged volumetric SRS were 7, 20, 28 and 36% at 3, 4, 5 and 10 years, respectively. In a subset of patients with more than 4 years of follow-up (n = 33), the obliteration rates after the initial 2-staged volumetric SRS were 9, 25, 32 and 40% at 3, 4, 5 and 10 years, respectively. In multivariate analysis a higher margin dose was the only significant factor. Higher margin dose was associated with a greater total obliteration rate (using MRI, p = 0.002, hazard ratio, 3.04, 95% confidence interval, CI, 1.52–6.08; using angiography p = 0.027, hazard ratio, 2.95, 95% CI, 1.13–7.68). Eight patients (17%) developed AVM hemorrhages after volumetric staged SRS and 5 patients died (at 0.4, 13, 14, 48 and 131 months). An annual hemorrhage rate was 6.5% in the latency interval. The cumulative rates of AVM hemorrhage after SRS were 4.3, 8.6, 8.6, 13.5 and 36.0% at 1, 2, 3, 5 and 10 years, respectively. In multivariate analyses, the number of prior hemorrhages was the only factor associated with an increased hemorrhage rate after volume-staged SRS (p = 0.017, hazard ratio, 1.68, 95% CI, 1.10–2.56).

A third SRS procedure was performed in 17 patients with a residual AVM at a median of 5 years (range, 33–113 months) after the second-stage SRS. This resulted in total obliteration in 6 additional patients at a median of 37 months after repeat SRS (range, 27–40 months). The median follow-up after repeat SRS was 39 months (range, 13–93 months). The obliteration rates after repeat SRS (n = 16) were 14, 31 and 66% at 3, 4 and 5 years, respectively. At the final follow-up, 11 of 47 patients who underwent initial volume staged SRS had total obliteration and 6 of 17 patients who underwent additional SRS had total obliteration. The actuarial rates of total obliteration after staged and additional SRS were 18, 45 and 56% at 5, 7 and 10 years after staged SRS, respectively (95% CI, 73.71–125.09 months). Three of 16 retreated patients suffered a fatal AVM hemorrhage at 18, 25 and 34 months after the third procedure. Two of these patients had suffered 2 hemorrhages before their initial volumetric staged SRS.

AREs were noted in 3 of 15 patients who had a third procedure at 11, 13 and 21 months afterwards. No patients developed a delayed cyst formation or a radiation-related neoplasm during the follow-up interval. One patient underwent surgery for an anterior communicating artery aneurysm 27 months after staged SRS. One patient underwent embolization 84 months after staged SRS but suffered 2 hemorrhages 2 and 6 weeks after embolization.

Discussion

Large AVMs pose a challenge for surgical resection, embolization and radiosurgery. Although AVM embolization prior to radiosurgery has been used for patients with large AVMs, recanalization was observed in 14–15% of patients. The obliteration rate after fractionated radiotherapy (2–4 Gy per fraction to a total dose of up to 50 Gy) is low and associated with significant side effects [4]. Redekop et al. [5] studied 15 patients with large AVMs treated with conventional fractionated external beam radiation therapy using 40 Gy in 15–28 fractions. These authors reported a 17% rate of total obliteration at a mean follow-up of 8 years. Kjellberg et al. [6] managed large AVMs using stereotactic Bragg peak proton beam therapy and found a complete obliteration rate of only 19% of patients. However, they postulated that some protection from further hemorrhage was achieved. Inoue and Ohye [7] in a study of large AVMs (larger than 10 cm^3) reported an obliteration rate of 36% and a hemorrhage rate of 36%.

Within 5 years of our initial experience using SRS (i.e. 1992), we became convinced that the narrow window between dose/response and complications required innovative thinking about the potential ways to improve outcomes for larger-volume (>10 cm^3) symptomatic, surgically untreatable AVMs. Our goal for prospective volume staging of large AVMs was to deliver a higher radiation dose to the entire AVM volume without compromising on the safety. Based on our previous experience that higher radiation doses increase AVM obliteration rates [1–3], our hypothesis was that staged-volume radiosurgery will enhance obliteration rates and thereby reduce intracranial hemorrhage risks. There was a concern that subtotal AVM SRS spaced over 3–6 months might increase the hemorrhage risk by altering the blood flow pattern within the AVM to nonirradiated nidus volume, and thus, the unprotected regions. In a linear accelerator-based SRS study, the hemorrhage risk for partially treated AVMs was noted to be higher (26%) in comparison to completely irradiated AVMs (5%) [8]. In our experience, only 1 patient had a hemorrhage from an untreated part of AVM at 4 months after the first procedure.

Embolization has been a part of multimodality management for large-volume AVM. Embolization however has limited curative potential and can be associated with higher morbidity as multiple embolization procedures are needed [9–12]. Improved obliteration rates have been reported with the use of a recently developed embolic agent (Onyx®, ev3, Irvine, Calif., USA), which may allow for safer and more effective deployment of embolic material. Onyx is a radiopaque, nonadhesive embolic fluid which precipitates upon contact with blood. Complications of embolization of AVMs have been reported in 6–14% of cases; the majority of complications are minor problems related to vascular access, but hemorrhage, stroke and death have also been reported [13, 14]. The purpose of pre-SRS embolization is to permanently obliterate a distinct part of the nidus and thus reduce its volume that is subsequently treated by radiosurgery. Our initial experience suggested that SRS targeting was more difficult after embolization. In addition, recanalization of previously embolized components may have led to late treatment failures, since embolized AVM volumes were not included in the SRS treatment volume.

Total AVM Obliteration

In a subgroup of 48 patients with AVMs larger than 15 ml, Pan et al. [15] found an obliteration rate of 25% after 40 months. In their single radiosurgery strategy, the average margin dose was 17.7 Gy for AVM volumes 10–20 ml and 16.5 Gy for volumes more than 20 ml. In their follow-up examinations, they observed 37% moderate and 12% severe AREs in patients with AVMs larger than 10 cm^3. Yang et al. [16] reported that AVM obliteration was achieved in 11 (33%) of 33 patients with AVMs of >14 cm^3 nidus volume after a single-session SRS with a mean margin dose of 14.1 Gy (range, 10–20 Gy) at a mean follow-up of 78 months (range, 34–166 months). Three of 4 patients after repeat SRS showed total obliteration. Miyawaki et al. [17] reported that the obliteration rate in patients with AVMs larger than 14 ml treated using linear accelerator radiosurgery was 22%. Inoue and Ohye [7] reported an obliteration rate of 36.4% and hemorrhage rate of 35.7% in the subgroup of AVMs larger than 10 ml treated by radiosurgery. It became clear to us that in the narrow corridor between dose response and complication, the chances to achieve a high obliteration rate with a low complication rate for large AVM radiosurgery are slim. For this reason, radiosurgical volume staging was developed as an option to manage large AVMs [18].

Hemorrhage after SRS

Pan et al. [15] reported a 9.2% risk of hemorrhage after single-session SRS for large AVMs (>10 cm^3) with a 3.9% risk of permanent morbidity. Chung et al. [19] studied 6 patients who underwent staged SRS for AVMs of >40 cm^3 and reported that 1 suffered hemorrhages within 8 months after the second-stage radiosurgery. Yang et al. [16] reported an annual hemorrhage rate of 2.9% after single-session SRS for AVMs >14 cm^3 in the hemorrhage group (n = 17) and 3.1% in the nonhemorrhage group (n = 29). These authors noted that pre-SRS embolization increased the risk of hemorrhage for the nonhemorrhage group, whereas embolization had no effect on the hemorrhage group. In our experience the number of prior hemorrhages was significantly associated with a higher rate of hemorrhage after staged SRS. Pre-SRS embolization was not associated with a change in hemorrhage rate after staged SRS.

Complications of SRS

Single-session SRS for AVMs is associated with a 2–3% risk of AREs resulting in a permanent neurological deficit [2, 20, 21]. Pollock et al. [18] studied the radiation dosimetry of staged-volume AVM radiosurgery and compared it with single-session procedures using 10 large AVMs (median volume of 17.4 cm^3, range, 7.4–53.3 cm^3). These authors reported an average of 11% (range, 4.9–21%: $p < 0.001$) reduction in the 12-Gy volume with staged-volume radiosurgery. There was also a significant reduction by an average of 27% (range, 12.5–51.3%; $p < 0.001$) in 12-Gy volume outside the AVM. This study suggested that staged-volume radiosurgery of large AVMs results in less radiation exposure to the adjacent brain. In our experience, the incidence of AREs was low, only 1 patient (2%) developed temporary symptomatic AREs after the first-stage SRS and 2 patients (4%) developed symptomatic AREs after the second-stage SRS. Three of 17 patients who underwent repeat SRS after failed staged SRS developed symptomatic AREs.

Future Directions

The obliteration rates for larger-volume AVMs are significantly lower than the obliteration rates after SRS for smaller-volume AVMs eligible for single-procedure SRS. In fact larger AVMs will require more than 2 SRS procedures to increase the total obliteration rates to approximately two thirds of patients. The time to obliteration is significantly longer in patients who undergo multistage SRS for larger-volume AVMs. In selected cases, staged radiosurgery may reduce the AVM volume to make a previously inoperable AVM suitable for resection [22]. At present we are not enthusiastic about the role of embolization prior to SRS, since permanent volume reduction after embolization could not be achieved in most patients, and we are not convinced that embolization alone reduces hemorrhage risks. However, the fact is that unless the embolization is attempted in many cases it would not be clear if a volume reduction could be obtained. We believe that partial AVM embolization makes SRS targeting and dosimetry more difficult. One strategy could be to reverse the timing of embolization and SRS. Thus volumetric SRS for the entire nidus can be completed first followed by embolization. Perhaps in such cases early flow reduction will enhance both the rate and the completeness of eventual obliteration. In addition, more aggressive treatment of AVM fistulas and proximal aneurysms may reduce the latency interval bleeding risks. Another attractive approach would be to use embolization for injection of radiation-sensitizing agents for the luminal endothelium during the SRS procedure itself. Thus, SRS immediately after embolization might more likely lead to earlier or more complete obliteration. In our 20-year experience, we have seen a variety of embolic materials such as polyvinyl alcohol, silk threads, coils and polymerizing cyanoacrylates. The data analysis for the present study was concluded prior to the introduction of Onyx which is a potentially improved embolic agent. Our subsequent clinical experience suggests that Onyx rarely results in exclusion of a volume of the AVM, thereby reducing the SRS target volume. In addition Onyx embolization has also resulted in significant MRI artifact that makes axial plan AVM visualization suboptimal. We believe that post-SRS embolization may provide greater benefit. In the future, prospective volume-staged SRS followed by innovative embolization strategies (to reduce flow, obliterate fistulas and occlude associated aneurysms) may further reduce the risk of hemorrhage.

Prospective volume-staged SRS for large AVMs has potential benefit but often requires multiple procedures spread over time. Our data supports the concept that larger-volume AVMs may require more than 2 procedures in order to improve the eventual obliteration rates to as high as 66% at 10 years.

Acknowledgements

The work described in this report was funded by a research grant to Dr. Kano from AB Elekta, Stockholm, Sweden.

Disclosure Statement

Drs. Lunsford, Kondziolka and Novotny are consultants for AB Elekta, and Dr. Lunsford is a stockholder.

References

1 Flickinger JC, Pollock BE, Kondziolka D, Lunsford LD: A dose-response analysis of arteriovenous malformation obliteration after radiosurgery. Int J Radiat Oncol Biol Phys 1996;36:873–879.

2 Liscak R, Vladyka V, Simonova G, Urgosik D, Novotny J Jr, Janouskova L, Vymazal J: Arteriovenous malformations after Leksell gamma knife radiosurgery: rate of obliteration and complications. Neurosurgery 2007;60:1005–1014, discussion 1015–1016.

3 Pollock BE, Flickinger JC, Lunsford LD, Maitz A, Kondziolka D: Factors associated with successful arteriovenous malformation radiosurgery. Neurosurgery 1998;42:1239–1244, discussion 1244–1247.
4 Karlsson B, Lindqvist M, Blomgren H, Wan-Yeo G, Soderman M, Lax I, Yamamoto M, Bailes J: Long-term results after fractionated radiation therapy for large brain arteriovenous malformations. Neurosurgery 2005;57:42–49.
5 Redekop GJ, Elisevich KV, Gaspar LE, Wiese KP, Drake CG: Conventional radiation therapy of intracranial arteriovenous malformations: long-term results. J Neurosurg 1993;78:413–422.
6 Kjellberg RN, Hanamura T, Davis KR, Lyons SL, Adams RD: Bragg-peak proton-beam therapy for arteriovenous malformations of the brain. N Engl J Med 1983;309:269–274.
7 Inoue HK, Ohye C: Hemorrhage risks and obliteration rates of arteriovenous malformations after gamma knife radiosurgery. J Neurosurg 2002;97: 474–476.
8 Colombo F, Pozza F, Chierego G, Casentini L, De Luca G, Francescon P: Linear accelerator radiosurgery of cerebral arteriovenous malformations: an update. Neurosurgery 1994;34:14–20, discussion 20–21.
9 Gobin YP, Laurent A, Merienne L, Schlienger M, Aymard A, Houdart E, Casasco A, Lefkopoulos D, George B, Merland JJ: Treatment of brain arteriovenous malformations by embolization and radiosurgery. J Neurosurg 1996;85:19–28.
10 Ogilvy CS, Stieg PE, Awad I, Brown RD Jr, Kondziolka D, Rosenwasser R, Young WL, Hademenos G: Recommendations for the management of intracranial arteriovenous malformations: a statement for healthcare professionals from a special writing group of the Stroke Council, American Stroke Association. Circulation 2001;103:2644–2657.
11 Paulsen RD, Steinberg GK, Norbash AM, Marcellus ML, Marks MP: Embolization of basal ganglia and thalamic arteriovenous malformations. Neurosurgery 1999;44:991–996, discussion 996–997.
12 Sinclair J, Kelly ME, Steinberg GK: Surgical management of posterior fossa arteriovenous malformations. Neurosurgery 2006;58:ONS-189–201, discussion ONS-201.
13 Friedlander RM: Clinical practice. Arteriovenous malformations of the brain. N Engl J Med 2007;356: 2704–2712.
14 Weber W, Kis B, Siekmann R, Kuehne D: Endovascular treatment of intracranial arteriovenous malformations with Onyx: technical aspects. AJNR Am J Neuroradiol 2007;28:371–377.
15 Pan DH, Guo WY, Chung WY, Shiau CY, Chang YC, Wang LW: Gamma knife radiosurgery as a single treatment modality for large cerebral arteriovenous malformations. J Neurosurg 2000;93(suppl 3):113–119.
16 Yang SY, Kim DG, Chung HT, Paek SH, Park JH, Han DH: Radiosurgery for large cerebral arteriovenous malformations. Acta Neurochir (Wien) 2009;151:113–124.
17 Miyawaki L, Dowd C, Wara W, Goldsmith B, Albright N, Gutin P, Halbach V, Hieshima G, Higashida R, Lulu B, Pitts L, Schell M, Smith V, Weaver K, Wilson C, Larson D: Five year results of LINAC radiosurgery for arteriovenous malformations: outcome for large AVMs. Int J Radiat Oncol Biol Phys 1999;44:1089–1106.
18 Pollock BE, Kline RW, Stafford SL, Foote RL, Schomberg PJ: The rationale and technique of staged-volume arteriovenous malformation radiosurgery. Int J Radiat Oncol Biol Phys 2000;48:817–824.
19 Chung WY, Shiau CY, Wu HM, Liu KD, Guo WY, Wang LW, Pan DH: Staged radiosurgery for extra-large cerebral arteriovenous malformations: method, implementation, and results. J Neurosurg 2008;109(suppl):65–72.
20 Lunsford LD, Kondziolka D, Flickinger JC, Bissonette DJ, Jungreis CA, Maitz AH, Horton JA, Coffey RJ: Stereotactic radiosurgery for arteriovenous malformations of the brain. J Neurosurg 1991;75:512–524.
21 Pollock BE, Meyer FB: Radiosurgery for arteriovenous malformations. J Neurosurg 2004;101:390–392, discussion 392.
22 Firlik AD, Levy EI, Kondziolka D, Yonas H: Staged volume radiosurgery followed by microsurgical resection: a novel treatment for giant cerebral arteriovenous malformations: technical case report. Neurosurgery 1998;43:1223–1228.

L. Dade Lunsford, MD, FACS
Lars Leksell Distinguished Professor of Neurological Surgery
University of Pittsburgh, Suite B-400, UPMC Presbyterian
200 Lothrop Street
Pittsburgh, PA 15213 (USA)
Tel. +1 412 647 6781, E-Mail lunsfordld@upmc.edu

Niranjan A, Kano H, Lunsford LD (eds): Gamma Knife Radiosurgery for Brain Vascular Malformations.
Prog Neurol Surg. Basel, Karger, 2013, vol 27, pp 81–88 (DOI: 10.1159/000341643)

Endovascular Embolization in Combination with Radiosurgery for Treatment of Arteriovenous Malformations

Robert A. Miller · Brian Jankowitz

Department of Neurological Surgery, University of Pittsburgh, Pittsburgh, Pa., USA

Abstract

There are several options for the treatment of patients with arteriovenous malformations (AVMs). Surgical resection, radiosurgery and endovascular embolization can be used alone or in conjunction. In patients with AVMs not amenable to surgical resection due to large size or location, radiosurgery can address some but not all of these issues as cure rates remain low for volumes >10 cm^3. Combining endovascular embolization with stereotactic radiosurgery allows potential volume reduction and reduction of risks related to factors that may increase bleeding risks during the latency interval after radiosurgery. The benefit of increased cure rates and possibly lower hemorrhage rates in the latency period may justify the added risk of embolization.

Complete surgical resection when feasible remains the gold standard for the successful treatment of arteriovenous malformations (AVMs), as it offers a high rate of cure with immediate elimination of hemorrhagic risk. However, open surgical risks are significant and numerous risk factors exist, including those associated with large AVM volumes, eloquent locations, deep venous drainage or patient comorbidities such as hypertension or cardiac disease. Radiosurgery addresses some but not all of these shortcomings with reduced morbidity and less concern for venous drainage or location. Radiosurgery has less success in large-volume AVMs. In addition patients remain at risk for hemorrhage during the latency interval until obliteration occurs. Endovascular embolization has the potential to work synergistically with radiosurgery to surmount these problems.

Combining endovascular embolization with stereotactic radiosurgery to treat AVMs allows potential volume reduction and elimination of high-risk features. Gobin et al. [1] and others [2, 3] described the first large series utilizing this technique in 125 patients. In this series, the AVMs varied from grade II to VI on the Spetzler-

Martin [4] scale with a mean grade of IV. Radiosurgery after embolization resulted in a 65% obliteration rate. This was higher in the group with a residual nidus of <2 cm, in which cases the obliteration rate increased to 79%. They also reported that no patients with completely occluded AVMs had a subsequent bleeding event during the mean follow-up interval of 40 months. Complications from embolization included a morbidity rate of 12.8% and a mortality rate of 1.6%. Additional studies indicate that the combination of these two modalities offers new options for the care of patients with otherwise difficult to treat AVMs.

Indications for Embolization in Conjunction with Gamma Knife Radiosurgery

Volume Reduction

AVMs that are greater than 3 cm in maximum diameter or whose volume is greater than 10–15 cm^3 are classified as large, and have historically been difficult to obliterate effectively with stereotactic radiosurgery alone [2, 5, 6]. Several studies have shown that in AVMs with a volume of 10–15 cm^3 treated with stereotactic Gamma Knife radiosurgery (GKRS), the obliteration rates ranged from 25 to 77%. AVMs with volumes greater than 15 cm^3 had consistently lower cure rates of less than 50% [7–9]. Furthermore, when large AVMS are located in eloquent locations (brainstem, sensorimotor cortex, thalamus, basal ganglia), radiation doses >12 Gy to the surrounding brain increase the risk of adverse radiation effects [10]. Targeting larger volumes allows more radiation to reach brain structures surrounding the AVM. Flickinger et al. [11] eloquently demonstrated this by relating the risk of adverse radiation effects to the volume of surrounding brain receiving 12 Gy or more.

While staged radiosurgery is an option, obliteration rates remain low. Sirin et al. [12] published a prospective study evaluating the results of AVMs greater than 15 cm^3 treated with GKRS. The total obliteration rate was 50% in 28 patients with a median follow-up of 50 months. Two patients received 3 procedures, and all others received 2 [12]. A recent paper discussed the importance of reducing the AVM volume prior to radiosurgery. Endovascular embolization reduced the volume from a mean of 20.1 cm^3 to a mean of 8.9 cm^3, resulting in an overall volume reduction of 56% and an AVM obliteration rate of 81% [13]. Blackburn et al. [13] were able to achieve this high cure rate by focusing on volume reduction as opposed to flow reduction. The distinction is subtle, but important. Endovascular embolization performed in the standard manner of treating the most accessible arterial feeders may only haphazardly knock out pieces of a large puzzle, leaving behind the same size AVM with internal components missing. This does affect the volumetric radiosurgical treatment plan. Moreover, embolization of internal AVM components can make it more difficult to stereotactically target the lesion, raising concern that preradiosurgical embolization may actually reduce cure rates [14]. The ideal embolization of large AVMs would selectively target peripheral feeders to yield a compact volume suitable for radiosurgery [15]. Blackburn et al. [13] reported that multisession segmental embolization was able to reduce the entire volume of the AVM. This is in contrast to prior techniques that were designed to reduce flow through the AVM, a result that does not decrease the volume necessary for GKRS nor improve cure rates [15]. In contrast, such an approach may improve the safety of microsurgical removal.

A consistent volumetric goal of embolization has been to reduce the eventual radiosurgical target to less than 11 cm^3 (fig. 1) [1–3, 6]. The radiographic obliteration rates of the AVMs in these series have ranged from 38 to 84%. Mizoi et al. [3] using polyvinyl alcohol embolization followed by GKRS reported a 38% obliteration rate in 29 patients with AVMs greater than 3 cm in diameter. They reported an associated 11% morbidity secondary to embolization. No complications were reported after radiosurgery [2]. Mathis et al. [2] described a 50% obliteration rate in 24 patients with a mean AVM volume of 37 cm^3 embolized with N-butylcyanoacrylate (NBCA) followed by GKRS. Their embolization morbidity was reported as 0%. They reported a 4% complication rate after radiosurgery [2]. Blackburn et al. [13] reported a series of 21 patients who had AVMs that averaged 4.2 cm in diameter. All underwent NBCA embolization followed by GKRS; the final obliteration rate was 81%. Postembolizaton morbidity was noted in 19% although there were no major permanent neurological deficits. They reported a 5% complication rate after radiosurgery [13].

Since complication rates of embolization are significant when compared to radiosurgery, combination of both procedures may ultimately improve obliteration rates and reduce hemorrhage risks during the latency interval after radiosurgery. Studies by Back et al. [16] and Sirin et al. [12] evaluating staged radiosurgery alone for large AVMs noted bleed rates of 21 and 14% with 3- and 4-year follow-up, respectively. In studies of embolization followed by radiosurgery, the latency interval hemorrhage rates were lower, ranging from 0 to 4% during the first 2–3 years of follow-up.

Elimination of High-Risk Features

Certain anatomical elements within AVMs have been shown to be more resistant to radiosurgical treatment, such as high flow arteriovenous fistulas and intranidal aneurysms [17]. Both are features of AVMs that may increase the risk of hemorrhage, neurological injury and other complications [18]. Recent reports have shown that treating these features with embolization prior to other modalities may reduce such risks [12]. Associated AVM aneurysms require special consideration that include coiling a proximal aneurysm (and leaving the AVM for radiosurgical treatment), or embolization of the arterial pedicle feeding the aneurysm and potentially eliminating distal flow. Care must be taken to make sure that a liquid embolic agent fills the aneurysm as it can still fill retrogradely if not embolized. High-flow fistulas can also be embolized selectively, taking special care to avoid occlusion of draining veins.

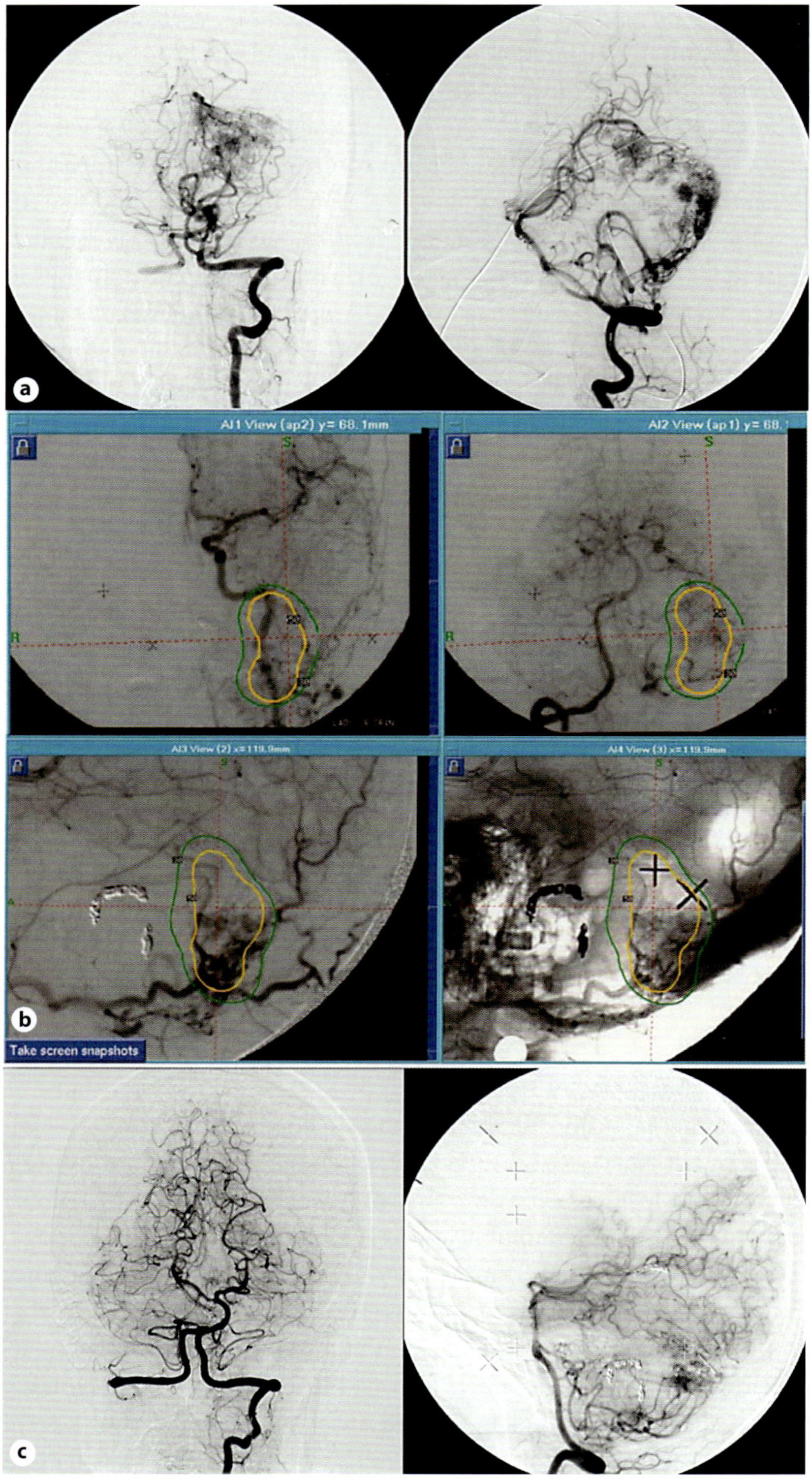
a
AI1 View (ap2) y= 68.1mm
AI2 View (ap1) y= 68.
AI3 View (2) x=119.9mm
AI4 View (3) x=119.9mm
b
Take screen snapshots
c

Technique

Embolization before GKRS versus Embolization after GKRS

The goal of embolization prior to GKRS is to reduce the AVM nidus volume to render a smaller target suitable for radiosurgery. If performed prior to GKRS, volume reduction is obtained by targeting arterial feeders at the periphery of the AVM to create a fixed, concise and hopefully permanently excluded volume. Embolization has also been used to treat AVMs after GKRS in patients who have a residual nidus. Marks et al. [19] reported 6 patients with persistent AVMs 2–4 years after radiosurgery. Embolization resulted in complete obliteration in 1 patient, volume reduction amenable to further radiosurgery in 2 and complete resection in 3 [19].

Another paradigm that deserves further study involves radiosurgery prior to embolization. It potentially allows the benefit of volumetric planning with full visualization of the AVM, before the artifact and typical piecemeal results of embolization. In such patients subsequent treatment may reduce flow and successfully treat associated aneurysms. Hypothetically this may reduce the risk of bleeding during the latency interval and improve the rate as well at the completeness of eventual AVM closure. Such an approach also reduces the possibility of subtotal target treatment by radiosurgery, caused by postembolization artifacts that obscure the remaining treatment volume. Partial AVM embolization leaving a significant artifact behind poses the worst of both scenarios, as the AVM is possibly obscured by the embolization agent and yet the treatment volume was not significantly reduced.

Embolization after radiosurgery arguably exposes the patient to the potential of complications from both treatment techniques. This approach may be most valuable when the treatment goal includes eliminating an aneurysm or fistulae, particularly in smaller AVMs where volume reduction is less important. Also, this technique may be considered in AVMs of borderline size (7–15 cm^3) which may be treated in one session without embolization, albeit at the cost of lower obliteration rates.

Agents

As technology in the field of embolization has been advanced, different options for treatment have become available. Liquid agents have become standard practice for embolization techniques. NBCA was the most commonly used agent in the USA. Its attributes include rapid polymerization that can be tailored to avoid early or late polymerization. The polymerization rate is dictated by the addition of Ethiodol, which

Fig. 1. **a** Posteroanterior and lateral vertebral artery angiograms of a 37-year-old female with prior hemorrhage showing a left cerebellar AVM. She underwent partial endovascular embolization using polyvinyl alcohol. GKRS was performed for residual AVM. **b** GKRS dose plan showing complete coverage of residual AVM seen on posteroanterior and lateral vertebral angiograms and lateral external carotid artery angiogram. **c** Anterior and lateral vertebral artery angiograms obtained 3 years after stereotactic radiosurgery showing the absence of a nidus and early venous drainage.

prolongs the time to form a polymer cast. Studies have shown that AVMs completely obliterated with NBCA usually do not recanalize [20, 21].

Limitations of this agent include the need for extensive training and experience, as the subjective formulation for time to polymerization can be over- or underestimated. The newest embolic agent on the US market is Onyx (EV3), which is a premixed liquid comprised of an ethylenevinyl alcohol copolymer, tantalum powder for radiopacity and dimethylsulfoxide. There are properties to Onyx that have been described as advantageous over NBCA. It is cohesive as opposed to adhesive, which theoretically reduces its adherence to foreign bodies, such as the injection catheter. It solidifies more slowly, thus allowing more controlled injection rates. This may decrease the risk of the agent refluxing too proximally in the arterial feeders or too distally in the venous circulation. The long-term recanalization rates for Onyx have yet to be determined, but appear to be low. Saatci et al. [22] have recently published their experience of treating 179 patients with Onyx for grade I–II AVMs, resulting in a recanalization rate of 1.1% after a mean follow-up of 3.9 years with a minimum of 1 year.

Regarding new advances in embolization treatment, detachable catheters now allow longer injection times and prevent the catheter from being glued in the artery. This allows interventionalists to focus on and maximize embolic penetration to one pedicle at a time, resulting in less piecemeal embolization patterns. This is of paramount importance as embolizing only one pedicle as opposed to knocking out every accessible pedicle provides the highest chance of segmental volume reduction.

Timing between Embolization and GKRS

Although intuitional practices vary, the timing between embolization and GKRS is generally greater than 4 weeks and reported up to 6 months. Although there is no clear consensus, allowing for resolution of postembolization magnetic resonance imaging changes, such as brain edema, may facilitate better targeting using magnetic resonance sequences.

Areas of Consideration

One of the concerns of this dual modality treatment is the potential for decreased rates of obliteration of the AVM when embolization is done prior to GKRS as compared to GKRS alone [23]. Back et al. [16] reported AVM obliteration rates of 75.9% in unstaged GKRS compared to 60% in a staged embolization followed by GKRS procedure. They also reported 73.7% obliteration in staged GKRS alone compared to 66.7% in embolization prior to staged GKRS [16]. However, they also note that the difference in rates failed to reach statistical significance in the four groups. Recanalization after embolization could account for this finding, although the most recent reports show a very low rate of renewed flow through previously embolized segments. Difficulty in radiosurgical targeting is also a concern after embolization, which can be surmounted by precise, segmental embolization or even radiosurgery prior to embolization. It has also been postulated that the molecular constitution of the liquid embolic agents decreases the radiation dose received by the AVM tissue. This has been supported by a few recent studies which proposed that the liquid embolic agents result in reduced radiation to the targeted tissue (i.e. beam attenuation) because the embolic agents absorb some of the radiation. The amount of radiation absorbed depends on the type of radiation. Using X-rays (i.e. a linear accelerator), total dose reduction through an embolic agent (cyanoacrylate in these studies) was up to 10–15% [24, 25]. In comparison, a recent study using γ-rays specifically from radioactive cobalt, the total dose reduction through Onyx as well as NBCA was <0.01–0.2% [26].

Conclusion

Patients that have large AVMs present a difficult challenge to treat. Although there is an added risk of injury by including embolization prior to radiosurgery, in selected series this increases the obliteration rate of the AVM by as much as 30%. Other reports emphasize that embolization prior to radiosurgery may reduce the obliteration rates for similar volume AVMs. Recent advances in endovascular techniques and materials have reduced recanalization rates, increased volume reduction and decreased morbidity and mortality from the procedure itself. In the array of options to treat AVMs, the combined use of embolization with radiosurgery can be an effective dual modality in appropriately selected patients.

References

1 Gobin YP, Laurent A, Merienne L, Schlienger M, Aymard A, Houdart E, Casasco A, Lefkopoulos D, George B, Merland JJ: Treatment of brain arteriovenous malformations by embolization and radiosurgery. J Neurosurg 1996;85:19–28.

2 Mathis JA, Barr JD, Horton JA, Jungreis CA, Lunsford LD, Kondziolka DS, Vincent D, Pentheny S: The efficacy of particulate embolization combined with stereotactic radiosurgery for treatment of large arteriovenous malformations of the brain. AJNR Am J Neuroradiol 1995;16:299–306.

3 Mizoi K, Jokura H, Yoshimoto T, Takahashi A, Ezura M, Kinouchi H, Nagamine Y, Boku N: Multimodality treatment for large and critically located arteriovenous malformations. Neurol Med Chir (Tokyo) 1998;38(suppl):186–192.

4 Spetzler RF, Martin NA: A proposed grading system for arteriovenous malformations. J Neurosurg 1986; 65:476–483.

5 Chang JH, Chang JW, Park YG, Chung SS: Factors related to complete occlusion of arteriovenous malformations after gamma knife radiosurgery. J Neurosurg 2000;93(suppl 3):96–101.

6 Ellis TL, Friedman WA, Bova FJ, Kubilis PS, Buatti JM: Analysis of treatment failure after radiosurgery for arteriovenous malformations. J Neurosurg 1998; 89:104–110.

7 Pan DH, Guo WY, Chung WY, Shiau CY, Chang YC, Wang LW: Gamma knife radiosurgery as a single treatment modality for large cerebral arteriovenous malformations. J Neurosurg 2000;93(suppl 3): 113–119.

8 Pollock BE, Gorman DA, Coffey RJ: Patient outcomes after arteriovenous malformation radiosurgical management: results based on a 5- to 14-year follow-up study. Neurosurgery 2003;52:1291–1296, discussion 1296–1297.

9 Yamamoto Y, Coffey RJ, Nichols DA, Shaw EG: Interim report on the radiosurgical treatment of cerebral arteriovenous malformations. The influence of size, dose, time, and technical factors on obliteration rate. J Neurosurg 1995;83:832–837.
10 Flickinger JC, Kondziolka D, Lunsford LD, Kassam A, Phuong LK, Liscak R, Pollock B: Development of a model to predict permanent symptomatic postradiosurgery injury for arteriovenous malformation patients. Int J Radiat Oncol Biol Phys 2000;46: 1143–1148.
11 Flickinger JC, Pollock BE, Kondziolka D, Lunsford LD: A dose-response analysis of arteriovenous malformation obliteration after radiosurgery. Int J Radiat Oncol Biol Phys 1996;36:873–879.
12 Sirin S, Kondziolka D, Niranjan A, Flickinger JC, Maitz AH, Lunsford LD: Prospective staged volume radiosurgery for large arteriovenous malformations: indications and outcomes in otherwise untreatable patients. Neurosurgery 2006;58:17–27.
13 Blackburn SL, Ashley WW Jr, Rich KM, Simpson JR, Drzymala RE, Ray WZ, Moran CJ, Cross DT 3rd, Chicoine MR, Dacey RG Jr, Derdeyn CP, Zipfel GJ: Combined endovascular embolization and stereotactic radiosurgery in the treatment of large arteriovenous malformations. J Neurosurg 2011;114: 1758–1767.
14 Pollock BE, Kondziolka D, Lunsford LD, Bissonette D, Flickinger JC: Repeat stereotactic radiosurgery of arteriovenous malformations: factors associated with incomplete obliteration. Neurosurgery 1996;38: 318–324.
15 Heros RC: Editorial: large arteriovenous malformations (published online February 18, 2011). Miami, University of Miami, Miller School of Medicine, Department of Neurological Surgery, DOI: 10.3171/2010.11.JNS101892.
16 Back AG, Vollmer D, Zeck O, Shkedy C, Shedden PM: Retrospective analysis of unstaged and staged Gamma Knife surgery with and without preceding embolization for the treatment of arteriovenous malformations. J Neurosurg 2008;109(suppl):57–64.
17 Yuki I, Kim RH, Duckwiler G, Jahan R, Tateshima S, Gonzalez N, Gorgulho A, Diaz JL, De Salles AA, Viñuela F: Treatment of brain arteriovenous malformations with high-flow arteriovenous fistulas: risk and complications associated with endovascular embolization in multimodality treatment. J Neurosurg 2010;113:715–722.
18 Haw CS, ter Brugge K, Willinsky R, Tomlinson G: Complications of embolization of arteriovenous malformations of the brain. J Neurosurg 2006;104: 226–232.
19 Marks MP, Lane B, Steinberg GK, Fabrikant JI, Levy RP, Frankel KA, Phillips MH: Endovascular treatment of cerebral arteriovenous malformations following radiosurgery. AJNR Am J Neuroradiol 1993; 14:297–303.
20 Debrun GM, Aletich V, Ausman JI, Charbel F, Dujovny M: Embolization of the nidus of brain arteriovenous malformations with N-butyl cyanoacrylate. Neurosurgery 1997;40:112–120, discussion 120–121.
21 Wikholm G: Occlusion of cerebral arteriovenous malformations with N-butyl cyano-acrylate is permanent. AJNR Am J Neuroradiol 1995;16:479–482.
22 Saatci I, Geyik S, Yavuz K, Cekirge HS: Endovascular treatment of brain arteriovenous malformations with prolonged intranidal Onyx injection technique: long-term results in 350 consecutive patients with completed endovascular treatment course. J Neurosurg 2011;115:78–88.
23 Pollock BE, Flickinger JC, Lunsford LD, Maitz A, Kondziolka D: Factors associated with successful arteriovenous malformation radiosurgery. Neurosurgery 1998;42:1239–1244, discussion 1244–1247.
24 Andrade-Souza YM, Ramani M, Scora D, Tsao MN, ter Brugge K, Schwartz ML: Embolization before radiosurgery reduces the obliteration rate of arteriovenous malformations. Neurosurgery 2007;60:443–451, discussion 451–452.
25 Andrade-Souza YM, Ramani M, Beachey DJ, Scora D, Tsao MN, ter Brugge K, Schwartz ML: Liquid embolisation material reduces the delivered radiation dose: a physical experiment. Acta Neurochir (Wien) 2008;150:161–164, discussion 164.
26 Mamalui-Hunter M, Jiang T, Rich KM, Derdeyn CP, Drzymala RE: Effect of liquid embolic agents on Gamma Knife surgery dosimetry for arteriovenous malformations. J Neurosurg 2011;115:364–370.

Brian Jankowitz, MD
Department of Neurological Surgery, UPMC Presbyterian, Suite B-400
200 Lothrop Street
Pittsburgh, PA 15213 (USA)
Tel. +1 412 647 3920, E-Mail janowitzbt@upmc.edu

Niranjan A, Kano H, Lunsford LD (eds): Gamma Knife Radiosurgery for Brain Vascular Malformations.
Prog Neurol Surg. Basel, Karger, 2013, vol 27, pp 89–96 (DOI: 10.1159/000341646)

Stereotactic Radiosurgery after Embolization for Arteriovenous Malformations

Hideyuki Kano[a,c] · Douglas Kondziolka[a,c] · John C. Flickinger[b,c] · Kyung-Jae Park[a,c] · Aditya Iyer[d] · Huai-che Yang[a,c,e] · Xiaomin Liu[a,c,f] · Edward A. Monaco III[a] · Ajay Niranjan[a,c] · L. Dade Lunsford[a,c]

Departments of [a]Neurological Surgery and [b]Radiation Oncology, [c]Center for Image-Guided Neurosurgery and [d]University of Pittsburgh School of Medicine, Pittsburgh, Pa., USA; [e]Department of Neurosurgery, Taipei Veterans General Hospital, Taipei, Taiwan, ROC; [f]Department of Neurosurgery and Gamma Knife Center, 2nd Hospital of Tianjin Medical University, Tianjin, PR China

Abstract

We sought to define the long-term benefits and risks of stereotactic radiosurgery (SRS) for arteriovenous malformation (AVM) patients who underwent prior embolization. Between 1987 and 2006, we performed Gamma Knife® SRS on 120 patients with AVM who underwent embolization followed by SRS. Sixty-four patients (53%) had at least 1 prior hemorrhage. The median number of embolizations varied from 1 to 5. The median target volume was 6.6 cm^3 (range, 0.2–26.3 cm^3). The median margin dose was 18 Gy (range, 13.5–25 Gy). After embolization, 25 patients (21%) developed symptomatic neurological deficits. The overall rates of total obliteration documented by either angiography or magnetic resonance imaging were 35, 53, 55 and 59% at 3, 4, 5 and 10 years, respectively. Nine patients (8%) had a hemorrhage during the latency interval and 7 patients died due to hemorrhage. The actuarial rates of AVM hemorrhage after SRS were 0.8, 3.5, 5.4, 7.7 and 7.7% at 1, 2, 3, 5 and 10 years, respectively. Permanent neurological deficits due to adverse radiation effects developed in 3 patients (2.5%) after SRS. Using a case-match control technique, we found that embolization prior to SRS was associated with a lower rate of total obliteration ($p = 0.028$) in comparison to radiosurgery alone. In this 20-year experience, we found that prior embolization reduced the rate of total obliteration after SRS and latency interval hemorrhage risks were not affected by prior embolization. In the future, the role of embolization after SRS should be explored.

Cerebral arteriovenous malformations (AVMs) are responsible for 2% of all hemorrhagic strokes [1]. The natural history of AVMs suggests a 2–5% annual overall risk of a spontaneous hemorrhage [2–5]. The average mortality from untreated AVMs varies from 0.7 to 1.0% per year [3, 5]. Rebleeding rates after initial hemorrhage have been reported to vary between 6 and 18% per year [4, 6–9]. Morbidity resulting from hemorrhage has been reported to vary between 53 and 81%, whereas mortality has ranged from 10 to 18% [4, 10]. The goal of treatment in cerebral AVMs is to completely eliminate the risk of intracranial hemorrhage and prevent new neurological deficits [11, 12]. The eradication of the hemorrhage risk often requires the use of multimodality management that includes microsurgical resection, endovascular embolization and stereotactic radiosurgery (SRS).

Endovascular embolization has been advocated as a primary therapy by some investigators [13]. However, most reports indicate that embolization has limited curative potential and may add to management morbidity [14–17]. Embolization complication rates range from 3 to 11% per procedure [18–25]. Embolization prior to microsurgery can lead to flow reduction, reduce eventual surgical blood loss and occlude vessels that may be difficult to reach during surgery [26]. Embolization prior to SRS is often employed to reduce the nidus size of larger brain AVMs, and thereby increase the benefit of subsequent SRS. Optimal embolization prior to SRS permanently reduces the treatable nidus volume.

Pittsburgh Experience

Between 1987 and 2006, 996 patients with brain AVMs underwent SRS; 120 patients underwent embolization followed by SRS. The median patient age was 33 years (range, 3–67 years). In this series, 64 patients (53%) had at least 1 prior hemorrhage. The AVMs were classified as Spetzler-Martin grade I in 4 (3%), grade II in 21 (18%), grade III in 54 (45%), grade IV in 27 (23%), grade V in 0 and grade VI in 14 patients (12%). In this subset of patients the median interval between embolization and SRS was 9.9 months (range, 4.2–217 months). The median number of embolizations varied from 1 to 5. Sixty-nine patients (57%) underwent 1 embolization before SRS. Thirty-seven patients (31%) had 2 embolization procedures, 9 (8%) had 3 embolizations, 2 (2%) had 4 embolizations, and 3 (3%) had 5 embolizations before SRS. A variety of embolization agents were used. These included polyvinyl alcohol particles (n = 20, 17%), N-butylcyanoacrylate (n = 38, 32%), isobutyl-2-cyanoacrylate (n = 14, 12%) and microcoils (n = 10, 8%). The embolization agents were not recorded in 38 patients (32%). Twenty-five patients (21%) developed complications after 1 or more embolization procedures. The complications of embolization included hemiparesis (n = 16, 13%), visual field deficit (n = 7, 6%) and dysphasia (n = 2, 2%). This report does not include patients who have undergone embolization using Onyx (ev3, Irvine, Calif., USA), a product available at our center since late 2006. The median target volume was 6.6 cm^3 (range, 0.2–26.3 cm^3). The median margin dose was 18 Gy (range, 13.5–25 Gy).

The overall rates of total obliteration documented by either angiography or magnetic resonance imaging were 35, 53, 55 and 59% at 3, 4, 5 and 10 years, respectively. Factors associated with a higher rate of AVM obliteration were smaller target volume, smaller maximum diameter, higher margin dose and timing of embolization during the most recent 10-year interval. Nine patients (8%) had a hemorrhage during the latency interval and 7 patients died due to hemorrhage. The overall annual hemorrhage rate was 2.7%. The actuarial rates of 1-, 2-, 3-, 5- and 10-year hemorrhage rates after SRS were 0.8, 3.5, 5.4, 7.7 and 7.7%, respectively. Factors associated with a higher risk of hemorrhage after SRS were a larger target volume and a greater number of prior hemorrhages. Three patients (2.5%) developed permanent neurological deficits due to adverse radiation effects (AREs). No patient died due to ARE. One patient developed a delayed cyst 210 months after SRS. A larger 12-Gy volume was associated with a higher risk of symptomatic AREs.

Of the 996 AVM patients who underwent single-stage SRS at our center between 1987 and 2006, 682 AVM patients without prior embolization who underwent SRS were eligible to serve as potential case control matches. For the purpose of analysis, these AVM patients who underwent prior embolization (n = 120, case cohort) were matched (identical sex, similar age, similar hemorrhage history, similar maximum nidus diameter, similar target volume, similar margin dose, similar Spetzler-Martin grade, similar Pollock-Flickinger score and similar follow-up duration) with 120 AVM patients who did not undergo embolization (controls).Using a case-match control technique, we found that embolization prior to SRS was associated with a lower rate of total obliteration ($p = 0.028$) in comparison to SRS alone (fig. 1). The rate of post-SRS hemorrhage was not statistically different between the two groups ($p = 0.756$). Embolization did not reduce the rate of hemorrhage during the latency interval after SRS. There was no significant difference in the rate of AREs between the two groups ($p = 0.820$).

Discussion

Endovascular embolization of AVM is a helpful adjunct to resection because partial embolization can significantly reduce intraoperative bleeding. The purpose of embolization prior to microsurgery of large AVMs is to reduce the nidus volume, to occlude feeding vessels and to diminish nidal blood flow. Complete obliteration of AVM is rarely achieved by embolization alone [14, 27–32]. The aim of embolization for large AVMs before SRS is to permanently obliterate a distinct volume of the AVM and thereby reduce the target volume for radiosurgery. Our experience initially suggested that embolization made SRS targeting more difficult, perhaps because flow reduction was a more likely outcome than volume reduction. In addition, recanalization of previously embolized components may have contributed to treatment failures, since such volumes were not included in the SRS target volume. For large AVMs, embolization can reduce the volume of the nidus to make it amenable to SRS. Similarly, the risk of hemorrhage may be reduced by embolizing feeding artery or intranidal aneurysms, while awaiting the delayed occlusion achieved by SRS [10]. However, our analysis did not find any protective benefit for pre-SRS embolization. Embolization

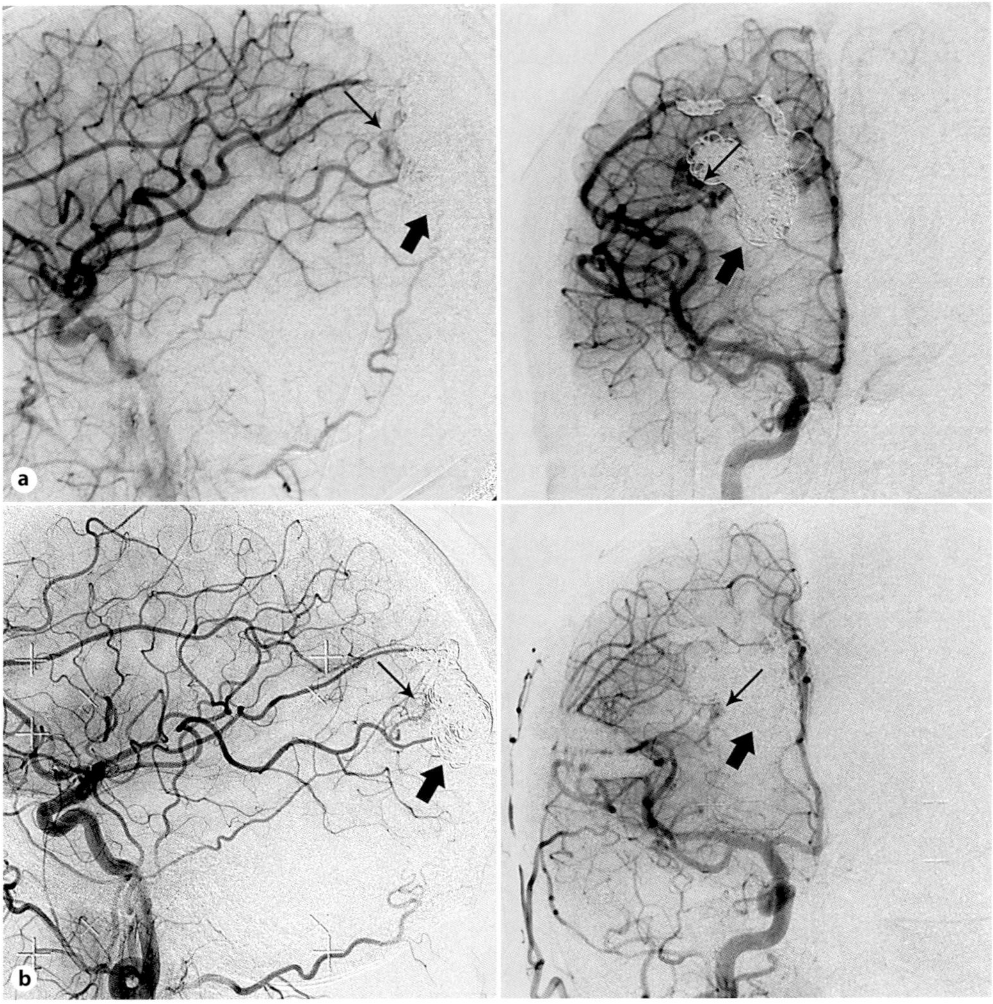

Fig. 1. **a** An 11-year-old girl presented with large occipital AVM. Anterior and lateral vertebral artery angiograms documenting the right occipital AVM at the time of SRS. She underwent coil embolization 5 months before SRS. The thick arrow shows the coil and the thin arrow the nidus. **b** Seven years after SRS, anterior and lateral vertebral artery angiograms showing residual nidus in the SRS field. The thick arrow shows the coil and the thin arrow the nidus.

may also make dose planning more difficult by also altering the 3-dimensional shape of the nidus, resulting potentially in a more irregular volume or one that has been divided into multiple compartments.

Embolization Followed by SRS for AVMs

The combined treatment modality of embolization followed by SRS has been used for medium- and large-size AVMs. Dawson et al. [33] in an initial report noted that only 2 of 7 patients had obliteration of the AVM at a follow-up of 2 years. Gobin et al. [14] studied 125 patients with AVM who underwent embolization before linear accelerator-based SRS. Total obliteration was achieved in 11% of AVMs by embolization alone. The nidus volume was reduced in 76% of their AVMs to a volume that facilitated SRS. Sixty-five percent of the partially embolized AVMs were obliterated following SRS. Preradiosurgery embolization was most effective for AVMs of 4–6 cm in size, with approximately 90% of them reduced to a size amenable to SRS. These authors noted a mortality rate of 1.6% and a morbidity rate of 12.8% related to embolization. No complications were associated with SRS. Izawa et al. [34] studied 15 patients who underwent embolization followed by SRS. In this series 10 patients were found to have a complete obliteration of AVMs in the follow-up, whereas 3 patients demonstrated more than 50% reduction in AVM nidal volume. Henkes et al. [35] reported a total obliteration rate of about 47%, although these lesions were of very high grade.

Andrade-Souza et al. [36] studied 61 patients who underwent embolization before linear accelerator-based SRS and performed analysis using case-match controls. These authors reported that SRS preceded by embolization reduced the obliteration rate of intracranial AVMs. The group that had embolization followed by SRS was noted to have a 47% total obliteration rate compared with 70% in those treated with SRS alone ($p = 0.036$). The risk of hemorrhage was 4 and 11%, respectively but was not significant ($p = 0.2$). In our analysis, prior embolization was associated with a lower rate of total obliteration ($p = 0.028$) but was not associated with any change in the hemorrhage rate after SRS ($p = 0.756$). The morbidity rate after 1 or more embolizations was 21% and after SRS it was 8.3% (permanent: 2.5%, temporary: 5.8%). In our experience, embolization performed during the second 10-year experience was significantly associated with a higher rate of total obliteration on magnetic resonance imaging or angiography. It should be noted that in these patients the nidus volume was significantly smaller ($p < 0.001$) and the margin dose was significantly higher ($p = 0.011$) compared to patients who underwent embolization during the first 10 years. No patients with AVM underwent Onyx embolization before SRS in the present series. Improved obliteration rates of approximately 20% have been reported for the use of this recently developed liquid embolic agent which may allow for safer and more effective deployment [37, 38]. Onyx embolization before SRS may make SRS target definition more challenging because of the dense cast visible on computed tomography and the artifacts left on both magnetic resonance imaging and angiography.

The risk of recanalization remains, because the embolized nidus may not be included within the SRS target volume. In our institution we performed volume-staged SRS for selected large-volume AVMs (>15 cm^3) [39]. Prospective volume-staged SRS for large AVMs has potential benefit but often requires multiple procedures spread over time. A potential treatment algorithm for patients with AVM based on nidus volume is suggested in figure 2.

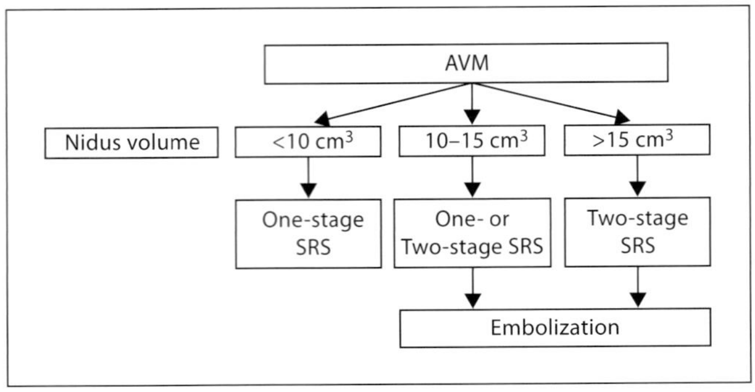

Fig. 2. A treatment algorithm proposed for the management of AVMs.

Conclusions

In our 20-year experience, we found that prior embolization reduced the rate of total obliteration after SRS although hemorrhage risks were unchanged. For patients who were embolized to volumes smaller than 8 cm^3, success was significantly improved. A marginal dose $\geq$18 Gy also improved obliteration rates. The value of liquid embolic agents remains to be determined in a larger study. For larger-volume AVMs, we prefer staged SRS. Prospective volume-staged SRS for large AVMs has potential benefit but often requires multiple procedures.

In the future, prospective volume-staged SRS in conjunction with innovative embolization strategies (to reduce flow, obliterate fistulas and occlude associated aneurysms) may further reduce the risk of hemorrhage.

Acknowledgements

The work described in this report was funded by a research grant to Dr. Kano from AB Elekta, Stockholm, Sweden, and the Osaka Medical Research Foundation for Incurable Diseases.

Disclosure Statement

Drs. Lunsford, Kondziolka, Niranjan and Novotny are consultants for AB Elekta, and Dr. Lunsford is a stockholder.

References

1 Brown RD Jr, Wiebers DO, Torner JC, O'Fallon WM: Frequency of intracranial hemorrhage as a presenting symptom and subtype analysis: a population-based study of intracranial vascular malformations in Olmsted County, Minnesota. J Neurosurg 1996; 85:29–32.

2 Auger RG, Wiebers DO: Management of unruptured intracranial arteriovenous malformations: a decision analysis. Neurosurgery 1992;30:561–569.

3 Brown RD Jr, Wiebers DO, Forbes G, O'Fallon WM, Piepgras DG, Marsh WR, Maciunas RJ: The natural history of unruptured intracranial arteriovenous malformations. J Neurosurg 1988;68:352–357.

4 Graf CJ, Perret GE, Torner JC: Bleeding from cerebral arteriovenous malformations as part of their natural history. J Neurosurg 1983;58:331–337.

5 Ondra SL, Troupp H, George ED, Schwab K: The natural history of symptomatic arteriovenous malformations of the brain: a 24-year follow-up assessment. J Neurosurg 1990;73:387–391.

6 Forster DM, Steiner L, Hakanson S: Arteriovenous malformations of the brain. A long-term clinical study. J Neurosurg 1972;37:562–570.

7 Fults D, Kelly DL Jr: Natural history of arteriovenous malformations of the brain: a clinical study. Neurosurgery 1984;15:658–662.

8 Itoyama Y, Uemura S, Ushio Y, Kuratsu J, Nonaka N, Wada H, Sano Y, Fukumura A, Yoshida K, Yano T: Natural course of unoperated intracranial arteriovenous malformations: study of 50 cases. J Neurosurg 1989;71:805–809.

9 Pollock BE, Flickinger JC, Lunsford LD, Bissonette DJ, Kondziolka D: Factors that predict the bleeding risk of cerebral arteriovenous malformations. Stroke 1996;27:1–6.

10 Yashar P, Amar AP, Giannotta SL, Yu C, Pagnini PG, Liu CY, Apuzzo ML: Cerebral arteriovenous malformations: issues of the interplay between stereotactic radiosurgery and endovascular surgical therapy. World Neurosurg 2011;75:638–647.

11 Lunsford LD, Kondziolka D, Flickinger JC, Bissonette DJ, Jungreis CA, Maitz AH, Horton JA, Coffey RJ: Stereotactic radiosurgery for arteriovenous malformations of the brain. J Neurosurg 1991;75:512–524.

12 Starke RM, Komotar RJ, Otten ML, Hahn DK, Fischer LE, Hwang BY, Garrett MC, Sciacca RR, Sisti MB, Solomon RA, Lavine SD, Connolly ES, Meyers PM: Adjuvant embolization with N-butyl cyanoacrylate in the treatment of cerebral arteriovenous malformations: outcomes, complications, and predictors of neurologic deficits. Stroke 2009; 40:2783–2790.

13 Hartmann A, Pile-Spellman J, Stapf C, Sciacca RR, Faulstich A, Mohr JP, Schumacher HC, Mast H: Risk of endovascular treatment of brain arteriovenous malformations. Stroke 2002;33:1816–1820.

14 Gobin YP, Laurent A, Merienne L, Schlienger M, Aymard A, Houdart E, Casasco A, Lefkopoulos D, George B, Merland JJ: Treatment of brain arteriovenous malformations by embolization and radiosurgery. J Neurosurg 1996;85:19–28.

15 Ogilvy CS, Stieg PE, Awad I, Brown RD Jr, Kondziolka D, Rosenwasser R, Young WL, Hademenos G: Recommendations for the management of intracranial arteriovenous malformations: a statement for healthcare professionals from a special writing group of the Stroke Council, American Stroke Association. Circulation 2001;103:2644–2657.

16 Paulsen RD, Steinberg GK, Norbash AM, Marcellus ML, Marks MP: Embolization of basal ganglia and thalamic arteriovenous malformations. Neurosurgery 1999;44:991–996, discussion 996–997.

17 Sinclair J, Kelly ME, Steinberg GK: Surgical management of posterior fossa arteriovenous malformations. Neurosurgery 2006;58:ONS189–201, discussion ONS201.

18 Cockroft KM, Hwang SK, Rosenwasser RH: Endovascular treatment of cerebral arteriovenous malformations: indications, techniques, outcome, and complications. Neurosurg Clin North Am 2005; 16:367–380.

19 Hartmann A, Mast H, Mohr JP, Pile-Spellman J, Connolly ES, Sciacca RR, Khaw A, Stapf C: Determinants of staged endovascular and surgical treatment outcome of brain arteriovenous malformations. Stroke 2005;36:2431–2435.

20 Haw CS, ter Brugge K, Willinsky R, Tomlinson G: Complications of embolization of arteriovenous malformations of the brain. J Neurosurg 2006;104: 226–232.

21 Jayaraman MV, Marcellus ML, Hamilton S, Do HM, Campbell D, Chang SD, Steinberg GK, Marks MP: Neurologic complications of arteriovenous malformation embolization using liquid embolic agents. AJNR Am J Neuroradiol 2008;29:242–246.

22 Kim LJ, Albuquerque FC, Spetzler RF, McDougall CG: Postembolization neurological deficits in cerebral arteriovenous malformations: stratification by arteriovenous malformation grade. Neurosurgery 2006;59:53–59, discussion 53–59.

23 Ledezma CJ, Hoh BL, Carter BS, Pryor JC, Putman CM, Ogilvy CS: Complications of cerebral arteriovenous malformation embolization: multivariate analysis of predictive factors. Neurosurgery 2006;58:602–611.
24 Meisel HJ, Mansmann U, Alvarez H, Rodesch G, Brock M, Lasjaunias P: Effect of partial targeted N-butyl-cyano-acrylate embolization in brain AVM. Acta Neurochir (Wien) 2002;144:879–887, discussion 888.
25 Taylor CL, Dutton K, Rappard G, Pride GL, Replogle R, Purdy PD, White J, Giller C, Kopitnik TA Jr, Samson DS: Complications of preoperative embolization of cerebral arteriovenous malformations. J Neurosurg 2004;100:810–812.
26 Brown RD Jr, Flemming KD, Meyer FB, Cloft HJ, Pollock BE, Link ML: Natural history, evaluation, and management of intracranial vascular malformations. Mayo Clin Proc 2005;80:269–281.
27 Deruty R, Pelissou-Guyotat I, Amat D, Mottolese C, Bascoulergue Y, Turjman F, Gerard JP: Complications after multidisciplinary treatment of cerebral arteriovenous malformations. Acta Neurochir (Wien) 1996;138:119–131.
28 Fournier D, ter Brugge KG, Willinsky R, Lasjaunias P, Montanera W: Endovascular treatment of intracerebral arteriovenous malformations: experience in 49 cases. J Neurosurg 1991;75:228–233.
29 Frizzel RT, Fisher WS 3rd: Cure, morbidity, and mortality associated with embolization of brain arteriovenous malformations: a review of 1,246 patients in 32 series over a 35-year period. Neurosurgery 1995;37:1031–1039, discussion 1039–1040.
30 Hurst RW, Berenstein A, Kupersmith MJ, Madrid M, Flamm ES: Deep central arteriovenous malformations of the brain: the role of endovascular treatment. J Neurosurg 1995;82:190–195.
31 Wikholm G, Lundqvist C, Svendsen P: Transarterial embolization of cerebral arteriovenous malformations: improvement of results with experience. AJNR Am J Neuroradiol 1995;16:1811–1817.
32 Wikholm G, Lundqvist C, Svendsen P: Embolization of cerebral arteriovenous malformations. I. Technique, morphology, and complications. Neurosurgery 1996;39:448–457, discussion 457–459.
33 Dawson RC 3rd, Tarr RW, Hecht ST, Jungreis CA, Lunsford LD, Coffey R, Horton JA: Treatment of arteriovenous malformations of the brain with combined embolization and stereotactic radiosurgery: results after 1 and 2 years. AJNR Am J Neuroradiol 1990;11:857–864.
34 Izawa M, Chernov M, Hayashi M, Iseki H, Hori T, Takakura K: Combined management of intracranial arteriovenous malformations with embolization and gamma knife radiosurgery: comparative evaluation of the long-term results. Surg Neurol 2009; 71:43–52, discussion 52–53.
35 Henkes H, Nahser HC, Berg-Dammer E, Weber W, Lange S, Kuhne D: Endovascular therapy of brain AVMs prior to radiosurgery. Neurol Res 1998;20: 479–492.
36 Andrade-Souza YM, Ramani M, Scora D, Tsao MN, ter Brugge K, Schwartz ML: Embolization before radiosurgery reduces the obliteration rate of arteriovenous malformations. Neurosurgery 2007;60:443–451, discussion 451–452.
37 Friedlander RM: Clinical practice. Arteriovenous malformations of the brain. N Engl J Med 2007;356: 2704–2712.
38 Weber W, Kis B, Siekmann R, Kuehne D: Endovascular treatment of intracranial arteriovenous malformations with Onyx: technical aspects. AJNR Am J Neuroradiol 2007;28:371–377.
39 Sirin S, Kondziolka D, Niranjan A, Flickinger JC, Maitz AH, Lunsford LD: Prospective staged volume radiosurgery for large arteriovenous malformations: indications and outcomes in otherwise untreatable patients. Neurosurgery 2006;58:17–27.

L. Dade Lunsford, MD, FACS
Lars Leksell Distinguished Professor of Neurological Surgery
University of Pittsburgh, Suite B-400, UPMC Presbyterian
200 Lothrop Street
Pittsburgh, PA 15213 (USA)
Tel. +1 412 647 6781, E-Mail lunsfordld@upmc.edu

Niranjan A, Kano H, Lunsford LD (eds): Gamma Knife Radiosurgery for Brain Vascular Malformations.
Prog Neurol Surg. Basel, Karger, 2013, vol 27, pp 97–106 (DOI: 10.1159/000341771)

Long-Term Side Effects of Radiosurgery for Arteriovenous Malformations

Masaaki Yamamoto · Takuya Kawabe · Bierta E. Barfod

Katsuta Hospital Mito Gamma House, Ibaraki, Japan

Abstract

In this report, our experiences with 181 consecutive patients who underwent Gamma Knife radiosurgery (GKRS) for arteriovenous malformations (AVMs) during an approximately quarter century period from 1978 to 2002 will be summarized along with much of what we have learned from a wealth of already published data. During the mean post-GKRS follow-up period of 10.2 years (range, 5.4–30.6), 15 (8.3%) of our 181 patients experienced stereotactic radiosurgery-related, symptomatic complications. Among these 15 patients, 12 manifested complications 5 years or more after GKRS. Furthermore, in 5 of these 12, the complications were seen 10 or more years after GKRS. In the present series, the actuarial complication rates computed using the Kaplan-Meier method were 2.3% at the fifth, 8.2% at the tenth, 15.2% at the fifteenth and 31.1% at the twentieth post-GKRS year. AVM volumes, Pollock-Flickinger AVM scores, the initial presentation of bleeding and centrally located AVMs were demonstrated to be significantly associated with the risk of delayed complications after GKRS ($p < 0.05$). There was a significant difference in complication rates between two patient groups, based on whether dose planning was performed using the older (Kula) or the modern (Gamma Plan) system (18.0 vs. 4.6%, χ^2 $p = 0.0002$). Although GKRS is undoubtedly an alternative to microsurgical resection for appropriately selected AVMs, we must weigh treatment results against complication risks which are not negligibly low.

With recent advances in both preoperative and intraoperative neuroimaging, as well as microsurgical instruments and techniques, neurosurgeons can resect many arteriovenous malformations (AVMs) completely with an acceptably low morbidity rate. Although this is unquestionably ideal, some AVMs cannot be resected safely even by the most experienced neurosurgeon because they are located within or near a critical brain structure or because the patient has contraindications for general anesthesia. The role of embolization as radical treatment is considered to be relatively limited in the management of AVM patients because only 10–20% of AVMs are completely curable using this technique alone [1, 2]. Instead, embolization is widely used as a presurgical or preradiosurgical procedure to reduce both nidus size and blood flow [3]. In contrast, stereotactic radiosurgery (SRS) is widely accepted as an alternative

Table 1. Incidences and latency periods of complications after irradiation

Authors	Patients n	Patients with complications n	Latency periods months
Linear accelerator system			
Colombo et al. [6]	180	9 (5.0%)	2–18
Friedman et al. [8]	158	5 (3.2%)	11–15
Gamma Knife			
Steiner et al. [17]	1,000	35 (3.5%)	4–56 (mean, 9.9)
Lunsford et al. [11]	227	10 (4.4%)	4–18
Yamamoto et al. [18]	121	6 (5.0%)	less than 60[1]
Yamamoto et al. [19]	885	24 (2.7%)	4–24 (mean, 12.2)
Liscak et al. [20]	330	24 (7.3%)	6–57 (median, 13.5)
Present study	181	15 (13.6%)	9–215 (mean, 105)[2]

[1] Although the latency period was not available, the maximum follow-up period in this series was 60 months.
[2] In 1 patient who experienced radiation-induced injury of the pons 19 months after radiosurgery, a second ictus occurred 81 months after Gamma Knife radiosurgery.

to microsurgery in the treatment of relatively small AVMs, particularly in deep brain locations (i.e. brainstem, basal ganglia or thalamus) or critical lobar areas (i.e. sensorimotor, speech or visual cortex) [4–18]. Since the historical reports by Steiner et al. [17] followed by those of Lunsford et al. [11], Colombo et al. [5, 6] and Friedman and Bova [7] as well as ours [19], complication rates after SRS for AVMs have long been accepted as relatively low, 3–5%, as shown in table 1. Recently, based on 330 AVM patients treated by Gamma Knife radiosurgery (GKRS), Liscak et al. [20] reported a complication rate of 7.3%. However, we recently documented that complication rates, particularly during the longer-term follow-up period after SRS, are not as low as previously thought [21]. In this report, our experiences with 181 consecutive patients who underwent GKRS for AVMs during an approximately quarter century period from 1978 to 2002 will be summarized along with much of what we have learned from a wealth of already published data. In particular, the authors address complications occurring many years after SRS as well as their pathogeneses.

Histopathological Changes after Stereotactic Radiosurgery and Pathogenesis of Complications

Although SRS-induced histopathological changes resulting in AVM obliteration with a 2- to 3-year latency period are detailed in the next report, we will briefly summarize them here to facilitate understanding of the pathogenesis of post-SRS complications.

The SRS-induced changes within an AVM are considered to occur as follows: a beam of ionizing radiation initially injures the endothelial cells of vessels, thereby inducing, as a reparative process, a gradual thickening of connective tissue, which leads to accumulation of myofibroblasts, histiocytes, collagen and variable amounts of fibrin within the vessel wall. This process eventually obstructs the lumina of the AVM vessels [22]. Szeifert et al. [23] reported that these stromal cells demonstrated marked immunohistochemical positivity for smooth muscle actin (SMA) while being somewhat less positive for vimentin and desmin. Therefore, Szeifert et al. concluded, based in part on electron-microscopic observations, that the contractile activity of myofibroblasts could be relevant to the process of shrinkage and eventual occlusion of AVMs after radiosurgery. However, we previously found that, despite the remarkable positivity for SMA demonstrated immunohistochemically in patent vessels, completely obliterated vessels within the treated nidus showed no SMA staining whatsoever [24, 25]. The role of myofibroblasts, which appear to play a major part in postradiosurgical nidus obliteration, was therefore considered to be limited to the early stage of the nidus obliteration process.

Schneider et al. [26] categorized obliteration processes in radiosurgically treated AVMs into three stages: 'endothelial or subendothelial damage', 'proliferation of intimal smooth muscle cells' and 'cellular degeneration and increased matrix'. The first stage was evidenced by a denuded endothelium or by disruption and separation of the endothelial lining from the underlying vessel walls. In the second stage, proliferation of smooth muscle cells around most or the entire wall circumference produced concentric or eccentric narrowing of the vessel lumina. The proliferative zone was immunohistochemically positive for SMA and collagen type IV (basement membrane type) while being negative for collagen types I and III (fibrillary structure types). In the third stage, cellular degeneration was evidenced by nuclear pyknosis and decreased cell number, most vessels had undergone obliteration of the entire vascular structure, with more or less uniformly dense hyalinization, and these changes were accompanied by loss of SMA and collagen type IV immunoreactivities. Our observations support their results; similar findings were obtained, particularly in the second and third stages [24, 25].

As described above, angiographically confirmed AVM obliteration does not mean total elimination of the nidus in the irradiated area; rather, it is SRS-induced tissue degeneration, consisting mostly of collagen fibers, which remains [24]. Such tissues are considered to gradually undergo liquefaction necrosis, resulting in vacuolation or collapse in most SRS-treated AVMs. However, although the underlying mechanism has not yet been fully clarified, this collagen tissue lesion persists and can even grow for many years after SRS in some cases. Usually, such a lesion is detected as a long-existing enhanced area on magnetic resonance images. Also, these lesions exude serous fluid into the surrounding normal brain tissue, thereby producing perilesional edema and/or cyst formation. Furthermore, this type of lesion undergoes neovascularization characterized by fragile vessel walls and repeated hemorrhage. This is considered to be the pathogenesis of chronic encapsulated hematoma or symptomatic hemorrhage occurring after complete nidus obliteration has been confirmed [27].

Table 2. List of patients with long-term complications after GKRS

No.	Age years	Sex	Location	Volume cm^3	P-F score	S-M grade	Doses, Gy max.	Doses, Gy min.	Post-GK results	Re-GK
1	14	M	occipital lobe	0.52	0.33	1	36.00	25.00	partial	no
2	10	F	temporal lobe	1.40	0.34	2	30.00	15.00	complete	no
3	32	F	midbrain	0.78	1.02	3	50.00	35.00	partial	no
4	16	F	splenium	1.51	0.47	2	50.00	14.00	partial	yes
5	11	M	midbrain	1.05	0.63	3	35.00	30.00	complete	no
6	30	F	pons	0.68	0.97	3	24.00	22.00	complete	no
7	9	M	pons	3.14	0.79	3	32.00	16.00	partial	yes
8	28	M	parietal lobe	24.15	2.98	3	70.00	7.00	complete	no
9	26	F	thalamus	3.17	1.14	3	50.00	15.00	partial	yes
10	38	F	thalamus	1.27	1.19	3	31.40	22.00	complete	no
11	14	F	thalamus	13.80	1.96	4	36.00	7.20	partial	yes
12	41	M	hypothalamus	3.20	1.44	3	33.33	16.70	partial	yes
13	48	M	temporal lobe	7.92	1.75	2	40.00	20.00	complete	no
14	63	M	temporal lobe	2.60	1.52	2	50.00	25.00	partial	no
15	62	M	frontal lobe	1.00	1.34	2	44.00	22.00	n.a.	no

P-F = Pollock-Flickinger; S-M = Spetzler-Martin; GK = Gamma Knife; n.a. = not available; CT = computed tomography; RT = radiotherapy; PCA = posterior cerebral artery.

As described above, SRS-induced histopathological changes of the intranidal angioarchitecture have been studied extensively. In contrast, knowledge of the histopathological changes affecting irradiated perinidal vessels is limited. We previously reported, based on an autopsy study of a patient who died due to a pulmonary artery embolism immediately after the second post-SRS year follow-up angiography, that remarkable intimal hypertrophy and fragmentation of the elastic laminae were observed even in nidus-unrelated pial arteries [28]. This finding indicates that, despite the abnormal vessels of an AVM being perhaps more susceptible to the effects of a high-dose single-fraction irradiation, normal surrounding blood vessels may also be affected. We speculate that such changes would progress for many years after SRS, eventually producing radiation necrosis of the normal brain in some cases.

Long-Term Side Effects of Stereotactic Radiosurgery for Arteriovenous Malformations

During the mean post-GKRS follow-up period of 10.2 years (range, 5.4–30.6), 15 (8.3%) of our 181 patients experienced GKRS-related, symptomatic complications, as listed in table 2. Among these 15 patients, 12 manifested complications 5

Post-re-GK results	Intervals years	Symptoms	Neuroimaging findings	Treatment	Symptom changes
	6.0	hemianopsia	cyst	surgical	recovery
	15.7	headache, vomiting	hemorrhage	surgical	recovery
	5.0	hemi-Parkinson	T_2-weighted hyperintensity	medical	unchanged
	12.0	headache, hemiparesis	enhanced mass, cyst, hemorrhage	surgical	recovery
complete	14.8	consciousness disturbance	enhanced mass, cyst	surgical	unchanged
	1.6	dizziness, vomiting	T_2-weighted hyperintensity	medical	recovery
	6.8	facial nerve palsy	T_2-weighted hyperintensity	medical	unchanged
complete	17.9	facial nerve palsy	T_2-weighted hyperintensity	medical	unchanged
	8.8	hemiparesis	enhanced mass, low density (CT)	medical	unchanged
	17.1	headache, hemiparesis	enhanced mass, cyst	surgical, RT	progressed
	0.8	headache, hemiparesis	hemorrhage	medical	recovery
complete	9.8	headache, hemiparesis	hemorrhage	medical	recovery
complete	5.4	hemianopsia	T_2-weighted hyperintensity	medical	unchanged
	4.0	hemiparesis	infarct due to PCA occlusion	medical	unchanged
	8.1	dementia	enhanced mass, cyst	surgical	recovery
	6.7	hemiparesis	T_2-weighted hyperintensity	medical	recovery

years or more after GKRS. Furthermore, in 5 of these 12, the complications were seen 10 or more years after GKRS. In the present series, the actuarial complication rates computed using the Kaplan-Meier method were 2.3% at the fifth, 8.2% at the tenth, 15.2% at the fifteenth and 31.1% at the twentieth post-GKRS year (fig. 1). In 1 (case No. 6 in table 2) of the 15 patients, who experienced radiation-induced injury of the pons 1.6 years after SRS, a second ictus occurred 6.8 years after GKRS. Fifteen of 16 ictuses, excluding 1 (case 8) in whom magnetic resonance imaging was contraindicated such that only a computed tomographic scan was obtained, were checked by magnetic resonance imaging. A gradually enlarging mass showing enhancement with cyst formation was demonstrated in 4, and in 1 of these 4 there was accompanying hemorrhage. In the remaining 11, T_2-weighted hyperintense areas were demonstrated in 6, hemorrhage after angiographically confirmed nidus obliteration in 3 and cyst formation and cerebral infarction due to posterior cerebral artery occlusion (radiation-induced vasculopathy) in 1 each. For the total of 16 ictuses, medical treatment was performed in 10, surgery in 5 and surgery followed by fractionated radiotherapy in 1 (case No. 9). The latter patient, whose pathology was anaplastic oligodendroglioma, died 18.3 years after the first SRS. After medical treatment, symptoms subsided in 4 patients but were

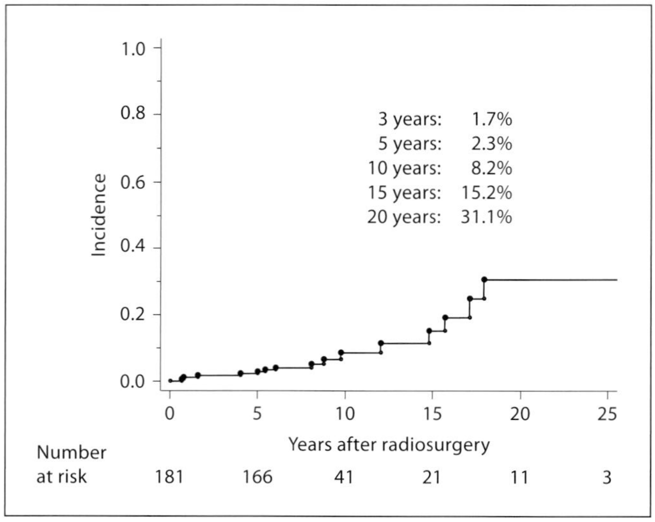

Fig. 1. Cumulative incidences of radiation-induced complications after GKRS.

Table 3. Clinical factors influencing GKRS-induced complications: continuous variables

	Multivariate	Univariate
Age	0.0516	0.6240
Volume	0.0360	0.8016
Pollock-Flickinger AVM score	0.0448	0.6897
Peripheral dose	0.2006	0.1592
Central dose	0.8253	0.8071
Follow-up period	0.6959	0.5897
Interval from GKRS to obliteration	0.8674	0.6541

unchanged in the other 6. Among the 5 patients who underwent surgery only, no tumor cells were found in the resected tissues and symptoms resolved in 4 and were unchanged in 1.

As shown in table 3, while none of the 7 clinical factors (continuous variables) examined reached statistical significance on univariate analysis, multivariate analysis demonstrated AVM volumes and Pollock-Flickinger AVM scores to be significantly associated with the risk for delayed complications after SRS ($p < 0.05$). Table 4 summarizes the results of statistical analyses for 2-category variables. Although neither multivariate nor univariate analysis showed patient age to influence the risk of complications, the incidence of complications in pediatric patients was significantly higher than that in adolescents (χ^2 $p = 0.0129$, log rank $p = 0.0211$). In

Table 4. Clinical factors influencing GKRS-induced complications: two-categorical variables

Patients				p value	
				χ^2	log rank
Sex					
Female	7 (9.5%)/74	Male	8 (7.5%)/107	0.6343	0.8835
Initial presentations					
Bleeding	15 (13.0%)/115	Nonbleeding	0 (0%)/66	0.0022	n.a.
Locations					
Central	9 (18.0%)/50	Noncentral	6 (4.6%)/131	0.0034	0.0593
Infratentorial	4 (15.4%)/26	Supratentorial	11 (7.1%)/155	0.1560	0.0642
Dose planning systems					
Kula	11 (18.0%)/55	Gamma Plan	4 (4.6%)/126	0.0002	0.1424
Procedures					
Single	10 (6.8%)/147	Multiple	5 (14.7%)/34	0.1320	0.2995
Age category					
<15 years	5 (22.7%)/22	16–25 years	1 (2.6%)/38	0.0129	0.0211
16–25 years	1 (2.6%)/38	26–60 years	7 (9.9%)/71	0.1363	0.5058
26–60 years	7 (9.9%)/71	>60 years	2 (4.0%)/50	0.2265	0.3357

n.a. = Not available.

all 15 patients with complications, the initial presentation was bleeding; none of those whose initial presentation was not bleeding experienced delayed post-SRS complications (χ^2 p = 0.0022). The incidence of complications was significantly higher in patients with centrally located AVMs than in those with non-central AVMs (χ^2 p = 0.0034). There was a significant difference in complication rates between two patient groups based on whether dose planning was performed using the older (Kula) or the modern (Gamma Plan) system (18.0 vs. 4.6%, χ^2 p = 0.0002).

The authors also experienced 4 patients who, despite remaining asymptomatic to date, showed delayed cyst formation on neuroimaging studies between 5 and 10 years after SRS.

It is clear that angiographically demonstrated nidus obliteration eliminates the risk of hemorrhage in the vast majority of patients. However, as reported previously, we experienced 1 patient who likely suffered a symptomatic hemorrhagic stroke 5 years after 2-year postradiosurgical angiography had demonstrated complete obliteration [29]. Furthermore, we recently experienced 2 additional patients with intracerebral hemorrhages which developed, respectively, 12 and 15 years after GKRS despite post-GKRS angiography having shown complete nidus obliteration. The recently published results of Maruyama et al. [30] support our observations.

Brief Comments

Delayed radiation-induced complications reportedly occur in 3.2–7.3% of patients with radiosurgically treated AVMs [4–18] (table 1). It is widely accepted that the dose-volume relation is the most important factor influencing the risk for delayed complications after radiosurgery; the larger the nidus volume and/or the higher the doses used, the greater the increases in complication risks. Flickinger et al. [31] reported that, among 30 patients who sustained postradiosurgical complications, symptoms resolved in 58% within 27 months with a significantly greater proportion resolving in those receiving less than 20 Gy at the nidus periphery as compared with those receiving more than 20 Gy (89 vs. 36%, p = 0.006). The second major consideration is how much normal brain volume is included within the target volume. Flickinger et al. described a 12-Gy volume of the normal brain as being an important factor. Karlsson et al. [32] reported, based on 1,128 AVM patients who underwent GKRS, that a previous hemorrhage reduced the risk of complications. However, in our experiences as described above, delayed radiation-induced complications occurred exclusively in patients whose AVMs had manifested with hemorrhage. The underlying mechanism is unknown but we can reasonably speculate that perinidal brain tissues underwent reparative processes once or more due to hemorrhage, and that scar tissue, consisting of collagen fibers with neovascularization, had thus been present prior to SRS. Such hemorrhage-induced scar tissues would probably respond to irradiation. According to a multi-institutional analysis of complication outcomes reported by Flickinger et al. [31], significantly greater symptom resolution was observed in patients with no prior history of hemorrhage and in those with symptoms of minimal severity.

As reported herein, recent dose planning techniques allow us to avoid excess irradiation to the normal brain, such that we can anticipate significantly reduced risks of delayed complications. However, because SRS exposes tissues to irradiation, oncogenicity is an inescapable problem. Kaido et al. [33] presented an AVM patient who underwent GKRS and ultimately died due to glioblastoma multiforme that had initially appeared in the target area 6.5 years after irradiation. Berman et al. [34] recently reported a patient in whom glioblastoma multiforme developed 9 years after linear accelerator-based GKRS for an AVM. We have also experienced 1 patient in whom a malignant glioma developed after GKRS for an AVM, as described above. Nevertheless, Rowe et al. [35] recently reported, based on 4,877 patients including 2,615 AVM patients, that only 1 new astrocytoma was diagnosed, whereas national incidence figures would have predicted 2.47 cases.

Conclusions

Although GKRS is undoubtedly an alternative to microsurgical resection for appropriately selected AVMs, we must weigh treatment results against complication risks which are not negligibly low. The reader should keep in mind that approximately one third of the patients described herein had radiosurgery early in the 'learning curve'. It is now apparent that the currently used computerized dose planning system contributed to a reduction in the long-term complication rate. We can expect this risk to be further reduced with present and future advancement in both imaging and computer technologies.

References

1 Wikholm G, Lundqvist C, Svendsen P: Embolization of cerebral arteriovenous malformations. I. Technique, morphology, and complications. Neurosurgery 1996;39:448–459.

2 Lundqvist C, Wikholm G, Svendsen P: Embolization of cerebral arteriovenous malformations. II. Aspects of complications and late outcome. Neurosurgery 1996;39:460–469.

3 Andrade-Souza Y, Zadeh G, Ramani M: Embolization prior to radiosurgery reduces the obliteration rate for arteriovenous malformations. Annu Meet Am Assoc Neurol Surgeons, New Orleans, April 18, 2005.

4 Betti OO, Munari C, Rosler R: Stereotactic radiosurgery with the linear accelerator: treatment of arteriovenous malformations. Neurosurgery 1989; 24:311–321.

5 Colombo F, Benedetti A, Pozza F, Marchetti C, Chierego G: Linear accelerator radiosurgery of cerebral arteriovenous malformations. Neurosurgery 1989;24:833–840.

6 Colombo F, Pozza F, Chierego G, Casentini L, De Luca G, Francescon P: Linear accelerator radiosurgery of cerebral arteriovenous malformations: an update. Neurosurgery 1994;34:14–21.

7 Friedman WA, Bova FJ: Linear accelerator radiosurgery for arteriovenous malformations. J Neurosurg 1992;77:832–841.

8 Friedman WA, Bova FJ, Mendenhall WM: Linear accelerator radiosurgery for arteriovenous malformations: the relationship of size to outcome. J Neurosurg 1995;82:180–189.

9 Kawamoto S: Radiosurgery of arteriovenous malformations (in Japanese). No Shinkei Geka (Neurol Surg, Tokyo) 1994;22:403–420.

10 Loeffler JS, Alexander E III, Sidden RL, Saunders WM, Coleman CN, Winston KR: Stereotactic radiosurgery for intracranial arteriovenous malformations using a standard linear accelerator. Int J Radiat Oncol Biol Phys 1989;17:673–677.

11 Lunsford LD, Kondziolka D, Flickinger JC, Bissonette DJ, Jungreis CA, Maitz AH, Horton JA, Coffey RJ: Stereotactic radiosurgery for arteriovenous malformations of the brain. J Neurosurg 1991;75:512–524.

12 Pollock BE, Lunsford LD, Kondziolka D, Maitz A, Flickinger JC: Patient outcomes after stereotactic radiosurgery for 'operable' arteriovenous malformations. Neurosurgery 1994;35:1–8.

13 Pollock BE, Lunsford LD, Kondziolka D, Bissonette DJ, Flickinger JC: Stereotactic radiosurgery for postgeniculate visual pathway arteriovenous malformations. J Neurosurg 1996;84:437–441.

14 Sasaki T, Kurita H, Saito I, Kawamoto S, Nemoto S, Terahara A, Kirino T, Takakura K: Arteriovenous malformations in the basal ganglia and thalamus: management and results in 101 cases. J Neurosurg 1998;88:285–292.

15 Souhami L, Olivier A, Podgorsak EB, Pla M, Pike GB: Radiosurgery of cerebral arteriovenous malformations with the dynamic stereotactic irradiation. Int J Radiat Oncol Biol Phys 1990;19:775–782.

16 Steiner L: Treatment of arteriovenous malformation by radiosurgery; in Wilson CB, Stein BM (eds): Intracranial Arteriovenous Malformations. Baltimore, Williams & Wilkins, 1984, pp 295–313.

17 Steiner L, Lindquist C, Steiner M: Radiosurgery; in Symon L (ed): Advances and Technical Standards in Neurosurgery. Wien, Springer, 1992, pp 19–102.

18 Yamamoto Y, Coffey RJ, Nichols DA, Shaw EG: Interim report on the radiosurgical treatment of cerebral arteriovenous malformations: the influence of size, dose, time and technical factors on obliteration rate. J Neurosurg 1995;83:832–837.

19 Yamamoto M, Tanaka T, Boku N, Fukuoka S, Hosoda H, Hirai T, Inoue H, Hamazaki M, Fujino H, Izawa M, Tsuzuki T, Iwai Y, Kobayashi T, Jokura H: Gamma knife radiosurgery for cerebral arteriovenous malformations: a multi-institutional study in Japan; in Kondziolka D (ed): Radiosurgery. Basel, Karger, 1998, vol 2, pp 147–156.

20 Liscak R, Vladyka V, Simonova G, Urgosik D, Novotny J, Janouskova L, Janouskova L, Vymazal J: Artriovenous malformations after Leksell gamma knife radiosurgery: rate of obliteration and complications. Neurosurgery 2000;60:1005–1016.
21 Yamamoto M, Hara M, Ide M, Ono Y, Jimbo M, Saito I: Radiation-related adverse effects observed on neuro-imaging several years after radiosurgery for cerebral arteriovenous malformations. Surg Neurol 1998;49:385–398.
22 Chang SD, Shuster DL, Steinberg GK, Levy RP, Frankel K: Stereotactic radiosurgery of arteriovenous malformations: pathologic changes in resected tissue. Clin Neuropathol 1997;16:111–116.
23 Szeifert GT, Kemeny AA, Timperley WR, Forster DM: The potential role of myofibroblasts in the obliteration of arteriovenous malformations after radiosurgery. Neurosurgery 1997;40:61–77.
24 Yamamoto M, Jimbo M, Kobayashi M, Toyoda C, Ide M, Tanaka N, Lindquist C, Steiner L: Long-term results of radiosurgery for arteriovenous malformation: Neurodiagnostic imaging and histological studies of angiographically confirmed nidus obliteration. Surg Neurol 1992;37:219–230.
25 Yamamoto M: Gamma knife radiosurgery: technology, applications, and future directions. Neurosug Clin North Am 1999;10:181–202.
26 Schneider BF, Eberhard DA, Steiner LE: Histopathology of arteriovenous malformations after gamma knife radiosurgery. J Neurosurg 1997;87: 352–357.
27 Kurita H, Sasaki T, Kawamoto S, Taniguchi M, Kitanaka C, Nakaguchi H, Kirino T: Chronic encapsulated expanding hematoma in association with gamma knife stereotactic radiosurgery for a cerebral arteriovenous malformation. Case report. J Neurosurg 1996;84:874–878.
28 Yamamoto M, Jimbo M, Ide M, Kobayashi M, Toyoda C, Lindquist C, Karlson B: Gamma knife radiosurgery for cerebral arteriovenous malformations: an autopsy report focusing on irradiation-induced changes observed in nidus-unrelated arteries. Surg Neurol 1995;44:421–427.
29 Yamamoto M, Jimbo M, Hara M, Saito I, Mori K: Gamma knife radiosurgery for cerebral arteriovenous malformations: long-term follow-up results focusing on complications occurring more than 5 years after irradiation. Neurosurgery 1996;38:906–914.
30 Maruyama K, Kawahara N, Shin M, Tago M, Kishimoto J, Kurita H, Kawamoto S, Morita A, Kirino T: The risk of hemorrhage after radiosurgery for cerebral arteriovenous malformations. N Engl J Med 2005;352:146–153.
31 Flickinger JC, Kondziolka D, Lunsford LD, Pollock BE, Yamamoto M, Gorman DA, Schomberg PJ, Sneed P, Larson D, Smith V, McDermott MW, Miyawaki L, Chilton J, Morantz RA, Young B, Jokura H, Liscak R: A multi-institutional analysis of complication outcomes after arteriovenous malformation radiosurgery. Int J Radiat Oncol Biol Phys 1999;44:67–74.
32 Karlsson B, Lax I, Söderman M: Factors influencing the risk for complications following Gamma Knife radiosurgery of cerebral arteriovenous malformations. Radiother Oncol 1997;43:275–280.
33 Kaido T, Hoshida T, Uranishi R, Akita N, Kotani A, Nishi N, Sakaki T: Radiosurgery-induced brain tumor. Case report. J Neurosurg 2001;95:710–713.
34 Berman EL, Eade TN, Brown D, Weaver M, Glass J, Zorman G, Feigenberg SJ: Radiation-induced tumor after stereotactic radiosurgery for an arteriovenous malformation: case report. Neurosurgery 2007;61: 1099.
35 Rowe J, Grainger A, Walton L, Silcocks P, Radatz A, Kemeny A: Risk of malignancy after gamma knife radiosurgery. Neurosurgery 2007;60:60–66.

Masaaki Yamamoto, MD
Katsuta Hospital, Mito Gamma House
5125-2 Nakane, Hitachi-Naka
Ibaraki 312-0011 (Japan)
Tel. +81 29 271 0011, E-Mail BCD06275@nifty.com

Niranjan A, Kano H, Lunsford LD (eds): Gamma Knife Radiosurgery for Brain Vascular Malformations.
Prog Neurol Surg. Basel, Karger, 2013, vol 27, pp 107–118 (DOI: 10.1159/000341647)

Management of Adverse Radiation Effects after Radiosurgery for Arteriovenous Malformations

Edward A. Monaco III · Ajay Niranjan · Hideyuki Kano · John C. Flickinger · Douglas Kondziolka · L. Dade Lunsford

Center for Image-Guided Neurosurgery, Department of Neurological Surgery, University of Pittsburgh and University of Pittsburgh Medical Center, Pittsburgh, Pa., USA

Abstract

Over the last two decades, stereotactic radiosurgery (SRS) has become a mainstay in the management of arteriovenous malformations (AVMs) of the brain. An extensive collective experience has demonstrated that SRS is a minimally invasive technique that can produce excellent AVM obliteration rates with only a modest risk of permanent adverse radiation effects (AREs). Controversy remains regarding the optimal treatment approach for AVMs, with much of the debate centered upon the risk:benefit ratios of microsurgical resection versus SRS. Proponents of surgery suggest that for appropriate Spetzler-Martin grade AVMs microsurgery harbors minimal morbidity and immediate cure. In contrast, supporters of SRS argue that many AVMs cannot be treated by microsurgery with limited morbidity, and that despite the possibility of hemorrhage during the latency to obliteration, the risk profile of SRS is more favorable. Unfortunately, a randomized clinic trial comparing microsurgery and SRS is not likely, so clinicians and patients must use available data to make their own decisions. Much effort has been expended to identify factors associated with AREs, defining their impact and predicting which patients are likely to have complete AVM obliteration in the absence of new neurological deficits. Refinement in an AVM management algorithm on these bases should better educate clinicians and patients about risk profiles, improve patient selection for different treatment strategies, and increase the likelihood of good therapeutic outcomes. Herein, we give a definition to the term ARE and review the suspected mechanisms that lead to them.

What Are Adverse Radiation Effects?

Debate persists regarding the most appropriate treatment for arteriovenous malformations (AVMs) of the brain: microsurgery or stereotactic radiosurgery (SRS). A key point of contention between the proponents of the two techniques is the difference in the risk profile of each therapy. Surgical dogma has for years been driven by the Spetzler-Martin grading scale [1], which suggests that good grade AVMs can be immediately cured microsurgically with limited morbidity at centers with extensive cerebrovascular experience. In contrast, SRS can potentially be effective for all surgical grades of AVMs with low morbidity and is minimally invasive. However, the benefit involves a delay between the time of treatment and obliteration (the latency interval) during which time secondary adverse radiation effects (AREs) may be detected. One focus of ongoing investigation is understanding and potentially mitigating radiation-induced brain tissue injury. We define AREs as any unexpected or undesirable postradiosurgery imaging change, not related to the natural history of the treated lesion, regardless of whether they are clinically symptomatic. The most clinically important AREs are those associated with clinical symptoms since such events require treatment.

In general, the effects of radiation on the brain have been divided into early or delayed responses. Within hours to days of treatment, the early reaction of the brain to radiation likely results from disruption in the blood-brain barrier and associated vasogenic edema. This has been likened to the skin's response to radiation manifest by transient erythema and edema due to dermal capillary congestion [2]. These changes may lead to new symptoms or exacerbate existing ones as preexisting edema around an AVM can increase or the associated mass effect can worsen. Symptoms related to early radiation effects can include headache, neurological deficit and seizures. Early AREs are typically transient and reversible, usually resolving spontaneously or responding to a short course of corticosteroids. After weeks, months or even years following radiation therapy, the brain can manifest a delayed injury response. It is this late ARE that is most problematic for patients and their treating physicians because of the high risk of permanent neurological sequelae and the resistance to treatment with short courses of corticosteroids [3]. Delayed symptomatic AREs are the focus of this review as they have an important and calculable effect on the risk profile of SRS for AVMs.

Mechanisms of Delayed Adverse Radiation Effects

The precise details of the molecular underpinnings that produce AREs are not completely understood. It appears that cytokine release leads to inflammatory changes in the irradiated volume and the vascular permeability of the brain tissue. Pathological examination of brain tissue demonstrating AREs has revealed: edema, reactive gliosis, blood vessel dilation, endothelial cell enlargement with endothelial thickening, and disruption of capillary structures. In the worst case examples, frank coagulative necrosis is observed [4, 5]. Shortly after irradiation, increased levels of inflammatory molecules like tumor necrosis factor-α (TNF-α), interleukin-1β, intracellular adhesion molecule-1 and glial fibrillary acidic protein have been detected in brain tissue [6, 7]. Radiation has also been demonstrated to suppress cerebral glucose metabolism in an animal model, a phenomenon that can yield oxidative free radical production [8]. Although these transient changes in brain tissue following radiation likely correspond more to acute radiation injury [9], they can have persistent consequences that lead to delayed AREs. One potent mediator of this reaction is likely TNF-α. TNF-α has been reported to trigger vascular necrosis and ultimately reactive gliosis [10]. In addition, early increases in cytokine levels recruit macrophages to irradiated tissue. These powerful immune cells release fibroblastic or astrocytosis growth factors, factors that could be critical in the mechanism of the vasculopathy of delayed radiation toxicity in the brain [11]. Vascular endothelial growth factor (VEGF) is another signaling molecule suspected to have a role in delayed ARE. Increased VEGF expression seems to correspond temporally with delayed radiation-induced brain toxicity [12]. Moreover, VEGF is suspected as a mediator of blood-brain barrier disruption and decreased endothelial cell density [12]. In one small study, Kan et al. [13] demonstrated that patients who developed symptomatic AREs following SRS for meningiomas had increased VEGF secretion compared to patients without associated increased T_2-weighted hyperintensity on imaging. Overall, these data provide a framework for understanding the complex series of events that are put in motion following brain irradiation. They provide an initial basis for targeted therapy directed at preventing or ameliorating delayed AREs.

AREs occur after SRS treatment for a variety of lesions including AVMs, meningiomas, vestibular schwannomas, primary gliomas, parenchymal metastases and cavernous malformations. However, although the imaging abnormalities that result appear similar and result in similar symptoms, it is not clear as to whether the mechanisms of ARE are the same for all lesion types. Following SRS to a tumor, AREs may in part be related to the release of factors from dying tumor cells into the surrounding brain tissue. It has been hypothesized that the perilesional abnormalities that appear following SRS for cavernous malformations are related to radiation sensitization by iron deposited from previous microhemorrhages [14]. Finally, after treatment of AVMs by radiosurgery it remains unclear as to what role the changing hemodynamics of AVM obliteration play in the development of altered magnetic resonance imaging (MRI) signal surrounding the target and eventually AREs. Data to date suggests that multiple modalities are necessary to effectively evaluate and treat symptomatic AREs.

Diagnosis of Adverse Radiation Effects

Frequent surveillance following radiosurgery with a combination of history, clinical examination and imaging studies is necessary to identify the appearance of symptomatic AREs and to document the desired response of an AVM to SRS. MRI is the optimum modality to identify and follow the evolution of AREs. AREs have been described as new areas of imaging-defined perilesional brain signal change. These changes can include new contrast enhancement of the target, regions of abnormal enhancement somewhat distant from the original target site, or perilesional areas of speckled enhancement [15], all of which can occur with or without accompanying perilesional reactive changes or necrosis [16]. Depending on volume and dose delivered, new areas of increased T_2-weighted signal intensity may develop in the brain tissue surrounding the irradiated nidus (fig. 1a, b). These imaging abnormalities can develop in as many as 30% of patients within 2 years of SRS. Such changes may be symptomatic in one third of patients, thus leaving approximately 10% of patients who develop symptomatic delayed AREs [17–19].

Extensive analysis has been performed to try and better understand the incidence, as well as the treatment parameters that contribute to the development of AREs. The largest study of this kind was a multi-institutional study of complications following SRS for AVMs [19]. Of the 1,255 patients treated, 102 (8%) developed symptomatic AREs; a rate of that has been confirmed by several smaller studies (table 1). Eighty of these symptomatic patients demonstrated evidence of parenchymal radiation injury, 12 had isolated cranial neuropathies, and 10 had new or worsened seizures. AREs were characterized in terms of severity: 39 cases were defined as minimal, 40 were mild, 21 disabling, and 2 were fatal. Forty-percent of symptomatic patients had complete symptom resolution. Patients with minimally severe symptoms were the most likely to have greater symptom resolution.

Radiation injury of the brain following SRS is related to the dose and irradiated volume. The volume effect was first reported in the late 1970s. Kjellberg related the likelihood of radiation necrosis after Bragg peak proton SRS of AVMs to the treatment volume and the prescription dose [20]. His 1% dose-volume isoeffective line and the 3% dose-volume isoeffect curve, derived from the integrated logistic formula proposed by Flickinger et al. [21, 22] for predicting brain necrosis, provided the first risk analysis of AREs following SRS. Subsequently, this dose-volume relationship has been refined. Specifically, the volume of tissue receiving 12 Gy or more has been found to be strongly correlated with the risk of imaging changes arising following SRS [23]. However, this '12-Gy volume', which depends on target volume and dose delivered, is a parameter that reflects radiation injury risk only for similar distributions of radiation within a limited range of doses. The 12-Gy volume is not a true threshold dose. Moreover these dose-volume relationships are most strongly predictive of post-SRS imaging changes and less so for symptomatic AREs.

Intuitively, a factor strongly associated with symptomatic AREs is location. Flickinger et al. [24] showed that following SRS for AVM, a brainstem location was significantly associated with the development of neurological sequelae. This concept of location-related sensitivity to AREs has been refined [18, 25, 26], yielding a model

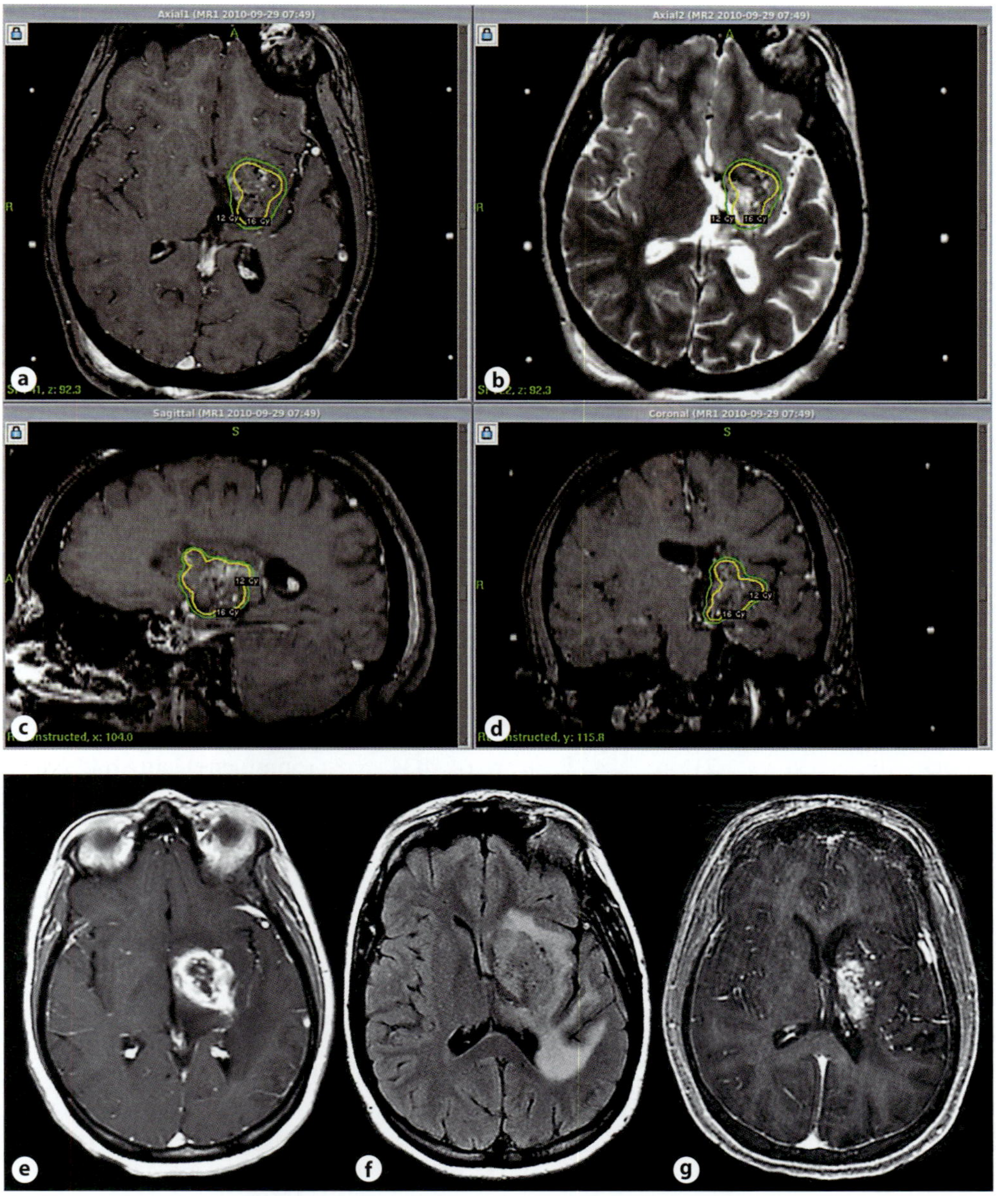

Fig. 1. a–d A 13-year-old girl underwent staged radiosurgery for a large left basal ganglia AVM. Five years later at the age of 18 years, she had second radiosurgery for residual AVM. A conformal radiosurgery dose plan was designed using contrast-enhanced spoiled gradient recalled acquisition in steady state (**a**) and T_2-weighted (**b**) images with sagittal (**c**) and coronal reconstruction (**d**). A margin dose of 18 Gy (maximum dose = 36 Gy) was prescribed to the 50% isodose line. **e–g** Nine months after radiosurgery, she presented with headache, word finding difficulty and right hemiparesis. MRI showed excessive contrast enhancement (**e**) of the lesion with severe surrounding edema (**f**). She was managed with high doses of corticosteroid. Her clinical condition gradually improved. A follow-up MRI performed 1 month later showed marked reduction in contrast enhancement as well as edema (**g**).

Table 1. The rate of symptomatic AREs following radiosurgery for AVMs reported by the University of Pittsburgh group

Reference	Patients n	Median margin dose Gy	Median AVM volume cm^3	AREs/patients	Notes
Wegner et al. [53]	293	20	3.3	39/293	validation of AVM score
Sirin et al. [54]	28	16	24.9	4/28	prospective staging of large AVMs
Maruyama et al. [55]	45	20	1.5	7/45	brainstem AVMs
Hadjipanayis et al. [56]	33	20	4.35	2/33	motor cortex AVMs
Maesawa et al. [57]	41	17	2.1	2/41	repeat SRS for AVMs
Flickinger et al. [19]	1,255	19	5.7	102/1,255	multi-institutional analysis of complications
Flickinger et al. [25]	332	20.9*	4.38*	30/332	effect of AVM location on complications
Pollock et al. [58]	34	21*	4.7*	4/34	postgeniculate AVMs
Pollock et al. [59]	65	21*	3.1*	1/65	'operable' AVMs
			Average	9.4%	

The asterisks indicate that only means (and not medians) were reported.

of risk assessment following SRS for AVMs: the modified Pollock-Flickinger AVM grading system [27]. Multivariate regression analysis modeling revealed that AVM volume, patient age and location were factors associated with outcome after SRS. This resulted in the following equation to predict which patients will undergo complete AVM obliteration without new neurological deficits: AVM score = (0.1)(volume, ml) + (0.02)(age, years) + (0.5)(location; hemispheric/corpus callosum/cerebellar = 0, basal ganglia/thalamus/brainstem = 1). Finally, the AVM microenvironment and individual variability in response to radiation may also be important. The reason why age is such an important factor in the AVM score is not clear, but may be reflective of changes in the ability of the brain's cellular machinery to repair radiation injury and respond to inflammation. Flickinger et al. [23] suggested that benign tumors (meningiomas or vestibular schwannomas) and AVMs had a higher risk of post-SRS imaging abnormalities, a finding that suggests there are differences in the tissue response of specific lesions that contribute to injury response.

Adverse Radiation Effect Therapies

Therapies for the delayed effects of SRS are difficult to study because of the time needed to manifest AREs. Because permanent SRS complications are infrequent, as well as multifactorial, there are few data on treatment strategies. Until recently, a patient manifesting an ARE following SRS had few therapeutic options. The mainstay in the treatment of symptomatic AREs is the administration of a course of high-dose anti-inflammatory corticosteroids followed by surgical excision (when feasible) in case of treatment failure [28]. The chronic use of corticosteroids is not trivial and can lead to weight gain, diabetes mellitus, immunosuppression, secondary infections and severe bone density loss. Surgical excision in refractory cases exposes the patient to the risks of surgery and general anesthesia.

As the molecular mechanisms of AREs are being identified, new therapies are being explored. Inflammation and immunomodulatory signaling molecules have been implicated in the body's response to irradiation. As these molecules are ubiquitous in injury response, great efforts have been made to modify their expression and activity. For example, pentoxifylline (PTX), a methylxanthine derivative used to treat conditions involving impaired regional microcirculation, has been shown to decrease the levels of TNF-α and interleukin-1, while also inhibiting the upregulation of VEGF following an inciting stimulus. Such cytokines have been implicated in the development of AREs [29, 30]. PTX also has been shown to improve regional blood flow while decreasing plasma fibrinogen levels and increasing fibrinolytic activity [11]. Clinically, PTX administration has been useful in ameliorating AREs in soft tissues following radiation therapy [29, 31–33].

α-Tocopherol, or vitamin E, may act as a scavenger of oxygen free radicals produced by cellular stress, an effect that can protect cell membranes from lipid peroxidation [29]. Several studies suggest vitamin E can facilitate normal tissue healing with limited scarring following radiation therapy [10, 29, 34]. In combination, PTX and vitamin E may have a synergistic action on extracellular matrix and cell regulation [34]. Indeed, a small clinical trial evaluating the combination of PTX and vitamin E in the treatment of chronic radiation injury to skin and soft tissue in patients who were treated with previous radiation showed that the combination reversed chronic radiotherapy damage [35]. Because of these encouraging results, Williamson et al. [16] treated 11 patients with suspected AREs following radiosurgery. Patients were treated with 400 mg of oral PTX and 400 IU of oral vitamin E, both twice a day. Three of the 11 patients had SRS for AVMs. Ten of the patients, including all 3 of the AVM patients, had a gradual reduction in AREs seen on serial MRIs following an average treatment of 6 months (range, 1.2–13.1 months). A single patient failed this management strategy but was found to have recurrent tumor at the time of a subsequent craniotomy. Overall, the combination of PTX and vitamin E was tolerated well as only 2 patients had side effects that included persistent nausea and vomiting. Although small, this study supports the hypothesis that in combination PTX and vitamin E may be useful in treating AREs following SRS. To make more concrete conclusions, a larger prospective randomized trial is needed.

PTX and vitamin E may possess indirect effects on VEGF to mitigate AREs. However, several investigators have hypothesized that direct inhibition of VEGF function may be an effective option for severe AREs [36–40]. Benoit et al. [40] used bevacizumab, a murine monoclonal antibody against VEGF, in 1 patient with brainstem and temporal lobe AREs and who previously failed long-term corticosteroid therapy. Following treatment much of the patient's symptomatology resolved coincident with improvement in lesional contrast enhancement and surrounding edema. One small randomized double-blind placebo-controlled trial of bevacizumab therapy for the treatment of AREs was performed in 14 patients with pathologically confirmed AREs following radiation therapy for several heterogeneous pathologies (i.e. meningioma, low-grade glioma, head and neck carcinoma) [41]. The patients who were treated with bevacizumab demonstrated both decreased lesional contrast-enhancement and perilesional edema on imaging. Only the bevacizumab-treated patients showed improvement in neurological symptoms. Although there are no definitive studies of the use of bevacizumab for the treatment of AREs resulting from SRS, anecdotal reports prompt consideration of the use of anti-VEGF therapies in the treatment of AREs. Clearly further study of bevacizumab in this setting is needed. Although no systematic study on the role of bevacizumab in managing AREs following AVM radiosurgery has been performed at our institution, we have used bevacizumab therapy to successfully manage ARE related to malignant brain tumors.

One final approach that is noteworthy because of its use in treating AREs following radiosurgery for AVMs is hyperbaric oxygen (HBO). HBO is typically used in the treatment of poorly healing wounds, infections and decompression sickness. The mechanism of HBO in healing is believed to be related to [7, 17, 24–26, 28]: increases in tissue oxygen levels, decreases in lactate concentrations, induction of fibroblastic activity and vasculogenesis, as well as leading to cerebral vasoconstriction and reducing vascular permeability [42–47]. Wanebo et al. [48] reviewed the use of HBO in the treatment of AREs following SRS for AVMs. In all reported cases, symptoms and radiographic evidence of AREs improved or completely resolved [48–52]. One patient required subsequent surgical decompression. Further study of HBO is necessary in the context, but its use could obviate the need for surgery in cases otherwise medically refractory. At the University of Pittsburgh, the management of symptomatic AREs includes frequent imaging surveillance in combination with a 2- to 4-week course of corticosteroids followed by PTX and vitamin E for 3 months. In refractory cases, surgical excision may be required (fig. 2).

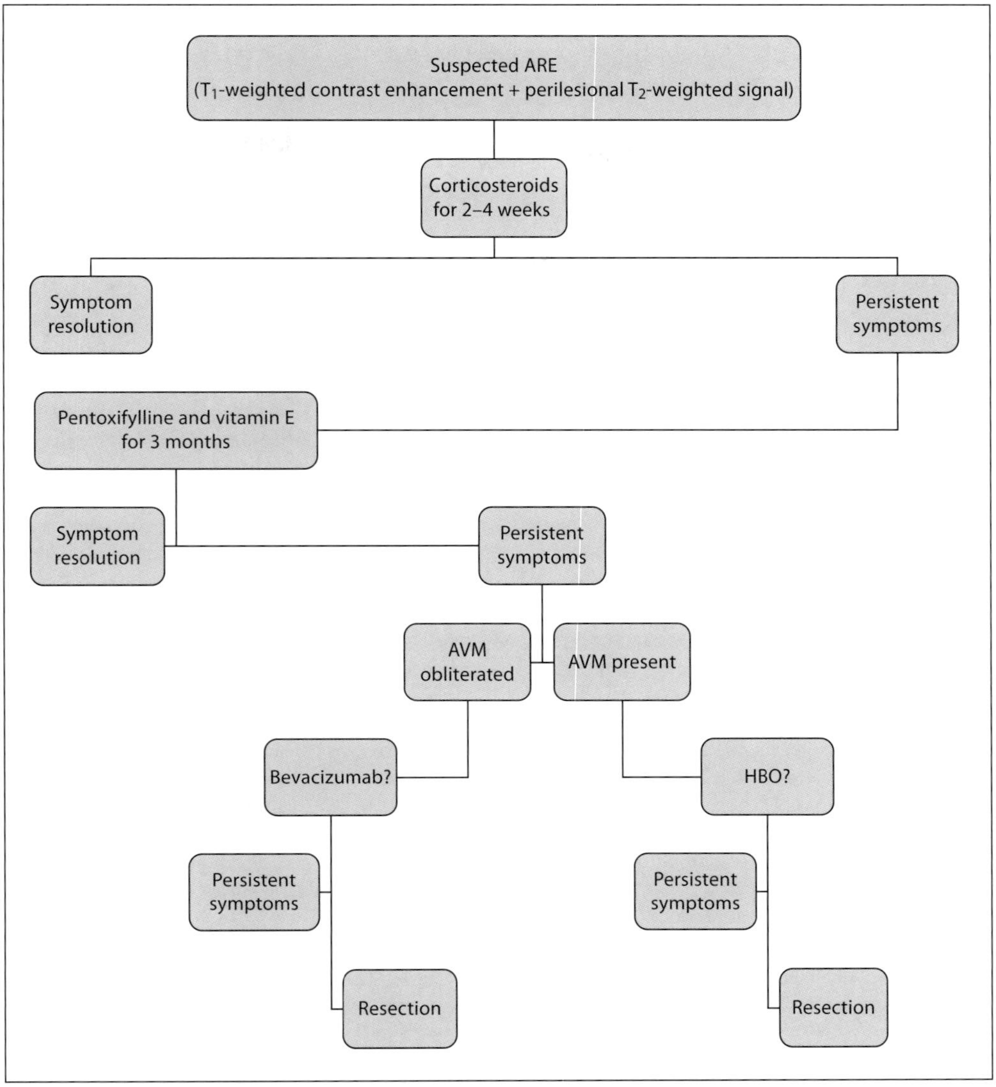

Fig. 2. Management algorithm for suspected AREs after SRS for AVM.

Conclusions

The optimum management strategy for AVMs remains controversial but options include microsurgical resection, embolization and SRS. In order to improve patient outcomes, continued work is necessary to study risk-benefit profiles as our technology and understanding improve. Although microsurgery can be used to cure some AVMs with low morbidity, SRS has proven to be a minimally invasive, safe and effective alternative, and it can be used to treat AVMs that are not reasonable surgical targets. Symptomatic AREs are uncommon but serious complications following radiosurgical management of AVMs and strategies to limit or treat their occurrence will benefit patients. Emerging evidence regarding the underlying mechanisms of AREs has yielded already produced investigations into directed therapies. Further study in radiosurgery patients is necessary in order to evaluate the safety and efficacy of these approaches.

References

1 Spetzler RF, Martin NA: A proposed grading system for arteriovenous malformations. J Neurosurg 1986; 65:476–483.

2 Moss CV, Brand WN, Battifora H: Radiation Oncology: Rationale, Technique and Results. St Louis, Mosby, 1973.

3 Kramer S, Lee KF: Complications of radiation therapy: the central nervous system. Semin Roentgenol 1974;9:75–83.

4 Munter MW, Karger CP, Reith W, Schneider HM, Peschke P, Debus J: Delayed vascular injury after single high-dose irradiation in the rat brain: histologic immunohistochemical, and angiographic studies. Radiology 1999;212:475–482.

5 Perry A, Schmidt RE: Cancer therapy-associated CNS neuropathology: an update and review of the literature. Acta Neuropathol 2006;111:197–212.

6 Hong JH, Chiang CS, Campbell IL, Sun JR, Withers HR, McBride WH: Induction of acute phase gene expression by brain irradiation. Int J Radiat Oncol Biol Phys 1995;33:619–626.

7 Sharp CD, Jawahar A, Warren AC, Elrod JW, Nanda A, Alexander JS: Gamma knife irradiation increases cerebral endothelial expression of intercellular adhesion molecule 1 and E-selectin. Neurosurgery 2003;53:154–160, discussion 160–161.

8 D'Avella D, Cicciarello R, Albiero F, Mesiti M, Gagliardi ME, Russi E, d'Aquino A, Princi P, d'Aquino S: Effect of whole brain radiation on local cerebral glucose utilization in the rat. Neurosurgery 1991;28:491–495.

9 Wood K, Jawahar A, Smelley C, Mullapudi S, De Laune A, Nanda A, Granger DN: Exposure of brain to high-dose, focused gamma rays irradiation produces increase in leukocytes-adhesion and pavementing in small intracerebral blood vessels. Neurosurgery 2005;57:1282–1288.

10 Prasad KN, Cole WC, Kumar B, Che Prasad K: Pros and cons of antioxidant use during radiation therapy. Cancer Treat Rev 2002;28:79–91.

11 Okunieff P, Augustine E, Hicks JE, Cornelison TL, Altemus RM, Naydich BG, Ding I, Huser AK, Abraham EH, Smith JJ, Coleman N, Gerber LH: Pentoxifylline in the treatment of radiation-induced fibrosis. J Clin Oncol 2004;22:2207–2213.

12 Tsao MN, Li YQ, Lu G, Xu Y, Wong CS: Upregulation of vascular endothelial growth factor is associated with radiation-induced blood-spinal cord barrier breakdown. J Neuropathol Exp Neurol 1999;58: 1051–1060.

13 Kan P, Liu JK, Wendland MM, Shrieve D, Jensen RL: Peritumoral edema after stereotactic radiosurgery for intracranial meningiomas and molecular factors that predict its development. J Neurooncol 2007;83:33–38.

14 Monaco EA, Khan AA, Niranjan A, Kano H, Grandhi R, Kondziolka D, Flickinger JC, Lunsford LD: Stereotactic radiosurgery for the treatment of symptomatic brainstem cavernous malformations. Neurosurg Focus 2010;29:E11.

15 Kumar AJ, Leeds NE, Fuller GN, Van Tassel P, Maor MH, Sawaya RE, Levin VA: Malignant gliomas: MR imaging spectrum of radiation therapy- and chemotherapy-induced necrosis of the brain after treatment. Radiology 2000;217:377–384.

16 Williamson R, Kondziolka D, Kanaan H, Lunsford LD, Flickinger JC: Adverse radiation effects after radiosurgery may benefit from oral vitamin E and pentoxifylline therapy: a pilot study. Stereotact Funct Neurosurg 2008;86:359–366.

17 Flickinger JC, Kondziolka D, Pollock BE, Maitz AH, Lunsford LD: Complications from arteriovenous malformation radiosurgery: multivariate analysis and risk modeling. Int J Radiat Oncol Biol Phys 1997;38:485–490.

18 Flickinger JC, Kondziolka D, Lunsford LD, Kassam A, Phuong LK, Liscak R, Pollock B: Development of a model to predict permanent symptomatic postradiosurgery injury for arteriovenous malformation patients. Arteriovenous Malformation Radiosurgery Study Group. Int J Radiat Oncol Biol Phys 2000; 46:1143–1148.

19 Flickinger JC, Kondziolka D, Lunsford LD, Pollock BE, Yamamoto M, Gorman DA, Schomberg PJ, Sneed P, Larson D, Smith V, McDermott MW, Miyawaki L, Chilton J, Morantz RA, Young B, Jokura H, Liscak R: A multi-institutional analysis of complication outcomes after arteriovenous malformation radiosurgery. Int J Radiat Oncol Biol Phys 1999;44:67–74.
20 Kjelberg RN: Isoeffective dose parameters for brain necrosis in relation to proton radiosurgical dosimetry; in Szilka G (ed): Stereotactic Cerebral Irradiation INSERM Symposium. Amsterdam, Elsevier Press, 1979, pp 157–166.
21 Flickinger JC: An integrated logistic formula for prediction of complications from radiosurgery. Int J Radiat Oncol Biol Phys 1989;17:879–885.
22 Flickinger JC, Schell MC, Larson DA: Estimation of complications for linear accelerator radiosurgery with the integrated logistic formula. Int J Radiat Oncol Biol Phys 1990;19:143–148.
23 Flickinger CJ, Kondziolka D, Kalend AM, Maitz AH, Lunsford LD: Radiosurgery-related imaging changes in surrounding brain: multivariate analysis and model evaluation. Radiosurgery 1996;1:229–236.
24 Flickinger JC, Lunsford LD, Kondziolka D, Maitz AH, Epstein AH, Simons SR, Wu A: Radiosurgery and brain tolerance: an analysis of neurodiagnostic imaging changes after gamma knife radiosurgery for arteriovenous malformations. Int J Radiat Oncol Biol Phys 1992;23:19–26.
25 Flickinger JC, Kondziolka D, Maitz AH, Lunsford LD: Analysis of neurological sequelae from radiosurgery of arteriovenous malformations: how location affects outcome. Int J Radiat Oncol Biol Phys 1998;40:273–278.
26 Pollock BE, Flickinger JC: A proposed radiosurgery-based grading system for arteriovenous malformations. J Neurosurg 2002;96:79–85.
27 Pollock BE, Flickinger JC: Modification of the radiosurgery-based arteriovenous malformation grading system. Neurosurgery 2008;63:239–243.
28 Plowman PN: Stereotactic radiosurgery. VIII. The classification of postradiation reactions. Br J Neurosurg 1999;13:256–264.
29 Delanian S, Porcher R, Balla-Mekias S, Lefaix JL: Randomized, placebo-controlled trial of combined pentoxifylline and tocopherol for regression of superficial radiation-induced fibrosis. J Clin Oncol 2003;21:2545–2550.
30 Amirkhosravi A, Meyer T, Warnes G, Amaya M, Malik Z, Biggerstaff JP, Siddiqui FA, Sherman P, Francis JL: Pentoxifylline inhibits hypoxia-induced upregulation of tumor cell tissue factor and vascular endothelial growth factor. Thromb Haemost 1998; 80:598–602.
31 Futran ND, Trotti A, Gwede C: Pentoxifylline in the treatment of radiation-related soft tissue injury: preliminary observations. Laryngoscope 1997;107: 391–395.
32 Nieder C, Zimmermann FB, Adam M, Molls M: The role of pentoxifylline as a modifier of radiation therapy. Cancer Treat Rev 2005;31:448–455.
33 Ozturk B, Egehan I, Atavci S, Kitapci M: Pentoxifylline in prevention of radiation-induced lung toxicity in patients with breast and lung cancer: a double-blind randomized trial. Int J Radiat Oncol Biol Phys 2004;58:213–219.
34 Lefaix JL, Delanian S, Vozenin MC, Leplat JJ, Tricaud Y, Martin M: Striking regression of subcutaneous fibrosis induced by high doses of gamma rays using a combination of pentoxifylline and alpha-tocopherol: an experimental study. Int J Radiat Oncol Biol Phys 1999;43:839–847.
35 Delanian S, Balla-Mekias S, Lefaix JL: Striking regression of chronic radiotherapy damage in a clinical trial of combined pentoxifylline and tocopherol. J Clin Oncol 1999;17:3283–3290.
36 Gonzalez J, Kumar AJ, Conrad CA, Levin VA: Effect of bevacizumab on radiation necrosis of the brain. Int J Radiat Oncol Biol Phys 2007;67:323–326.
37 Torcuator R, Zuniga R, Mohan YS, Rock J, Doyle T, Anderson J, Gutierrez J, Ryu S, Jain R, Rosenblum M, Mikkelsen T: Initial experience with bevacizumab treatment for biopsy confirmed cerebral radiation necrosis. J Neurooncol 2009;94:63–68.
38 Liu AK, Macy ME, Foreman NK: Bevacizumab as therapy for radiation necrosis in four children with pontine gliomas. Int J Radiat Oncol Biol Phys 2009; 75:1148–1154.
39 Wong ET, Huberman M, Lu XQ, Mahadevan A: Bevacizumab reverses cerebral radiation necrosis. J Clin Oncol 2008;26:5649–5650.
40 Benoit A, Ducray F, Cartalat-Carel S, Psimaras D, Ricard D, Honnorat J: Favorable outcome with bevacizumab after poor outcome with steroids in a patient with temporal lobe and brainstem radiation necrosis. J Neurol 2010;258:328–329.
41 Levin VA, Bidaut L, Hou P, Kumar AJ, Wefel JS, Bekele BN, Prabhu S, Loghin M, Gilbert MR, Jackson EF: Randomized double-blind placebo-controlled trial of bevacizumab therapy for radiation necrosis of the central nervous system. Int J Radiat Oncol Biol Phys 2011;79:1487–1495.

42 Davis JC, Dunn JM, Gates GA, Heimbach RD: Hyperbaric oxygen. A new adjunct in the management of radiation necrosis. Arch Otolaryngol 1979; 105:58–61.
43 Kapp JP, Phillips M, Markov A, Smith RR: Hyperbaric oxygen after circulatory arrest: modification of postischemic encephalopathy. Neurosurgery 1982;11:496–499.
44 Manson PN, Im MJ, Myers AM: Improved capillaries by hyperbaric oxygen in skin flaps. Surg Forum 1980;31:564–566.
45 Marx RE, Johnson RP, Kline SN: Prevention of osteoradionecrosis: a randomized prospective clinical trial of hyperbaric oxygen versus penicillin. J Am Dent Assoc 1985;111:49–54.
46 Mink RB, Dutka AJ: Hyperbaric oxygen after global cerebral ischemia in rabbits reduces brain vascular permeability and blood flow. Stroke 1995;26:2307–2312.
47 Regli F, Yamaguchi T, Waltz AG: Effects of inhalation of oxygen on blood flow and microvasculature of ischemic and nonischemic cerebral cortex. Stroke 1970;1:314–319.
48 Wanebo JE, Kidd GA, King MC, Chung TS: Hyperbaric oxygen therapy for treatment of adverse radiation effects after stereotactic radiosurgery of arteriovenous malformations: case report and review of literature. Surg Neurol 2009;72:162–167.
49 Chuba PJ, Aronin P, Bhambhani K, Eichenhorn M, Zamarano L, Cianci P, Muhlbauer M, Porter AT, Fontanesi J: Hyperbaric oxygen therapy for radiation-induced brain injury in children. Cancer 1997;80:2005–2012.
50 Leber KA, Eder HG, Kovac H, Anegg U, Pendl G: Treatment of cerebral radionecrosis by hyperbaric oxygen therapy. Stereotact Funct Neurosurg 1998; 70(suppl 1):229–236.
51 Lynn M, Friedman WA: Hyperbaric oxygen in the treatment of a radiosurgical complication: technical case report. Neurosurgery 2007;60:E579.
52 Takenaka N, Imanishi T, Sasaki H, Shimazaki K, Sugiura H, Kitagawa Y, Sekiyama S, Yamamoto M, Kazuno T: Delayed radiation necrosis with extensive brain edema after gamma knife radiosurgery for multiple cerebral cavernous malformations – case report. Neurol Med Chir (Tokyo) 2003;43: 391–395.
53 Wegner RE, Oysul K, Pollock BE, Sirin S, Kondziolka D, Niranjan A, Lunsford LD, Flickinger JC: A modified radiosurgery-based arteriovenous malformation grading scale and its correlation with outcomes. Int J Radiat Oncol Biol Phys 2011;79:1147–1150.
54 Sirin S, Kondziolka D, Niranjan A, Flickinger JC, Maitz AH, Lunsford LD: Prospective staged volume radiosurgery for large arteriovenous malformations: indications and outcomes in otherwise untreatable patients. Neurosurgery 2006;58:17–27.
55 Maruyama K, Kondziolka D, Niranjan A, Flickinger JC, Lunsford LD: Stereotactic radiosurgery for brainstem arteriovenous malformations: factors affecting outcome. J Neurosurg 2004;100:407–413.
56 Hadjipanayis CG, Levy EI, Niranjan A, Firlik AD, Kondziolka D, Flickinger JC, Lunsford LD: Stereotactic radiosurgery for motor cortex region arteriovenous malformations. Neurosurgery 2001; 48:70–76.
57 Maesawa S, Flickinger JC, Kondziolka D, Lunsford LD: Repeated radiosurgery for incompletely obliterated arteriovenous malformations. J Neurosurg 2000; 92:961–970.
58 Pollock BE, Lunsford LD, Kondziolka D, Bissonette DJ, Flickinger JC: Stereotactic radiosurgery for postgeniculate visual pathway arteriovenous malformations. J Neurosurg 1996;84:437–441.
59 Pollock BE, Lunsford LD, Kondziolka D, Maitz A, Flickinger JC: Patient outcomes after stereotactic radiosurgery for 'operable' arteriovenous malformations. Neurosurgery 1994;35:1–7.

Ajay Niranjan, MCh, MBA
Department of Neurological Surgery, University of Pittsburgh Medical Center, Suite B-400
200 Lothrop Street
Pittsburgh, PA 15213 (USA)
Tel. +1 412 647 6250, E-Mail niranjana@upmc.edu

Niranjan A, Kano H, Lunsford LD (eds): Gamma Knife Radiosurgery for Brain Vascular Malformations.
Prog Neurol Surg. Basel, Karger, 2013, vol 27, pp 119–129 (DOI: 10.1159/000341772)

Morphological Observations in Brain Arteriovenous Malformations after Gamma Knife Radiosurgery

György T. Szeifert[a,b] · Marc Levivier[c] · José Lorenzoni[c] · István Nyáry[b] · Ottó Major[b] · Andras A. Kemeny[d]

[a]Department of Neurotraumatology, Péterfy Traumatological Centre, and [b]Department of Neurological Surgery, Semmelweis University, Budapest, Hungary; [c]Centre Gamma Knife, Université Libre de Bruxelles, Brussels, Belgium; [d]National Centre for Stereotactic Radiosurgery, Sheffield, UK

Abstract

Morphological studies after Gamma Knife radiosurgery (GKRS) revealed endothelial destruction followed by spindle-shaped cell proliferation in the subendothelial region and in the connective tissue stroma of arteriovenous malformation (AVM) vessels. Histological, immunohistochemical and ultrastructural characteristics of this spindle-shaped cell population in the irradiated AVMs were reminiscent of those described as myofibroblasts in wound healing processes and pathological fibromatoses. These modified fibroblasts have contractile capacity, therefore this might contribute to the vessel occlusion, shrinking process and final volume reduction of AVMs after GKRS. Similar histopathological changes were observed in a cavernous malformation following high-dose irradiation.

Since the first report by Steiner et al. [1] in 1972, radiosurgery has become an effective and widespread primary or alternative management modality for selected cerebral arteriovenous malformations (AVMs). The goal of stereotactic radiosurgery in the treatment of brain AVMs is to obliterate the nidus completely to eliminate the risk of hemorrhage.

Pathologically, AVMs are considered hamartomatous lesions of the brain originating from embryonic maldevelopment [2, 3]. Histologically, they are characterized by clusters of abnormal arteries and arterialized veins with irregular vessel wall structure, and without an intervening capillary bed. Following Virchow's fundamental work on the pathological description of vascular brain lesions [4], the current histopathological classification of cerebral vascular malformations into AVMs, cavernomas, teleangiectasias and venous anomalies was elaborated by McCormick

[5]. Histology of abnormal vessels in AVMs had already been described extensively. The purpose of the present study is to demonstrate morphological changes in irradiated cerebral vascular malformations after Gamma Knife radiosurgery (GKRS).

Histopathological Observations

Incompletely (Subtotally) Obliterated AVMs

Surgical pathology material was obtained from 7 patients who had undergone GKRS for AVMs but they suffered rebleeding 10–52 months after treatment, therefore the AVMs were resected by open craniotomy. Specimens were fixed in 10% neutral buffered formaldehyde, processed routinely, and embedded in paraffin. Besides the routine hematoxylin-eosin (HE), elastic van Gieson and Masson trichrome staining, immunohistochemical reactions were performed on 5-μm sections to study desmin, vimentin, α-smooth muscle actin, S-100 protein, glial fibrillary acidic protein, CD34 and factor VIII-related antigens in the cell populations of malformations after irradiation. Double immunoenzymatic labeling with peroxidase and alkaline phosphatase for α-smooth muscle actin/vimentin, α-smooth muscle actin/desmin and vimentin/desmin was also performed to demonstrate the presence of both antigens in the same cell. Tissue samples from 5 resected AVMs which were not treated with GKRS served as nonirradiated controls. For transmission electron-microscopic investigations, the specimens were reembedded in Araldite from the original paraffin-embedded material, cut, and stained with uranyl acetate and lead citrate.

Light microscopy revealed different stages of tissue reactions apparently starting with endothelial destruction and granulation tissue formation, followed by a spindle-shaped cell infiltration, turning into scar tissue replacement and hyaline degeneration (fig. 1a). Vascular channels that had undergone incomplete obliteration were obstructed by fibrin thrombi (fig. 1b). In cases of total obliteration they were completely replaced by degenerated hyaline scar tissue, and only the vessels' contour was recognizable without any identifiable lumina. Immunohistochemical reactions demonstrated marked α-smooth muscle actin positivity in the spindle-shaped stromal cells (fig. 1c). The vimentin and desmin reactions were also positive but with less intensity compared to the α-smooth muscle actin activity. Using double labeling vimentin/desmin positivity was revealed on the same spindle cells. With the α-smooth muscle actin/vimentin and α-smooth muscle actin/desmin double reactions, only the α-smooth muscle actin positivity was detected, probably because of the vigorous intensity of this antigen masking the fainter desmin and vimentin antigen expression. The stromal spindle cell proliferation was closely related to the adventitial layer of the vessels. Vimentin positivity was more pronounced in the scar tissue areas. The antigen profile of the subendothelial proliferating spindle cells showed strong α-smooth muscle actin positivity, whereas activity of vimentin and desmin was less marked. Factor VIII-related antigen was expressed by the lining endothelial cells in a considerably reduced proportion of the vessels. A higher percentage of the vessels did not reveal any endothelial activity at all. Glial fibrillary acidic protein and S-100 protein were demonstrated in the glial cells of the surrounding brain parenchyma but not in the stromal cells or vessels of the AVMs. In the early stages after irradiation, granulation tissue formation and spindle cell proliferation were more prominent, whereas in the later stages, collagen production and hyalinization were more pronounced.

Electron microscopy demonstrated diverse ultrastructural characteristics in the spindle cell population. There were cells demonstrating features of typical conventional resting fibroblasts with oval nuclei and a smooth contour as well as cisterns of endoplasmic reticulum. These cell types were usually surrounded by massive bundles of collagen fibers in the extracellular matrix. Other cells with similar nuclear morphology contained abundant intracytoplasmic filaments and sometimes prominent nucleoli. Nuclear deformations were connected with well-developed rough endoplasmic reticulum. In modified fibroblasts with folds and indentations on the nuclear contour, a striking fibrillary system developed also within the cytoplasm. These ultrastructural characteristics reflect morphological consequences of a contractile activity.

Completely (Totally) Obliterated AVM with Rebleeding

A deep cerebral AVM presenting with recurrent hemorrhage 5 years following angiography-confirmed nidus obliteration was investigated 7 years after radiosurgery. Histological examination demonstrated that the majority of AVM vessels were replaced by scar tissue (fig. 2a). However, some of them still exhibited thrombus organization by granulation tissue 7 years after radiosurgery (fig. 2b). Factor VIII and CD34 reactions revealed vessel neoformation within thrombuses of the AVM channels (fig. 2c). Proliferating spindle-shaped cells with α-smooth muscle actin and vimentin expression were identified in the granulation tissue.

Cavernous Malformation

Stereotactic radiosurgery is a controversial treatment modality in the management of cerebral cavernous malformations [6–8]. Systematic pathological studies of irradiated specimens could probably help to resolve the controversy [9, 10]. Light-microscopic investigation of a surgically resected thalamic cerebral cavernous malformation 1 year after 40-Gy irradiation revealed endothelial cell destruction in the cavernous channels (fig. 3a), and marked fibrosis with scar tissue formation in the connective stroma of the lesion (fig. 3b). These histopathological findings were similar to those described in AVMs after GKRS, and suggest that an ionizing effect of radiation energy evokes vascular and connective tissue stroma changes in cerebral cavernous malformations as well.

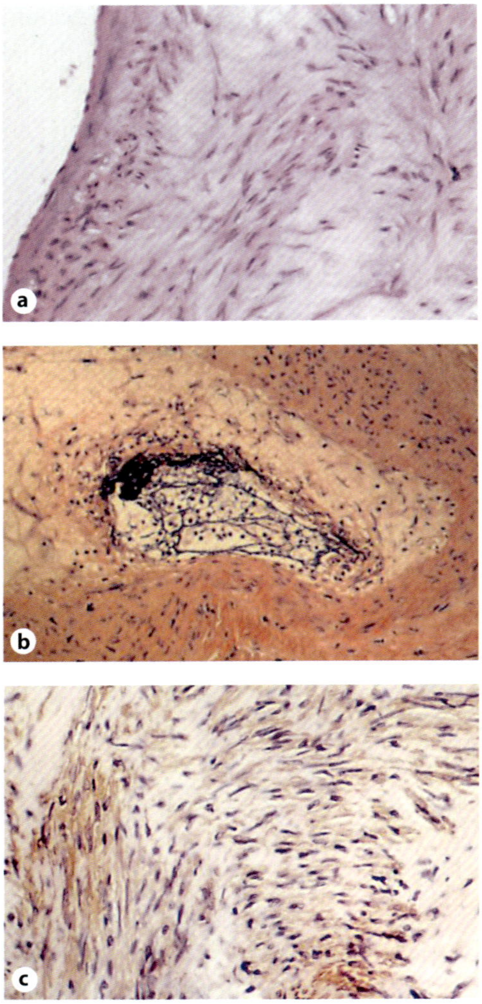

1

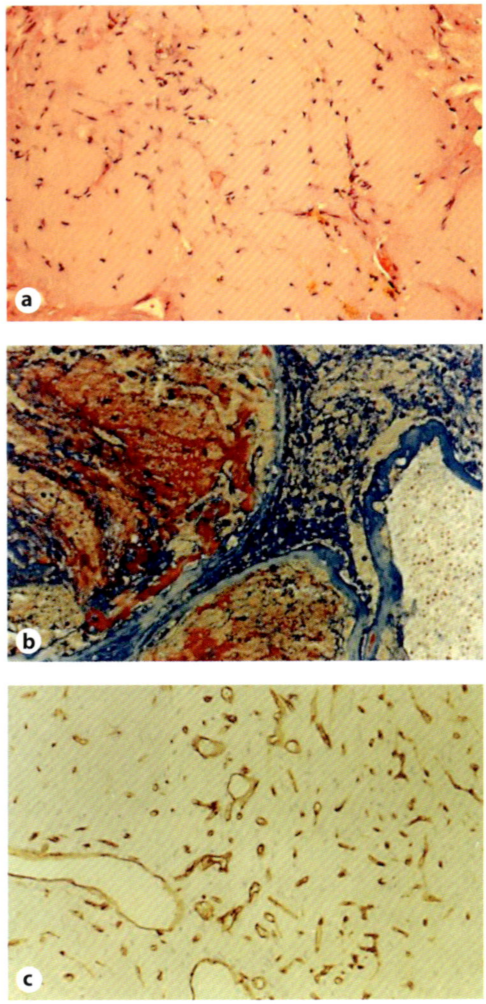

2

Fig. 1, 2. Human histological observations on irradiated AVMs.
1 Incompletely obliterated AVM. **a** Endothelial destruction and prominent spindle-shaped cell proliferation in the subendothelial region of an AVM vessel wall. HE. ×200. **b** An AVM vessel lumen obliterated by fibrin thrombi. Masson trichrome. ×100. **c** Immunohistochemical expression of α-smooth muscle actin in spindle-shaped stromal cells. ×200.
2 'Totally' obliterated AVM. **a** Scar tissue replacing AVM channels. Elastic van Gieson. ×100. **b** Organization of thrombi in AVM vessels. Masson trichrome. ×100. **c** Recanalization of thrombi in an AVM vessel. CD34 immunohistochemical reaction. ×100.

Experimental Observations

Experimental GKRS of rat middle cerebral arteries (fig. 4a, b) demonstrated that endothelial destruction of the vessel wall appears to be among the earliest histological changes following irradiation (fig. 4c, d). This process is accompanied by an increased apoptotic activity in the surrounding brain tissue (fig. 4e, f).

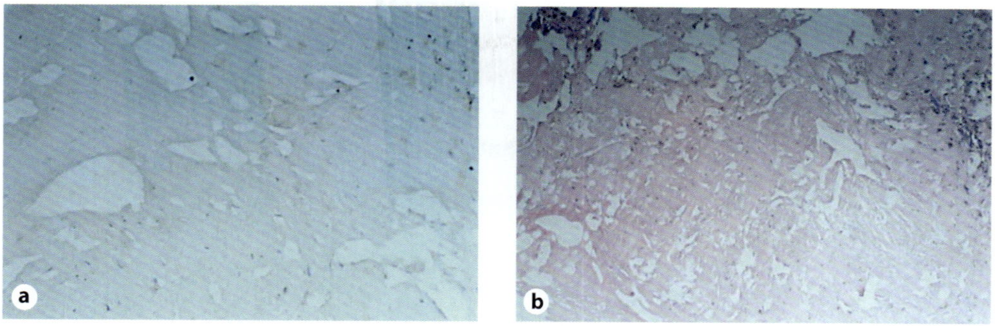

Fig. 3. 40-Gy-irradiated cavernous malformation. **a** Endothelial destruction in cavernous channels. CD34 reaction. ×200. **b** Prominent hyaline degenerated scar tissue formation in the stroma. HE. ×200.

In human AVM tissue culture experiments, immunohistochemistry revealed vigorous vimentin positivity in the nonirradiated control AVM cultures, which gradually decreased by time in the irradiated specimens. Smooth muscle α-actin positivity was prominent in the irradiated cultivated samples suggesting transformation of resting fibroblasts onto activated myofibroblastic elements with contractile capacity (fig. 5a). This transformation process was confirmed by the appearance of transforming growth factor-β activity in the irradiated AVM cell lines also (fig. 5b). These data support the hypothesis that one of the contributing factors to AVM shrinkage and obliteration after radiosurgery might be fibrocyte-to-myofibroblast cell transformation in the vessel wall.

Discussion

Radiosurgery was originally introduced to treat functional disorders [11]. Soon after its development AVMs became one of the major indications, providing a new tool for the treatment of brain lesions in regions where surgical access was unacceptably risky [12–14]. Magnetic resonance imaging and angiographic studies have documented that 65–87% of AVMs are obliterated, and that 75% shrink in volume 2–5 years after radiosurgery [15].

Although the histology of abnormal vessels in AVMs had been demonstrated previously [16], relatively little was known about the pathological response of AVMs to a single high-dose ionizing radiation treatment. Recently a few publications have described histopathological changes in the vessels of cerebral AVMs after radiosurgery [17–22]. It seems that the early reaction from the connective tissue stroma of an AVM is formation of granulation tissue infiltrated by chronic inflammatory cells. Later, a spindle-shaped cell population follows the granulation tissue and, in turn, is replaced by a hypocellular, hyaline degenerated scar tissue, which is the stable

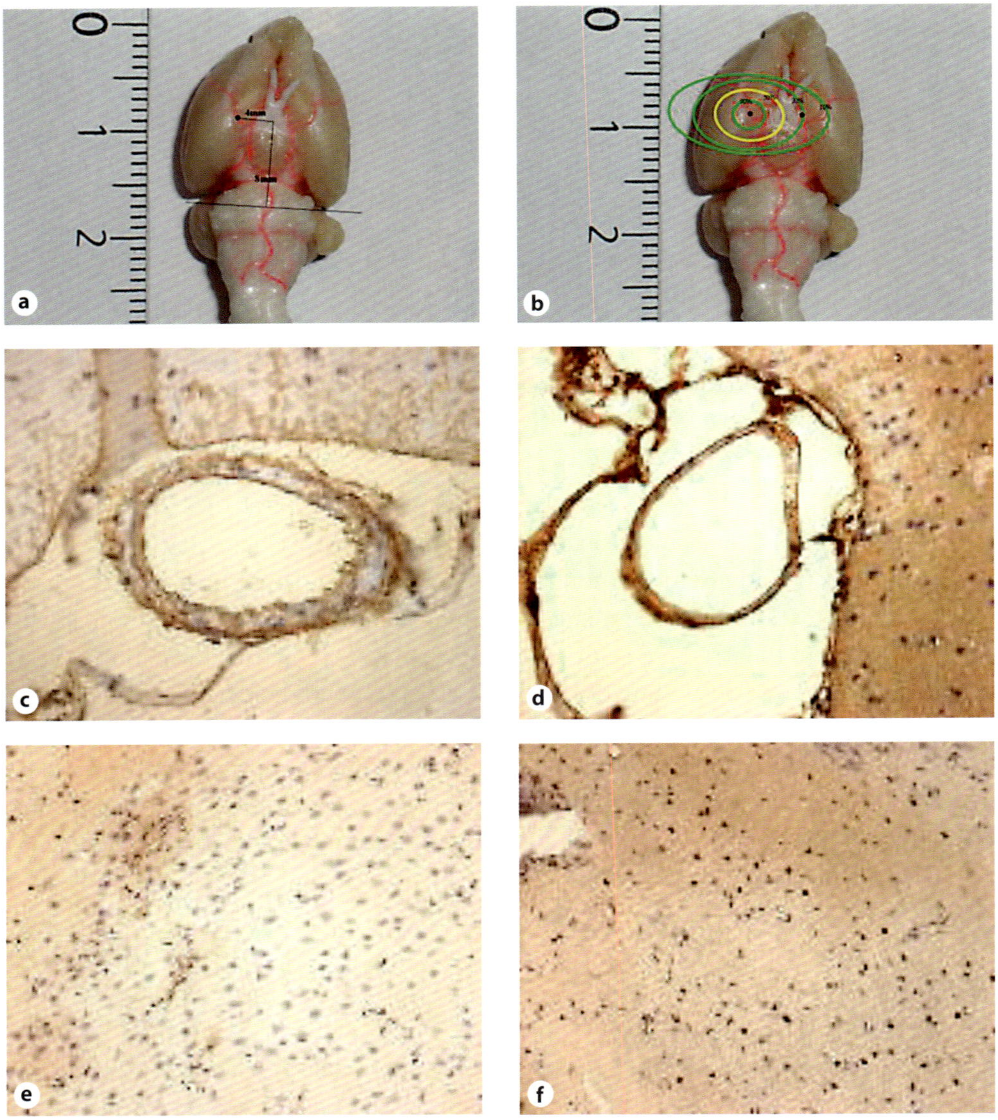

Fig. 4. Experimental observations on irradiated rat brains. **a** Angiography of cerebral base vessels and targeting of the right middle cerebral artery on rat brain. **b** Superposing of isodose curves for dose calculation. **c** Nonirradiated control AVM with lining endothelial cell layer. Factor VIII immune reaction. ×200. **d** Destruction of endothelial cells 2 months after 15-Gy irradiation. Factor VIII reaction. ×200. **e** Scattered apoptotic cells in nonirradiated control rat brain around the middle cerebral artery at 50% isodose. Caspase-3 immune reaction. ×200. **f** Enhanced apoptotic activity in rat brain at 50% isodose, 2 months after 15-Gy irradiation. Caspase-3 reaction. ×200.

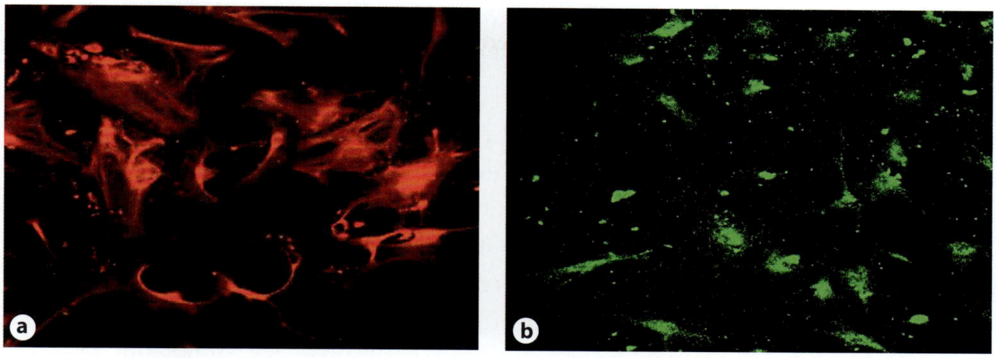

Fig. 5. **a** Vigorous α-smooth muscle actin positivity in 25-Gy-irradiated human AVM tissue culture cells. ×1,000. **b** Transforming growth factor-β activity was prominent as well. ×1,000.

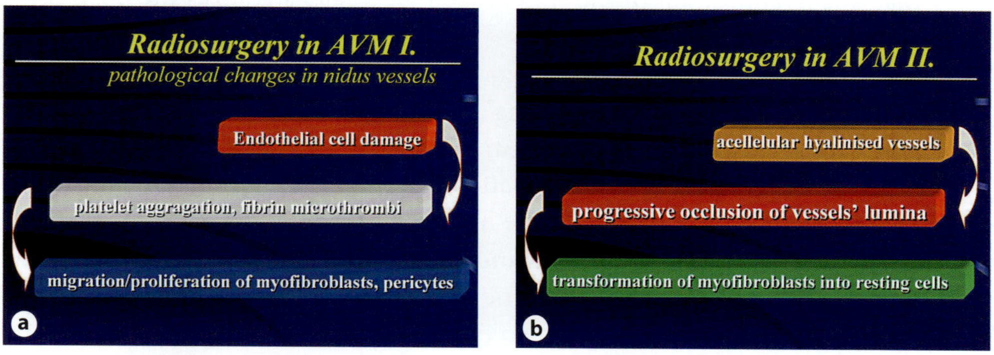

Fig. 6. Summary of pathological changes evoked by radiosurgery on AVM vessels.

end result of the obliteration process. The thrombo-obliterative course starts with endothelial destruction followed by subendothelial and perivascular spindle cell proliferation. These spindle cells express immunohistochemical, ultrastructural and experimental characteristics resembling those of myofibroblasts [23], and they have a contractile capacity through α-smooth-muscle actin production. In later stages conventional resting fibroblasts and fibrocytes produce collagen bundles to replace myofibroblasts. Collagen fibers undergo hyaline degeneration and form scar tissue, which supplements and stabilizes the AVM vessels, thus obliterating the lumina 'safely' (fig. 6a, b).

As stated previously, there is a latent interval of some years between treatment and occlusion of an AVM. It is still not clear from the different series whether there is a significant change in the risk of hemorrhage during the latency period. The risk is higher for larger AVMs and for older patients, and is lower when higher-dose radiation is used [24, 25]. Another issue is that the total obliteration of the nidus verified on negative angiography has been until recently considered definitive evidence of cure after radiosurgical treatment of an AVM [26, 27]. However, a few cases have been reported with recurrent hemorrhage after angiographic confirmation of AVM occlusion [28–30]. Indirectly, the results of the current study might suggest how this could happen. During the obliteration process there might be thrombus evolution, which plugs the lumen and precludes the filling of the vessel at the time of angiography (fig. 1b). This occlusion could be responsible for the normal angiogram, and the patient might be thought to be 'cured'; however, thrombi may undergo recanalization. The newly formed vessels usually possess an abnormal, disorganized, thin, fragile wall structure (fig. 2c) that might serve as a pathological basis for potential rupture and rebleeding contrary to the normal-appearing angiograms. Therefore, these vessels might be regarded as 'nonsafely' obliterated channels as long as organization of thrombi has not been completed by granulation tissue followed by scar tissue replacement. It is emphasized that it is hyalinization of the scar tissue that finally stabilizes the obstructed AVM vessels.

Regular neurological and radiological follow-up examination (contrast-enhanced magnetic resonance imaging and magnetic resonance angiography at 6-month intervals until the disappearance of contrast enhancement) is recommended for radiosurgery-treated patients with AVMs. The abundant capillary content of the granulation tissue probably supplies background for the arterial blush on control angiograms and for the contrast enhancement on the computerized tomography and magnetic resonance images as well. The proliferation of granulation tissue might also explain the increased metabolic activity of the AVM region after radiosurgery because an increase in activity has been detected by positron emission tomography [29]. Its disappearance indicates the maturation of the scar-forming reaction. The role of combined magnetic resonance imaging and positron emission tomography follow-up examinations should be considered in the future. This sensitive imaging technique provides independent metabolic data that are complementary to the anatomical information of angiography, computed tomography or magnetic resonance imaging [31, 32]. With these sophisticated methods we might be able to detect metabolic activity of angiographically occult, invisible, but as yet unsafe and only seemingly obliterated AVMs.

Conclusions

Histopathological findings suggest the role of recanalization in the recurrence of hemorrhage following radiosurgical obliteration of cerebral vascular malformations. Contribution of myofibroblastic elements with contractile capacity in the vessels' occlusion, shrinkage and final volume reduction of AVMs after GKRS was also explored.

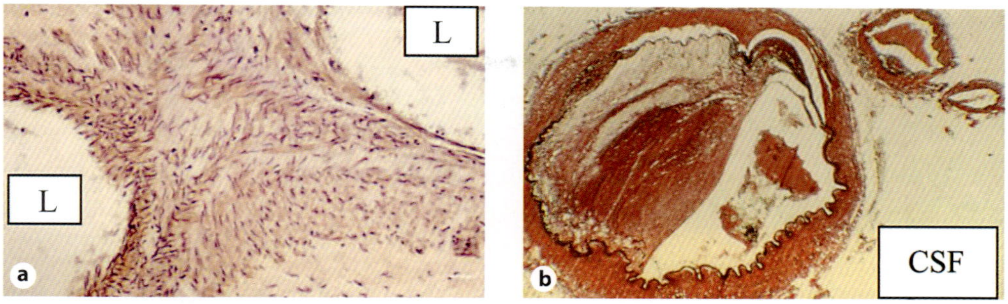

Fig. 7. a Abundant stromal spindle-shaped cells in a 50-Gy GKRS-treated AVM nidus. L = Lumina of AVM vessels. α-Smooth muscle actin immune reaction. ×200. **b** Partly thrombosed aneurysmal sac surrounded by cerebrospinal fluid space (CSF). Elastic van Gieson. ×50.

Quo Vadis?

Although radiosurgery and the Gamma Knife have obtained an outstanding role in the management of brain AVMs for the 21st century, it could not achieve any success in the treatment of berry aneurysms on cerebral vessels. Apart from sporadic anecdotes, no convincing scientific study exists in the literature demonstrating the obliteration effect of radiosurgery on these lesions. However, this problem includes great scientific and practical potential. Rupture of saccular aneurysms and subarachnoid hemorrhage constitute the most common pathology among cerebrovascular disorders. What is the reason for their radioresistance contrary to AVMs? One explanation might be the difference of their histological structure demonstrated by figure 7. The vessels of AVMs are embedded into a connective tissue stroma containing abundant spindle-shaped cells and myofibroblastic elements (fig. 7a) that seem to respond with proliferation and vessel obliteration to irradiation. In contrast, berry aneurysms are surrounded by cerebrospinal fluid spaces, without a connective tissue stroma (fig. 7b), therefore lacking the cellular pool that could react with the described pathological changes. The same mechanism may explain the relative radioresistance of direct arteriovenous fistulae [33]. The goal of radiosurgical research might be to search for a sensitizing agent to irradiation, thus promoting the activation of saccular-wall elements, and obliteration of the lumen of berry aneurysms with GKRS.

Acknowledgement

Dr. Szeifert was supported and wishes to thank for the encouragement (TONE 750531531204).

References

1 Steiner L, Leksell L, Greitz T, Forster DM, Backlund EO: Stereotaxic radiosurgery for cerebral arteriovenous malformations. Report of a case. Acta Chir Scand 1972;138:459–464.

2 Dandy W: Arteriovenous aneurysm of the brain. Arch Surg 1928;17:190–243.

3 Olivecrona H, Landenheim J: Congenital Arteriovenous Aneurysms of the Carotid and Vertebral Arterial Systems. Berlin, Springer, 1957.

4 Virchow R: Die krankhaften Geschwülste: Dreissig Vorlesungen, gehalten während des Wintersemesters 1862–1863 an der Universität zu Berlin. Berlin, Hirschwald, 1863.

5 McCormick WF: The pathology of vascular ('arteriovenous') malformations. J Neurosurg 1966;24: 807–816.

6 Karlsson B, Kihlstrom L, Lindquist C, Ericson K, Steiner L: Radiosurgery for cavernous malformations. J Neurosurg 1998;88:293–297.

7 Maesawa S, Kondziolka D, Lunsford LD: Stereotactic radiosurgery for management of deep brain cavernous malformations. Neurosurg Clin North Am 1999;10:503–511.

8 Hasegawa T, McInerney J, Kondziolka D, Lee JY, Flickinger JC, Lunsford LD: Long-term results after stereotactic radiosurgery for patients with cavernous malformations. Neurosurgery 2002;50:1190–1197, discussion 1197–1198.

9 Gewirtz RJ, Steinberg GK, Crowley R, Levy RP: Pathological changes in surgically resected angiographically occult vascular malformations after radiation. Neurosurgery 1998;42:738–742, discussion 742–743.

10 Nyáry I, Major O, Hanzely Z, Szeifert GT: Histopathological findings in a surgically resected thalamic cavernous hemangioma 1 year after 40-Gy irradiation. J Neurosurg 2005;102(suppl):56–58.

11 Leksell L: Cerebral radiosurgery. I. Gammathalamotomy in two cases of intractable pain. Acta Chir Scand 1968;134:585–595.

12 Lunsford LD, Kondziolka D, Flickinger JC, et al: Stereotactic radiosurgery for arteriovenous malformations of the brain. J Neurosurg 1991;75:512–524.

13 Maruyama K, Kondziolka D, Niranjan A, et al: Stereotactic radiosurgery for brainstem arteriovenous malformations: factors affecting outcome. J Neurosurg 2004;100:407–413.

14 Massager N, Regis J, Kondziolka D, et al: Gamma knife radiosurgery for brainstem arteriovenous malformations: preliminary results. J Neurosurg 2000;93(suppl 3):102–103.

15 Szeifert GT, Major O, Fazekas I, et al: Effects of radiation on cerebral vasculature: a review. Neurosurgery 2001;48:452–453.

16 Mandybur TI, Nazek M: Cerebral arteriovenous malformations: a detailed morphological and immunohistochemical study using actin. Arch Pathol Lab Med 1990;114:970–973.

17 Schneider BF, Eberhard DA, Steiner LE: Histopathology of arteriovenous malformations after gamma knife radiosurgery. J Neurosurg 1997;87: 352–357.

18 Szeifert GT: Radiosurgery and AVM histopathology. J Neurosurg 1998;88:356–357.

19 Szeifert GT, Kemeny AA, Timperley WR, et al: The potential role of myofibroblasts in the obliteration of arteriovenous malformations after radiosurgery. Neurosurgery 1997;40:61–65, discussion 65–66.

20 Yamamoto M, Jimbo M, Ide M, et al: Gamma knife radiosurgery for cerebral arteriovenous malformations: an autopsy report focusing on irradiation-induced changes observed in nidus-unrelated arteries. Surg Neurol 1995;44:421–427.

21 Yamamoto M, Jimbo M, Kobayashi M, et al: Long-term results of radiosurgery for arteriovenous malformation: neurodiagnostic imaging and histological studies of angiographically confirmed nidus obliteration. Surg Neurol 1992;37:219–230.

22 Asgari S, Bassiouni H, Gizewski E, Van de Nes JAP, Stolke D, Sandalcioglu IE: AVM resection after radiation therapy – clinico-morphological features and microsurgical results. Neurosurg Rev 2010;33: 53–61.

23 Gabbiani G, Ryan GB, Majno G: Presence of modified fibroblasts in granulation tissue and their possible role in wound contraction. Experientia 1971; 27:549–550.

24 Friedman WA, Blatt DL, Bova FJ, et al: The risk of hemorrhage after radiosurgery for arteriovenous malformations. J Neurosurg 1996;84:912–919.

25 Karlsson B, Lax I, Soderman M: Risk for hemorrhage during the 2-year latency period following gamma knife radiosurgery for arteriovenous malformations. Int J Radiat Oncol Biol Phys 2001;49: 1045–1051.

26 Levrier O, Manera L, Regis J, et al: Advances in the contributions of imaging to stereotaxic localization of cerebral arteriovenous malformations for radiosurgery. Neurochirurgie 2001;47:201–211.

27 Lindquist C, Steiner L: Stereotactic radiosurgical treatment of arteriovenous malformations; in Lunsford LD (ed): Modern Stereotactic Neurosurgery. Boston, Nijhoff, 1988, pp 491–505.

28 Lindqvist M, Karlsson B, Guo WY, et al: Angiographic long-term follow-up data for arteriovenous malformations previously proven to be obliterated after gamma knife radiosurgery. Neurosurgery 2000; 46: 803–808, discussion 809–810.

29 Szeifert GT, Salmon I, Baleriaux D, et al: Immunohistochemical analysis of a cerebral arteriovenous malformation obliterated by radiosurgery and presenting with re-bleeding. Case report. Neurol Res 2003;25:718–721.
30 Yamamoto M, Jimbo M, Hara M, et al: Gamma knife radiosurgery for arteriovenous malformations: long-term follow-up results focusing on complications occurring more than 5 years after irradiation. Neurosurgery 1996;38:906–914.
31 Levivier M, Wikier D, Goldman S, et al: Integration of the metabolic data of positron emission tomography in the dosimetry planning of radiosurgery with the gamma knife: early experience with brain tumors. Technical note. J Neurosurg 2000;93(suppl 3):233–238.
32 Levivier M, Wikler D Jr, Massager N, et al: The integration of metabolic imaging in stereotactic procedures including radiosurgery: a review. J Neurosurg 2002;97:542–550.
33 Hodgson TJ, Kemeny AA, Gholkar A, Deasy N: Embolization of residual fistula following stereotactic radiosurgery in cerebral arteriovenous malformations. Am J Neuroradiol 2009;30:109–110.

György T. Szeifert, MD, PhD
Department of Neurotraumatology, Péterfy Traumatological Centre and
Department of Neurological Surgery, Semmelweis University of Budapest
Fiumei út 17
HU–1081 Budapest (Hungary)
Tel. +36 306894150, E-Mail gszeifert@yahoo.co.uk

Niranjan A, Kano H, Lunsford LD (eds): Gamma Knife Radiosurgery for Brain Vascular Malformations.
Prog Neurol Surg. Basel, Karger, 2013, vol 27, pp 130–140 (DOI: 10.1159/000341773)

Stereotactic Radiosurgery Guideline for the Management of Patients with Intracranial Arteriovenous Malformations

Ajay Niranjan · L. Dade Lunsford

Department of Neurological Surgery, University of Pittsburgh, Pittsburgh, Pa., USA

Abstract

Our objective was to provide guidelines about the use of stereotactic radiosurgery in symptomatic patients with imaging-identified arteriovenous malformations (AVMs) of the brain. We reviewed evidence-based medicine and clinical experience with radiosurgery for AVM of the brain to develop guidelines and provide scientific foundation for patients and physicians. Major recommendations include the definition of AVM patients suitable for various management strategies ranging from observation to surgical excision to endovascular embolization and stereotactic radiosurgery. The optimal dose range for volumetric conformal AVM stereotactic radiosurgery has been largely established based on location and volume of the AVM. The relationship to prior embolization or prior surgery has been evaluated. The role of repeat radiosurgery has been assessed for those patients with incomplete obliteration of their AVM after 3 years have elapsed. The causes of failure of stereotactic radiosurgery have also been identified. A clinical algorithm for the potential role of stereotactic radiosurgery for a symptomatic brain AVM was defined. The guidelines provide a framework for professional judgment and treatment selection alternatives.

Once identified, arteriovenous malformations (AVMs) may be suitable for 1 or more of 4 management strategies: observation, endovascular embolization, surgical excision or stereotactic radiosurgery [1–5]. AVM management depends on the risk of subsequent hemorrhage, which is determined by the anatomical (magnetic resonance imaging, MRI, and angiography), historical and demographic features of the individual patient [6]. Young age, prior hemorrhage, small AVM size, deep venous drainage and high flow may make subsequent hemorrhage more likely. Observation may be most appropriate for large-volume AVMs (average diameter 4–5 cm), especially for patients who have never bled. Studies of the natural history of AVMs suggest an annual hemorrhage rate of 2–4% with an annual 1% mortality rate from AVM bleeding. A second strategy is endovascular embolization, which is often used as an adjunct preceding surgical removal of the AVM via craniotomy and at times before stereotactic radiosurgery [7–12]. Other vascular anomalies may be associated with AVMs including the presence of proximal intracranial or intranidal aneurysms. Such aneurysms may pose additional risk factors to patients. Surgical management is an option for patients with resectable AVMs, although incomplete surgical removal may prompt eventual radiosurgery. Embolization prior to radiosurgery is thought to be beneficial in some cases, but in other cases may lead to less reliable recognition of the target volume suitable for radiosurgery. Recanalization of embolized AVM components may require subsequent retreatment for portions of the AVM previously thought to be occluded by successful embolization. Stereotactic radiosurgery is considered for patients with unresectable AVMs.

Although there are several published reports on long-term outcomes after AVM radiosurgery [13–20], no guidelines are available for medical professionals to make an evidence-based decision. We developed a radiosurgery practice guideline that provides treatment recommendations for use by medical and public health professionals as well as patients with the diagnosis of brain or dural AVM.

Methods

Computerized searches of published literature (primary sources), hand searches of published literature (secondary sources) and searches of electronic clinical databases were performed. Medline and Pubmed searches were completed for the years 1971 to March 2011. Search terms included 'arteriovenous malformation', 'AVM', 'vascular malformation', 'stereotactic radiosurgery'. Bibliographies from recently published reviews were reviewed and relevant articles were retrieved.

Outcomes Considered

Total obliteration of the AVM within 3 years was the primary end point of interest. Additional outcome end points included resolution or an improvement in seizure disorders if present, resolution or reduction in vascular headache syndromes, prevention of bleeding risks from the AVM (estimated to vary between 1 and 10% per year depending upon prior bleeding history, location and volume). Improvement in the existing neurological deficits, maintenance of quality of life, employability and prevention of adverse radiation effects were also considered.

Major Recommmendations

Patient Selection

- Patients with intracranial AVM defined by modern neurodiagnostic imaging, including computed tomography (CT), MRI and cerebral angiography, should be considered for radiosurgery, surgical removal and endovascular embolization. AVM patients typically present with one or more of the following: brain hemorrhage (especially when located in deep anatomical locations of the brain), persistent seizures, vascular headaches or progressive neurological deficits.

- The selection of patients suitable for various management strategies is dependent on prior bleeding history, age of the patient, existing comorbidities, anatomical location and clinical history.
- Some patients may have had prior intracranial surgery for blood clot (hematoma) evacuation or partial AVM resection. The safe interval between surgery and stereotactic radiosurgery is not known, but it is reasonable to perform radiosurgery once the patient has achieved a stable neurological recovery or plateau (generally within 2–3 months after the intracranial hemorrhage or prior surgery).
- Some AVM patients will have been previously treated by embolization for volumetric reduction or flow reduction. The optimal time between prior embolization and radiosurgery is not known, but generally waiting for a period of several weeks is considered beneficial in order to reduce the likelihood of vascular ischemic complications or residual cerebral edema sometimes associated with embolization followed by early radiosurgery.

Treatment/Management

- AVMs are considered suitable for 4 management strategies alone or in combination: observation only, surgical excision, endovascular embolization (designed to reduce either a selected volume or flow through the AVM) and stereotactic radiosurgery.
- Stereotactic radiosurgery is typically employed alone but may also be employed in combination with prior surgery or embolization in selected circumstances [21]. Patients who undergo single-stage stereotactic radiosurgery most often have AVMs with an average diameter of 3 cm (0.1–10 cm^3). Prospective stereotactic radiosurgery volumetric staging is frequently performed for symptomatic patients with AVM volumes of 10–15 cm^3 in the absence of other acceptable risk management strategies [22].

Imaging for Radiosurgery

- High-resolution stereotactic MR images supplemented by cerebral angiography are optimal for dose planning (fig. 1). Some centers use CT angiograms instead of cerebral angiography.
- Aneurysms within the AVM or on feeding arteries may be identified occasionally. Intranidal aneurysms may increase the annual bleeding rate of an AVM, but the recognition of intranidal aneurysms is highly subjective. Patients with aneurysms proximal to the AVM should be considered for either clipping or coiling to prevent hemorrhage from aneurysm during the latency interval after AVM management. Although there is no consensus on the timing of coiling or clipping, our preference is to perform AVM radiosurgery first in order to reduce the impact of MR artifacts produced by clips or coils – if it is unclear what vascular anomaly bled.

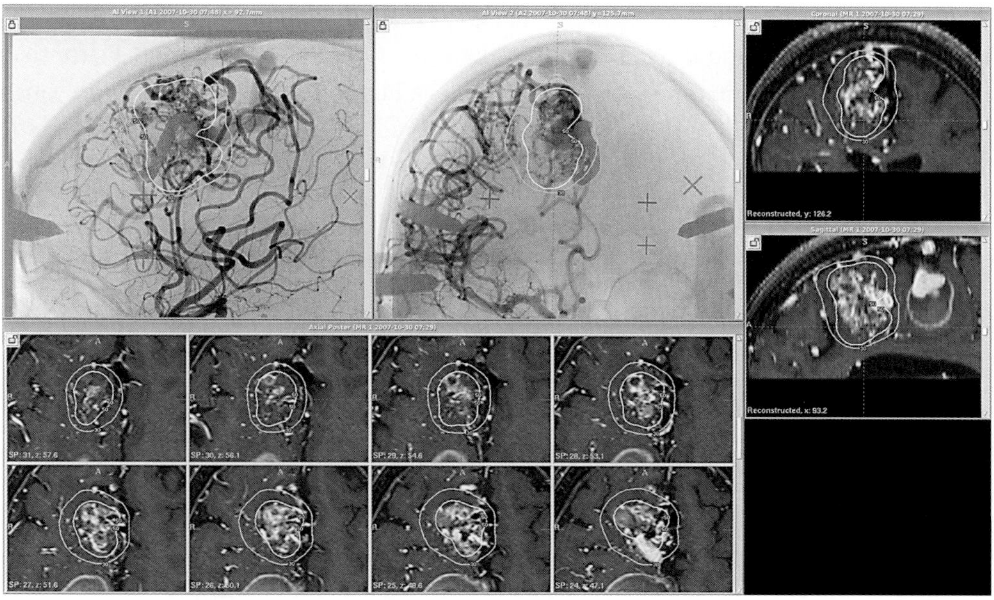

Fig. 1. A 62-year-old woman was diagnosed with right frontal AVM following an intracranial hemorrhage and seizure. She underwent partial embolization using Onyx. The residual AVM was treated with Gamma Knife radiosurgery. The radiosurgery dose plan projected onto the angiogram and MRI show complete coverage of residual AVM. A margin dose of 18 Gy was prescribed to the 50% isodose line.

Dose Selection

- The optimal dose range for volumetric conformal stereotactic AVM radiosurgery has been largely established based on location and volume of the AVM. Doses at the margin of the AVM typically range from 16 to 25 Gy in a single fraction, when the 3-dimensional volume of the AVM is defined by stereotactic guidance during the procedure itself [23–25]. Stereotactic volumetric axial plane imaging (MRI or CT) supplemented by conventional or digital subtraction angiography is usually necessary for complete conformal dose planning. AVM obliteration rates are significantly improved when the AVM marginal dose is ≥18 Gy.
- Dose selection depends on location, volume, estimated adverse radiation risks, preexisting neurological conditions and bleeding history. Depending upon the technology used, the margin of the AVM dose is usually 50–70% of the central target dose within the AVM. A sharp fall-off of the radiation dose outside of the target volume is required.

Medical Management

Patients usually receive a single dose (40 mg) of methylprednisolone at the conclusion of the radiosurgery procedure. They can continue to take their other medications (e.g. antiepileptics, analgesics) during and after the procedure as recommended by their physicians.

If a patient is receiving antiepileptic drugs to manage seizures, the blood levels of antiepileptic drugs should be checked on the day of radiosurgery to make sure that a therapeutic level is maintained at the time of radiosurgery. For patients with lobar location AVMs but with a history of seizures, it is advisable to give a loading dose of antiepileptic drugs so that they have a therapeutic level during radiosurgery. These drugs can be tapered off within a week.

Follow-Up Evaluations

Postradiosurgical clinical examinations and MR studies are requested at 6-month and then yearly intervals for the first 3 years in order to monitor the effects of radiosurgery on AVM (gradual obliteration). If MRI at the 3-year mark suggests complete disappearance of the AVM nidus, an angiogram is obtained to confirm the obliteration. If the MRI before 3 years suggests nidus obliteration, angiography is generally delayed until 3 full years have elapsed since no change in treatment recommendations is planned until 3 or more years of observation have passed (fig. 2). If angiography after 3 years demonstrates that the AVM nidus is not obliterated, repeat stereotactic radiosurgery may be considered as an additional strategy to obtain the desired final results, complete obliteration.

- Causes of failure of stereotactic radiosurgery include inadequate visualization of the target nidus, lack of intraoperative stereotactic 3-dimensional images (volumetric axial plane imaging), insufficient dose to achieve the obliterative response, compression of the AVM nidus by a prior hematoma or poor nidus visualization secondary to overlying vascular structures. In a few selected cases, radiobiological resistance of undetermined etiology may be the cause of obliteration failure.

Patients who have residual AVMs identified by neurodiagnostic imaging at 3 years (after radiosurgery) may be candidates for a second stereotactic radiosurgical procedure. Alternatively, patients with larger-volume AVMs (>10 cm^3) may be considered suitable for up-front volumetric staging of AVMs by treating different anatomical components of the AVM at intervals staged between 3 and 6 months. The interval for staging of radiosurgery prospectively is not established. Stereotactic radiosurgery should not be considered as the panacea for large-volume AVMs unsuitable for surgery or embolization. At selected centers with experience, estimated obliteration rates at 5 years after 2 or more radiosurgical procedures approach 60–70%. For smaller-volume AVMs (average diameters <3 cm^3), estimated complete obliteration rates at 3 years after a single procedure vary from 70 to 90%.

Postradiosurgery Imaging Changes

The probability of developing postradiosurgery imaging changes depends on marginal dose and treatment volume [26, 27]. The volume of tissue receiving 12 Gy or more (the 12-Gy volume) is the single factor that seems to have the closest correlation with the probability of developing imaging changes. Location does not seem to affect

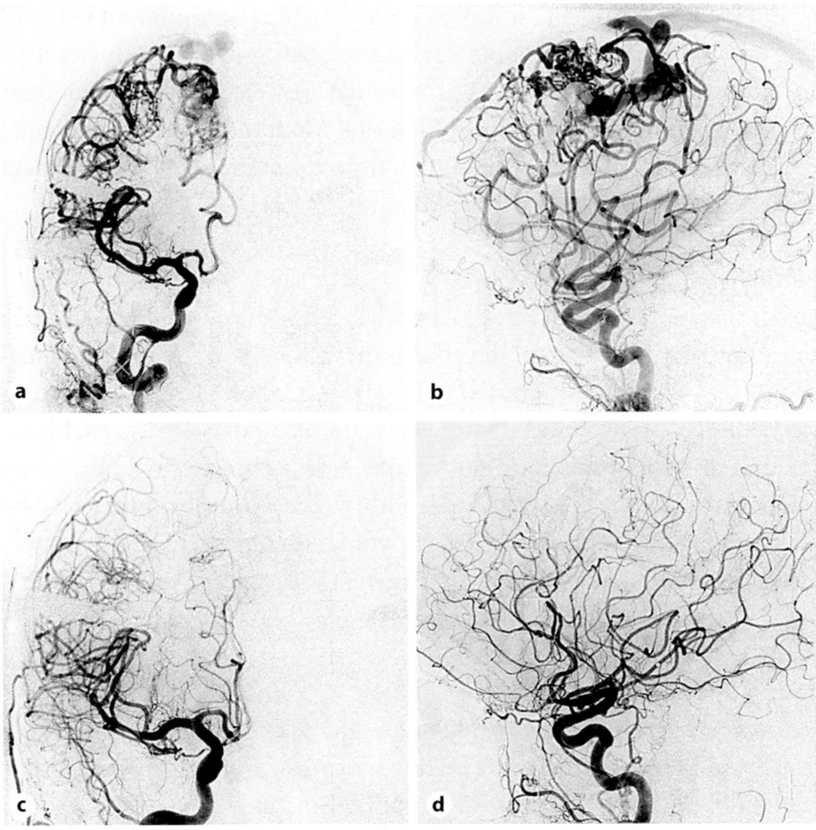

Fig. 2. Cerebral posteroanterior (**a**) and lateral angiograms (**b**) prior to radiosurgery show right frontal AVM. Follow-up angiograms (**c**, **d**) performed 3 years after radiosurgery show complete obliteration of the nidus.

the risk of developing imaging changes but has a marked effect on whether or not these changes are associated with symptoms. Postradiosurgery imaging changes (new areas of high T_2-weighted signal in brain surrounding the irradiated AVM nidus) develop in approximately 30% of patients 1–24 months after radiosurgery. Two thirds of such patients are asymptomatic, leaving approximately 10% of all patients who develop symptomatic postradiosurgery imaging changes. Patients with symptomatic imaging changes can usually be managed with corticosteroids for a limited interval of several weeks. Subsequently, some patients may benefit from a 3-month trial of Trental 400 mg twice per day and vitamin E 400 IU twice per day.

Late Complications after AVM Radiosurgery

Delayed complications of radiosurgery on AVMs include hemorrhage despite angiographically documented complete obliteration of the AVM, temporary or permanent radiation injury to the brain such as persistent edema, radiation necrosis, radiation-induced tumors and cyst formation [28, 29]. It is impossible to estimate the actual incidence of radiosurgery-associated neoplasms because the numerator (incidence) and denominator (total number of patients who underwent radiosurgery) are not available. We warn all our patients that the risk of radiation-associated tumor(s) may be as high as 1 in 1,000, although neither the Pittsburgh experience [30] nor the data from Sheffield, UK [31], confirm this increased theoretical risk.

Counseling for Sport-Related Activities

Patients are advised to resume normal activities after radiosurgery. Although there is no specific data available on the optimum level of activity, we recommend that pending documentation of AVM obliteration, patients refrain from high energy contact sports such as football, wrestling and boxing. They are also advised to avoid postures or positions that might put strain on the venous drainage from the brain (such has hanging upside down, roller coaster rides, upside down yoga positions, various gymnastics, and diving head first in the swimming pool). Noncontact sports are preferred. Patients are advised to avoid lifting or straining that requires excessive force, breath holding, grunting, or other strenuous weight lifting.

Management of Residual AVMs after Radiosurgery

Repeat radiosurgery is an option for most patients with residual or persistent nidus 3 years or more after initial radiosurgery. The dose-response curve for obliterating previously treated AVM seems similar to untreated AVM but because retreatment volumes are usually smaller than initial volumes, slightly higher marginal doses may be feasible. The rate of adverse effects is slightly higher than would be expected with no prior radiation [32].

Management of Large AVMs

Large AVMs pose a challenge for surgical resection, embolization or radiosurgery. Some may be treated using multimodal management but a population of patients with large AVMs remains 'untreatable'. Although AVM embolization prior to radiosurgery has been used for patients with large AVMs, recanalization was observed in 14–15% of patients. Single-stage radiosurgery of a large-volume AVM results in either unacceptable radiation-related risks (due to exposure of large volumes of normal surrounding tissue) or low obliteration efficacy.

The staged volume radiosurgery approach is recommended if the total treatment volume is expected to be more than 15 cm^3, and considered when the volume is between 10 and 15 cm^3 [22]. Usually after outlining the total volume of the AVM nidus on the MRI, the malformation is divided into two volumes (medial or lateral, superior or inferior components). Using the computer dose planning system, the AVM is divided into two approximately equal volumes. The volume designated for treatment with each stage is outlined at the time of the first procedure using tools available in the Gamma Plan software. Only the volume selected for the first procedure is treated. The second-stage radiosurgery procedure is performed 3–6 months after the first procedure. At the time of the second procedure, the previous radiosurgery plan (stage 1) is imported and coregistered with new stereotactic MR images. The outline of stage 1 and 2 nidus volume and the previous plan covering the stage 1 volume are projected onto new stereotactic images. A new treatment plan covering the stage 2 volume is designed and the dose is prescribed according to the volume being treated. The concept of volume staging with a margin dose selection at a minimum of 16 or preferably 18 Gy seems reasonably safe and effective. Longer follow-up duration is needed to assess the final outcome in these patients as some may take up to 5 years for nidus obliteration.

Role of Preradiosurgical Embolization

The purpose of embolizing large AVMs prior to radiosurgery is to permanently decrease the volume of the AVM which facilitates more effective radiosurgery [7, 9, 11, 33]. Embolization can only be an effective adjunct to radiosurgery if it results in permanent reduction of the nidus volume. Reduction in flow within the AVM does not improve radiosurgery results. The data suggest that the efficacy of combined embolization and radiosurgery is either comparable or inferior to radiosurgery alone. The combination of embolization and radiosurgery does not provide any additional protection against AVM hemorrhage during the latency period, with comparable risks of hemorrhage in treated and untreated AVMs. In short, the use of embolization prior to radiosurgery does not offer any advantages over radiosurgery alone at least in terms of success of radiosurgical obliteration. It may have benefit for the management of aneurysms associated with the AVM. Its role after radiosurgery requires further analysis.

Potential Benefits of Radiosurgery

All the published studies have shown a significant response of stereotactic radiosurgery for AVMs, including a high rate of AVM nidus obliteration, concomitant improvement in seizure control, headache resolution and a satisfactory (low) rate of adverse radiation effects that might lead to additional neurological deficits.

Potential successful outcomes include complete AVM obliteration, symptomatic relief, no new neurological deficits, no long-term complications and lifelong prevention of bleeding risks.

The literature has documented the cost savings benefit of stereotactic radiosurgery versus invasive surgical procedures and the lower risk potential of bleeding, anesthesia problems, infections and side effects which may result in transient or permanent disabilities from open surgery.

Subgroups Most Likely to Benefit

Radiosurgery may be especially suitable for the following groups of patients:
- patients in advanced age groups;
- patients with excessive medical comorbidity risk factors for surgical excision;

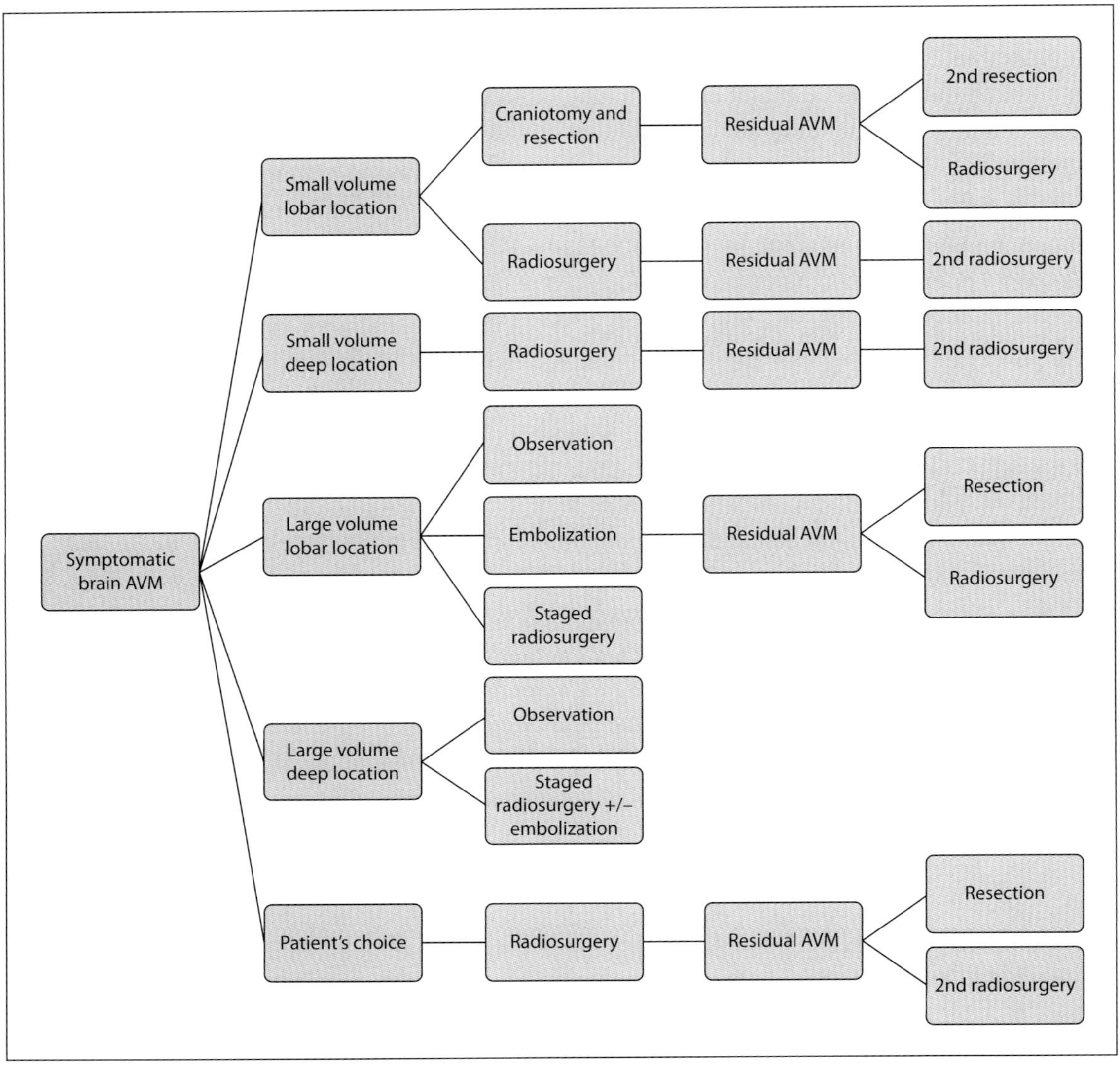

Fig. 3. Proposed management algorithm for patients with intracranial AVM.

- patients with AVMs located in eloquent areas of the brain where open surgery would likely result in severe neurological deficits;
- patients with AVMs considered unsuitable for complete obliteration by endovascular embolization.

Clinical Algorithm

A number of factors are considered in making a recommendation. These factors include:

1 patient's age;
2 patient's medical condition;

3 previous bleed;
4 prior procedures;
5 volume of AVM;
6 location of AVM;
7 presenting symptoms.

A broad outline of the management algorithm is shown in figure 3; however, the final recommendation is usually influenced by the recommending neurosurgeon's experience along with patient preference.

Qualifying Statements

This guideline is intended to provide the scientific foundation and initial framework for the management of intracranial AVM. The assessment and recommendations provided in this guideline represent the best professional judgment of authors at this time, based on research data and expertise currently available. This guideline is not intended as a substitute for professional medical advice and does not address specific procedures or conditions for any patient.

References

1 Sandalcioglu IE, Wanke I, Zappala V, Forsting M, Sure U: The management of arteriovenous malformations. J Neurosurg Sci 2011;55:57–69.
2 Darsaut TE, Guzman R, Marcellus ML, Edwards MS, Tian L, Do HM, et al: Management of pediatric intracranial arteriovenous malformations: experience with multimodality therapy. Neurosurgery 2011;69:540–556.
3 Chang SD, Marcellus ML, Marks MP, Levy RP, Do HM, Steinberg GK: Multimodality treatment of giant intracranial arteriovenous malformations. Neurosurgery 2003;53:1–11, discussion 12–13.
4 Ondra SL, Troupp H, George ED, Schwab K: The natural history of symptomatic arteriovenous malformations of the brain: a 24-year follow-up assessment. J Neurosurg 1990;73:387–391.
5 Richling B, Killer M, Al-Schameri AR, Ritter L, Agic R, Krenn M: Therapy of brain arteriovenous malformations: multimodality treatment from a balanced standpoint. Neurosurgery 2006;59:S148–S157, discussion S3–S13.
6 Pollock BE, Flickinger JC, Lunsford LD, Bissonette DJ, Kondziolka D: Factors that predict the bleeding risk of cerebral arteriovenous malformations. Stroke 1996;27:1–6.
7 Miyachi S, Negoro M, Okamoto T, Kobayashi T, Kida Y, Tanaka T, et al: Embolisation of cerebral arteriovenous malformations to assure successful subsequent radiosurgery. J Clin Neurosci 2000; 7(suppl 1):82–85.
8 Raymond J, Iancu D, Weill A, Guilbert F, Bahary JP, Bojanowski M, et al: Embolization as one modality in a combined strategy for the management of cerebral arteriovenous malformations. Intervent Neuroradiol 2005;11(suppl):57–62.
9 Andrade-Souza YM, Ramani M, Scora D, Tsao MN, ter Brugge K, Schwartz ML: Embolization before radiosurgery reduces the obliteration rate of arteriovenous malformations. Neurosurgery 2007;60:443–451, discussion 451–452.
10 Jahan R, Murayama Y, Gobin YP, Duckwiler GR, Vinters HV, Vinuela F: Embolization of arteriovenous malformations with Onyx: clinicopathological experience in 23 patients. Neurosurgery 2001; 48:984–995, discussion 995–997.
11 Henkes H, Nahser HC, Berg-Dammer E, Weber W, Lange S, Kuhne D: Endovascular therapy of brain AVMs prior to radiosurgery. Neurol Res 1998;20: 479–492.

12 Weber W, Kis B, Siekmann R, Kuehne D: Endovascular treatment of intracranial arteriovenous malformations with Onyx: technical aspects. AJNR Am J Neuroradiol 2007;28:371–377.
13 Pollock BE, Flickinger JC, Lunsford LD, Maitz A, Kondziolka D: Factors associated with successful arteriovenous malformation radiosurgery. Neurosurgery 1998;42:1239–1244, discussion 1244–1247.
14 Chang JH, Chang JW, Park YG, Chung SS: Factors related to complete occlusion of arteriovenous malformations after gamma knife radiosurgery. J Neurosurg 2000;93(suppl 3):96–101.
15 Pan DH, Guo WY, Chung WY, Shiau CY, Chang YC, Wang LW: Gamma knife radiosurgery as a single treatment modality for large cerebral arteriovenous malformations. J Neurosurg 2000;93(suppl 3):113–119.
16 Pollock BE, Gorman DA, Brown PD: Radiosurgery for arteriovenous malformations of the basal ganglia, thalamus, and brainstem. J Neurosurg 2004;100: 210–214.
17 Levy EI, Niranjan A, Thompson TP, Scarrow AM, Kondziolka D, Flickinger JC, et al: Radiosurgery for childhood intracranial arteriovenous malformations. Neurosurgery 2000;47:834–841, discussion 841–842.
18 Lunsford LD, Kondziolka D, Flickinger JC, Bissonette DJ, Jungreis CA, Maitz AH, et al: Stereotactic radiosurgery for arteriovenous malformations of the brain. J Neurosurg 1991;75:512–524.
19 Maruyama K, Kondziolka D, Niranjan A, Flickinger JC, Lunsford LD: Stereotactic radiosurgery for brainstem arteriovenous malformations: factors affecting outcome. J Neurosurg 2004;100:407–413.
20 Steiner L, Leksell L, Greitz T, Forster DM, Backlund EO: Stereotaxic radiosurgery for cerebral arteriovenous malformations. Report of a case. Acta Chir Scand 1972;138:459–464.
21 Kano H, Lunsford LD, Flickinger JC, Yang HC, Flannery TJ, Awan NR, et al: Stereotactic radiosurgery for arteriovenous malformations. 1. Management of Spetzler-Martin grade I and II arteriovenous malformations. J Neurosurg 2012;116:11–20.
22 Kano H, Kondziolka D, Flickinger JC, Park KJ, Parry PV, Yang HC, et al: Stereotactic radiosurgery for arteriovenous malformations. 6. Multistaged volumetric management of large arteriovenous malformations. J Neurosurg 2012;116:54–65.
23 Flickinger JC, Kondziolka D, Lunsford LD: Dose selection in stereotactic radiosurgery. Neurosurg Clin North Am 1999;10:271–280.
24 Flickinger JC, Kondziolka D, Maitz AH, Lunsford LD: An analysis of the dose-response for arteriovenous malformation radiosurgery and other factors affecting obliteration. Radiother Oncol 2002;63: 347–354.
25 Flickinger JC, Pollock BE, Kondziolka D, Lunsford LD: A dose-response analysis of arteriovenous malformation obliteration after radiosurgery. Int J Radiat Oncol Biol Phys 1996;36:873–879.
26 Ledezma CJ, Hoh BL, Carter BS, Pryor JC, Putman CM, Ogilvy CS: Complications of cerebral arteriovenous malformation embolization: multivariate analysis of predictive factors. Neurosurgery 2006;58: 602–611, discussion 611.
27 Flickinger JC, Kondziolka D, Pollock BE, Maitz AH, Lunsford LD: Complications from arteriovenous malformation radiosurgery: multivariate analysis and risk modeling. Int J Radiat Oncol Biol Phys 1997;38:485–490.
28 Hara M, Nakamura M, Shiokawa Y, Sawa H, Sato E, Koyasu H, et al: Delayed cyst formation after radiosurgery for cerebral arteriovenous malformation: two case reports. Minim Invasive Neurosurg 1998; 41:40–45.
29 Morihiro Y, Kato S, Imoto H, Nomura S, Harada K, Kajiwara K, et al: Cyst formation after radiosurgery for brain arteriovenous malformation treated with cystoperitoneal shunt. No Shinkei Geka Neurol Surg 2010;38:751–756.
30 Niranjan A, Kondziolka D, Lunsford LD: Neoplastic transformation after radiosurgery or radiotherapy: risk and realities. Otolaryngol Clin North Am 2009; 42:717–729.
31 Rowe J, Grainger A, Walton L, Silcocks P, Radatz M, Kemeny A: Risk of malignancy after gamma knife stereotactic radiosurgery. Neurosurgery 2007;60:60–65, discussion 65–66.
32 Kano H, Kondziolka D, Flickinger JC, Yang HC, Flannery TJ, Awan NR, et al: Stereotactic radiosurgery for arteriovenous malformations. 3. Outcome predictors and risks after repeat radiosurgery. J Neurosurg 2012;116:21–32.
33 Yen CP, Sheehan JP, Schwyzer L, Schlesinger D: Hemorrhage risk of cerebral arteriovenous malformations before and during the latency period after Gamma knife radiosurgery. Stroke 2011;42:1691–1696.

Ajay Niranjan, MCh, MBA
Department of Neurological Surgery, University of Pittsburgh Medical Center, Suite B-400
200 Lothrop Street
Pittsburgh, PA 15213 (USA)
Tel. +1 412 647 6250, E-Mail niranjana@upmc.edu

Niranjan A, Kano H, Lunsford LD (eds): Gamma Knife Radiosurgery for Brain Vascular Malformations.
Prog Neurol Surg. Basel, Karger, 2013, vol 27, pp 141–146 (DOI: 10.1159/000341774)

Cavernous Malformations and Hemorrhage Risk

Douglas Kondziolka · Edward A. Monaco III · L. Dade Lunsford

Department of Neurological Surgery and Center for Image-Guided Neurosurgery, University of Pittsburgh Medical Center, Pittsburgh, Pa., USA

Abstract

Widespread availability of magnetic resonance imaging has helped our understanding of the natural history of cavernous malformations (CMs) of the brain. CMs present with diverse clinical manifestations. Supratentorial CMs are often identified incidentally. The clinical presentation corresponds with lesion location. Symptomatic, hemorrhagic CMs of the brainstem pose a challenging clinical problem as they are often associated with high surgical morbidity. In order to study the natural history of CM, we performed a prospective analysis on a series of patients who were sent to us for management. During the mean prospective follow-up interval of 34 months, 9 hemorrhages occurred. History of prior hemorrhage was the most important risk factor for subsequent hemorrhage. The annual hemorrhage was 0.6% in patients who never had a symptomatic hemorrhage. Patients who had prior hemorrhage have a higher (4.5%) annual hemorrhage rate.

Cavernous malformations (CMs) of the brain present with a diverse set of clinical manifestations, and are often found in asymptomatic patients. When they occur in critical brain locations and cause hemorrhage, they can be the cause of neurological disability. While CMs of the brain occur in 0.1–4.0% of the population, they comprise 8–15% of all its vascular lesions [1]. These angiographically occult vascular abnormalities typically occur supratentorially; however, those isolated to the brainstem have been reported to account for 9–35% of all CMs [2, 3]. A number of etiologies have been identified for CMs, including: genetic, congenital, postsurgical and post-radiation effects [4, 5]. Up to one third of patients harboring CMs possess associated developmental venous anomalies [6].

The near ubiquity of magnetic resonance imaging (MRI) has increased the frequency with which CMs are diagnosed, and has better elucidated the epidemiology and natural history of these lesions [2, 4, 7–10]. Presentation symptoms correspond with lesion location and while supratentorial CMs are often identified incidentally or after seizures, those in the brainstem typically produce focal neurological deficits. Symptomatic, multiple hemorrhagic CMs of the brainstem present a vexing clinical problem, as they are often not amenable to surgical resection with acceptable risk. The annual hemorrhage risk has been estimated to be 0.1–2.5% per lesion-year and 0.25–16.5% per patient-year, but this risk is substantially higher (up to 34% annual risk) for patients with prior hemorrhagic events.

Clinical Presentation

Patient Populations

First, we performed a prospective analysis on a series of patients who were sent to us for management [9]. Because this set of patients was asymptomatic and had non-disabling symptoms with or without hemorrhage, they were followed without specific treatment. We entered all patients selected for conservative management into a registry designed to assess the prospective natural history of the disorder. Our goal was to obtain data regarding the outcome of CMs and their collective rates of symptomatic hemorrhage, seizure development and subsequent need for treatment. We planned to correlate recorded clinical criteria with the observed prospective outcome. Conservative management was recommended for 162 patients, all of whom were entered immediately into a prospective natural history registry. We recommended conservative treatment if: (1) the patient had an asymptomatic lesion; (2) the malformation was associated with a medically controlled seizure disorder; (3) the malformation was located in a critical brain region but the patient had only one hemorrhage or minimal symptoms; (4) the patient was elderly or medically infirm, or (5) the patient had multiple CMs and the actual symptomatic lesion could not be determined. In the registry we recorded patient age, sex, number of prior hemorrhages, the presence or absence of seizures or headache, brain location, type of diagnostic imaging performed, date, and the name and address of the referring physician [9].

We were able to collect data on 122 patients, with a mean age of 37 years. During the mean prospective follow-up interval of 34 months (range, 1–82 months), 9 hemorrhages occurred. Seven patients had 1 hemorrhage and 1 patient had 2 hemorrhages. Thus, 9 hemorrhages in 341.6 prospective years of observation equaled a 2.63% annual hemorrhage rate in the overall patient group. We found no difference in the hemorrhage rate between men and women, between patients with or without seizures ($p = 0.11$), between patients with or without headaches ($p = 0.06$), or between patients with solitary versus multiple lesions ($p = 0.15$). The most important risk factor for subsequent hemorrhage was the occurrence of a prior hemorrhage. Of the 61 patients who had never had a symptomatic hemorrhage, only 1 sustained a hemorrhage in the follow-up period (0.6% annual hemorrhage rate). In the 61 patients who sustained a hemorrhage before entry into the registry, 8 hemorrhages in 7 patients were found in the follow-up period (annual hemorrhage rate of 4.5%; $p = 0.028$).

Porter et al. [2] reported the University of Toronto prospective experience in 173 patients, again with a mean age of 37 years. Follow-up was available for 104 patients to a median of 41 months. Imaging found that an interval hemorrhage occurred in 7 patients (5 males and 2 females) during the 427 patient-years of observation, yielding an annual rate of 1.6%. All hemorrhages were symptomatic and all occurred in patients with deep lesions: 6 infratentorial (all brainstem) and 1 supratentorial (thalamus). The median time to hemorrhage during the follow-up period was 16 months. The main risk factor for subsequent hemorrhage was brain location (infratentorial having higher risk) rather than history of prior hemorrhage.

Second, we prospectively collected pre- and postradiosurgery data from 68 patients (whose brainstem CMs were treated between 1988 and 2005); they were retrospectively analyzed with the approval of the University of Pittsburgh Institutional Review Board [11]. The average age of patients in this analysis was 41.2 years (range, 5–79 years). All patients had previously experienced at least 2 hemorrhagic events, and 36.8% had suffered 3 or more bleeds (range, 3–12 bleeds). Bleeding events were defined as the development of a new neurological deficit with coexisting imaging evidence of new blood products in a newly discovered or previously identified CM. Information pertaining to clinical events was obtained via discussions with patients and/or their treating physicians combined with review of all available imaging studies. The diagnosis of a CM was made by computed tomography prior to 1990 and by MRI after 1990. Sixty-four patients (94.1%) presented with preexisting neurological deficits resulting from CM hemorrhages. Fifteen patients (22.1%) had previously undergone partial microsurgical resection. Half of the patients underwent angiography prior to stereotactic radiosurgery (SRS). These studies failed to identify a vascular abnormality. Only 1 patient (1.47%) was found to have an associated developmental venous anomaly.

Hemorrhage was defined as imaging evidence of a new area of blood density corresponding to a new neurological sign or symptom. The annual hemorrhage rate was calculated using the following formula: total number of hemorrhages in all patients/total number of patient-years observed. Hemorrhage rates were compared before and after SRS using a paired t test.

Pretreatment Hemorrhage Rate

Pretreatment observation comprised the time from the first symptomatic, image-documented hemorrhage to the time of SRS. Thus, a total of 386 patient-years were observed with a mean pretreatment observation period of 5.68 years (range, 1–38 years). There were 193 hemorrhages documented during this time (2.84 per patient). All patients had at least 2 hemorrhages prior to SRS (range, 2–12). After exclusion of the first hemorrhage (193 – 68 = 125 hemorrhages), the calculated annual hemorrhage rate was 32.38% (125 hemorrhages in 386 patient-years observed) [11].

It has been observed by our group [12], and by others, that symptomatic brainstem CMs have a high rate of rehemorrhage (up to a 60% annual risk) and corresponding neurological deficits. Indeed, CMs of the brainstem are of unique interest

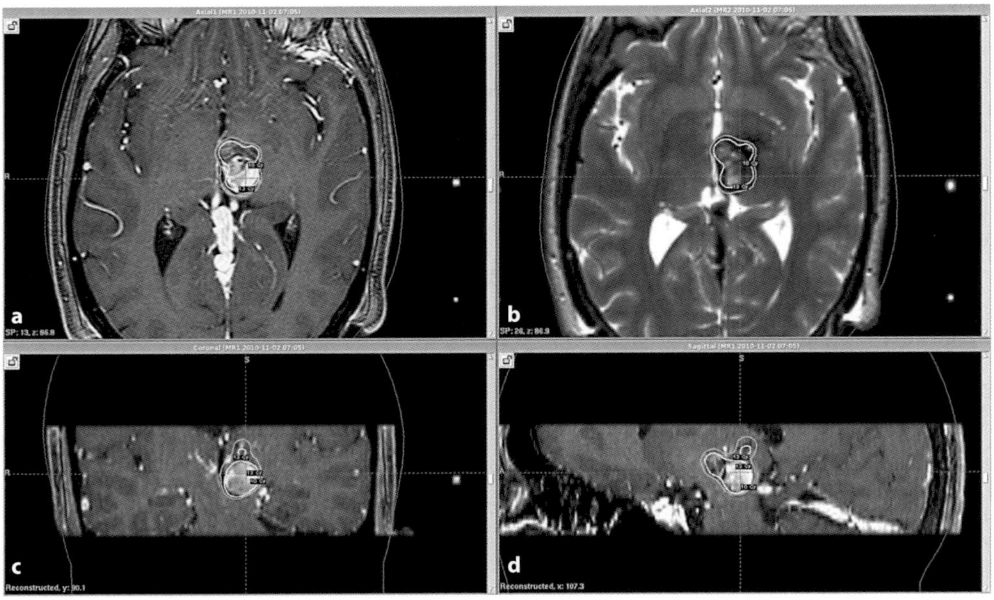

Fig. 1. A 38-year-old male presented with 2 symptomatic intracranial hemorrhages. MRI showed left thalamic CM. A conformal radiosurgery dose plan was designed using contrast-enhanced axial MR images (**a**, **b**) with sagittal (**c**) and coronal reconstruction (**d**). A margin dose of 14 Gy was prescribed to the 50% isodose line.

because even bleeding events too small to be resolvable with modern imaging can cause profound neurological sequelae. Multiple hemorrhagic, symptomatic CMs of the brainstem are admittedly a rare entity with only a few hundred patients presented in several retrospective series. As such, management of this neurologically devastating problem is not clearly defined. Herein, we have shown that in a highly selective group of patients with surgically high-risk symptomatic CMs of the brainstem, SRS is a reasonable alternative treatment with a safety profile similar or better than other treatment approaches.

Although the treatment of choice for most symptomatic CMs is microsurgical resection, when discovered in locations like the brainstem the risks are not trivial. Porter et al. [3] reviewed a series of 86 patients who underwent surgery for brainstem CMs. Fifty-two percent of the CMs in this series reached the pial surface. Following surgery, 33% of patients had new cranial nerve deficits, 30% demonstrated cerebellar findings, and 29% had new-onset weakness. The overall rate of temporary and/or permanent morbidity and mortality was 35%. Overall mortality was 8% and all-cause 30-day mortality was 3.5%. Twelve percent had permanent or severe deficits. Eleven patients required additional surgery to either retreat the target lesion or address a complication. For CM in high-risk locations for resection, SRS can be an important surgical approach that appears to significantly lower the hemorrhage risk (fig. 1, 2) [1, 11, 13].

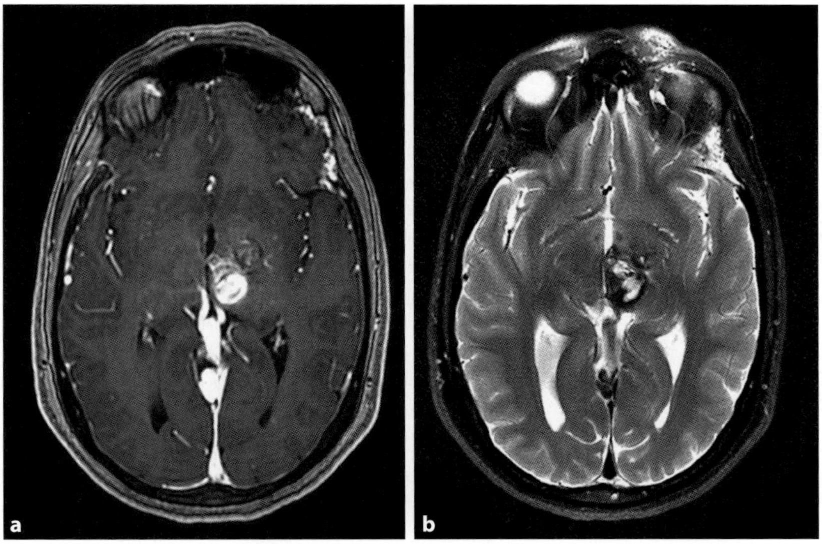

Fig. 2. One-year follow-up MRI after radiosurgery shows stable appearance of thalamic cavernous malformation on T_1- (**a**) and T_2-weighted (**b**) MRI, without evidence of new hemorrhage.

The natural history of brainstem CMs has not been fully elucidated. As such, our data, and those of others, cannot refute the possibility that some CMs may bleed repeatedly and then cease to bleed. This phenomenon has been referred to as 'temporal clustering', although data supporting this concept is limited.

Disclosure

Drs. Lunsford and Kondziolka are consultants with AB Elekta. Dr. Lunsford is also a stockholder in AB Elekta.

References

1 Hasegawa T, McInerney J, Kondziolka D, Lee JY, Flickinger JC, Lunsford LD: Long-term results after stereotactic radiosurgery for patients with cavernous malformations. Neurosurgery 2002;50:1190–1197, discussion 1197–1198.
2 Porter PJ, Willinsky RA, Harper W, Wallace MC: Cerebral cavernous malformations: natural history and prognosis after clinical deterioration with or without hemorrhage. J Neurosurg 1997;87:190–197.
3 Porter RW, Detwiler PW, Spetzler RF, Lawton MT, Baskin JJ, Derksen PT, et al: Cavernous malformations of the brainstem: experience with 100 patients. J Neurosurg 1999;90:50–58.
4 Labauge P, Brunereau L, Levy C, Laberge S, Houtteville JP: The natural history of familial cerebral cavernomas: a retrospective MRI study of 40 patients. Neuroradiology 2000;42:327–332.

5 Larson JJ, Ball WS, Bove KE, Crone KR, Tew JM Jr: Formation of intracerebral cavernous malformations after radiation treatment for central nervous system neoplasia in children. J Neurosurg 1998;88: 51–56.
6 McLaughlin MR, Kondziolka D, Flickinger JC, Lunsford S, Lunsford LD: The prospective natural history of cerebral venous malformations. Neurosurgery 1998;43:195–200, discussion 201.
7 Aiba T, Tanaka R, Koike T, Kameyama S, Takeda N, Komata T: Natural history of intracranial cavernous malformations. J Neurosurg 1995;83:56–59.
8 Del Curling O Jr, Kelly DL Jr, Elster AD, Craven TE: An analysis of the natural history of cavernous angiomas. J Neurosurg 1991;75:702–708.
9 Kondziolka D, Lunsford LD, Kestle JR: The natural history of cerebral cavernous malformations. J Neurosurg 1995;83:820–824.
10 Maraire JN, Awad IA: Intracranial cavernous malformations: lesion behavior and management strategies. Neurosurgery 1995;37:591–605.
11 Kondziolka D, Lunsford LD, Flickinger JC, Kestle JR: Reduction of hemorrhage risk after stereotactic radiosurgery for cavernous malformations. J Neurosurg 1995;83:825–831.
12 Mathiesen T, Edner G, Kihlstrom L: Deep and brainstem cavernomas: a consecutive 8-year series. J Neurosurg 2003;99:31–37.
13 Lunsford LD, Khan AA, Niranjan A, Kano H, Flickinger JC, Kondziolka D: Stereotactic radiosurgery for symptomatic solitary cerebral cavernous malformations considered high risk for resection. J Neurosurg 2010;113:23–29.

Douglas Kondziolka, MD, FACS
Peter J. Jannetta Professor of Neurological Surgery
Department of Neurological Surgery
UPMC Presbyterian, Suite B-400, 200 Lothrop Street
Pittsburgh, PA 15213 (USA)
Tel. +1 412 647 6782, E-Mail kondziolkads@upmc.edu

Niranjan A, Kano H, Lunsford LD (eds): Gamma Knife Radiosurgery for Brain Vascular Malformations.
Prog Neurol Surg. Basel, Karger, 2013, vol 27, pp 147–156 (DOI: 10.1159/000341781)

Radiosurgery of Brain Cavernomas – Long-Term Results

Roman Liscak

Na Homolce Hospital, Prague, Czech Republic

Abstract

The radiosurgery of cavernomas remains a controversial issue. The only way to verify the positive effect of the treatment is by clinical observation during a longer follow-up period, where a decreased annual risk of rebleeding should be observed after the latent interval inherent to radiosurgery. Besides this, an improvement in clinical symptoms (e.g. secondary epilepsy) and regression of the treated lesion might also be observed. In a group of 112 patients with brain cavernomas treated in our centre between 1992 and 2000 with the marginal dose of a median 16 Gy, the risk of bleeding decreased from 2% before the treatment to 0.5% after 2 years' latent interval (median follow-up 84 months). A decrease in the extent of the cavernoma was observed in 53% of cases and an increase in 6.4%. Epilepsy, if present before the treatment, improved in 45% of cases. The risk of temporary and permanent morbidity caused by radiosurgery was 14.6 and 0.9%, respectively. This morbidity can be reduced by a lower marginal dose, and future studies should show if repeated radiosurgery decreases the risks from a natural course of the disease in those cases where the initial radiosurgery failed.

A brain cavernoma is a controversial indication for radiosurgery, and readiness to treat this clinical entity varies among different radiosurgical centres. This controversy arises mainly from the frustrating fact that there is no direct diagnostic tool to verify the successful end point of the treatment compared to complete obliteration of the arteriovenous malformation (AVM) after radiosurgery as seen on angiography made after an appropriate latent interval from the time of treatment. The process of evaluating the clinical results of treating cavernomas is therefore ambiguous. Further, the behaviour of cavernomas crosses the borderline between hamartomas and tumours more frequently than that of AVMs – intracerebral cavernomas that appear and grow after birth have been observed and documented [1–4], or does this increase of cavernoma represent rebleeding without the clinical symptoms in functionally silent areas? Information about the natural course and predictive factors for cavernoma growth is incomplete. Cavernomas do not display uniform behaviour, and their status can vary from indolent, through bleeding, epileptogenic to growing lesions [1–7]. Nevertheless, the theoretical goal of radiosurgery of cavernomas is the same as that for AVMs that can be visualized by angiography – i.e. to prevent rebleeding from the lesion and improve the prognosis compared to that of the natural course of the disease.

Prague Experience at Na Homolce Hospital

As we have already published, 112 patients with brain cavernoma were treated by Leksell Gamma Knife in Prague between 1992 and 2000 [8]. The age of this group of patients ranged between 13 and 81 years, with a median of 42 years. All locations were represented – brainstem 33 patients, temporal 24, frontal 13, parietal 10, thalamus 9, basal ganglia 8 and occipital 7.

Half of the cavernomas were in deep, inoperable locations. The cavernoma was solitary in 99 patients and multilocular in 13. In cases of multiple cavernomas, the one causing symptomatic bleeding was treated. Seven patients had undergone previous partial microsurgical resection of the cavernoma, and Gamma Knife radiosurgery was the primary treatment in 94% of cases. The cavernomas evoked epilepsy in 44 patients. The neurodeficit (according to the anatomical localization) persisted before radiosurgery in 51 patients, and 30 patients complained of headaches.

There were 89 events reported in the case histories as bleeding in 59 patients before radiosurgery, in 23 of them repeatedly (max. 4 bleedings). The risk of bleeding before radiosurgery was calculated from the number of haemorrhages divided by the risk years from the birth of the patients (table 1). The volume of the cavernomas ranged from 0.06 to 12.5 cm^3, with a median of 0.9 cm^3. The maximum dose ranged from 16 to 50 Gy, with a median of 30 Gy. The marginal dose ranged from 9 to 36 Gy, with a median of 16 Gy, which was applied on a median 50% isodose.

Results

In an initial report [8], the follow-up covered 107 patients and ranged from 6 to 114 months, with a median of 48 months. At least 10 years have elapsed since this group of patients was treated and we have updated the follow-up. A clinical follow-up was available in all patients, a radiological one in 110 of them, and both had a range of 5–184 months, with a median of 84 months.

Rebleeding was reported in 7 patients in the initial report; this number increased to 11. These events were observed in 5–168 months, with a median of 24 months after radiosurgery. The annual risk of rebleeding was calculated from the number of events divided by the number of follow-up years (table 1). Rebleeding was associated with

Table 1. Annual risk of bleeding (%)

	Before GKS	≤2 years after GKS	>2 years after GKS
112 patients	2	3.2	0.5
59 patients, bleeding before GKS	3.7	5.3	0.2
53 patients, no bleeding before GKS	0	1	0.8

GKS = Gamma Knife surgery.

morbidity (impaired neurodeficit) in 7 patients (6.5%), which was temporary in 1 patient and persistent in 6 (2 patients with brainstem cavernoma died).

Radiological follow-up with at least 1 magnetic resonance imaging (MRI) was performed on the 110 patients and increased from a median 36 months in the initial report to a median 84 months after Gamma Knife treatment. In 58 patients (53%), a decrease in the cavernoma was observed 8–131 months (median 26 months) after radiosurgery, and in 7 patients the cavernoma increased (6.4%) 8–168 (median 86 months) after radiosurgery (fig. 1, 2). Detection of collateral oedema from the initial report was not different, and it was detected in 30 patients (27.3%) 3–49 months (median 11 months) after radiosurgery (fig. 2). In 17 of them (15.5%) oedema was symptomatic, and corticotherapy was administered to 16 patients for 1–12 months (median 2.5 months). Oedema resolved in 23 patients 8–40 months (median 18 months) after radiosurgery. Symptoms resolved in 16 patients 8–37 months (median 12 months) after radiosurgery, thus persistent morbidity caused by oedema remained in 1 patient (0.9%). Morbidity from the radiosurgery itself (symptomatic oedema) and the unaffected natural course of the disease (rebleeding) are shown in figure 3 (1 patient had symptomatic oedema associated with rebleeding).

Epileptic seizures before radiosurgery were observed in 44 patients. Improvement after radiosurgery was observed in 20 of these (45%) by 1–30 months (median 6 months) after radiosurgery. Impairment caused by collateral oedema was observed in 2 patients 6 and 8 months after radiosurgery, which resolved 12 months after radiosurgery. Persistent morbidity from epilepsy impairment was not observed.

In the initial paper [8], 4 patients were reported to have died. Two patients with brainstem cavernomas died 6 and 51 months after radiosurgery, and the cause of death was probably rebleeding in both patients, but neither MRI nor computed tomography or the autopsy results were available to prove it. The other 2 patients died from trauma and suicide. Since that time another 2 patients have died – 1 patient with brainstem cavernoma died 14 years after radiosurgery due to a gradual increase in the cavernoma; there was no ictal event classified as rebleeding. Another 61-year-old patient with temporal cavernoma died 5 years after radiosurgery for unknown reasons.

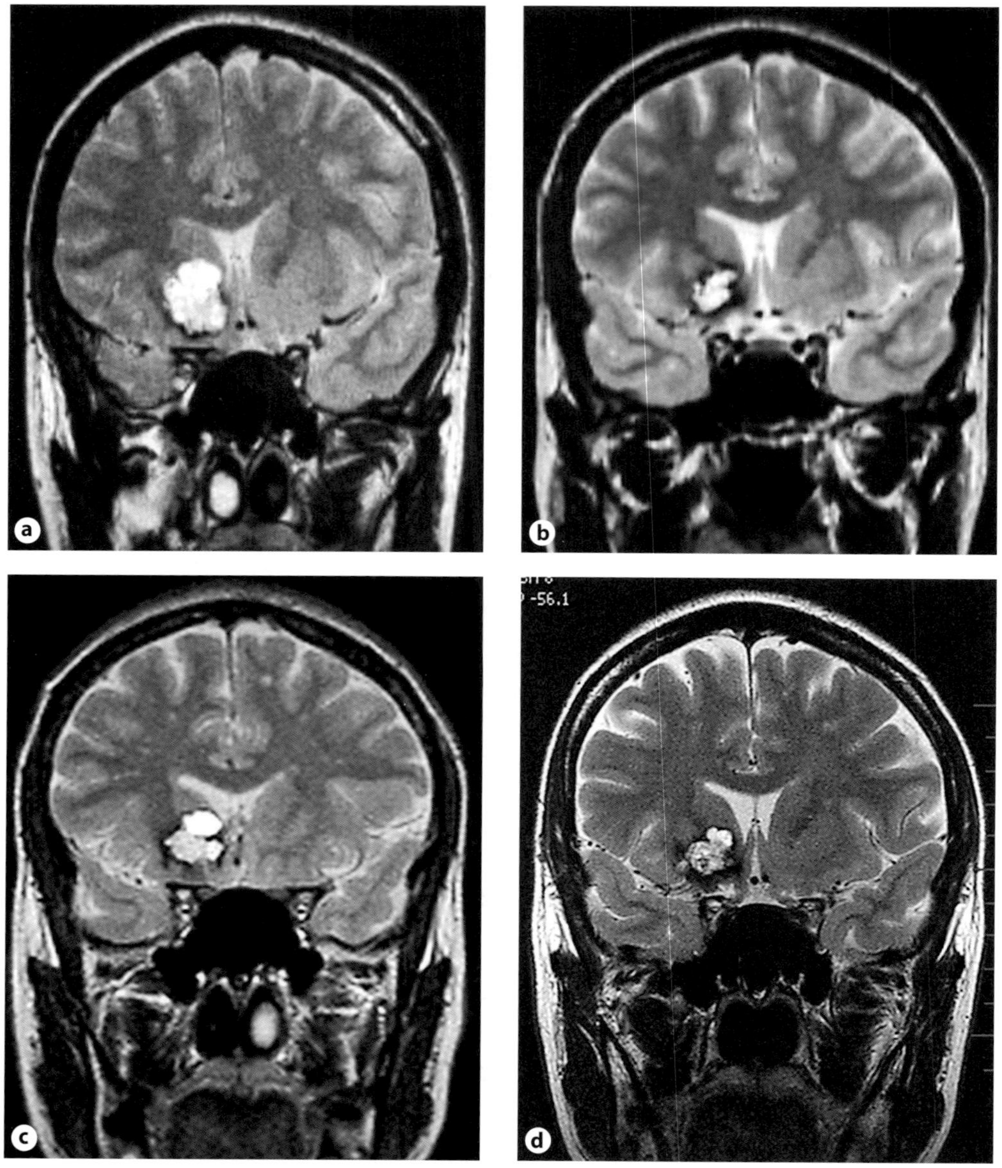

Fig. 1. **a** 28-year-old woman, with no history of bleeding, showing progressive visual impairment before the treatment and secondary epilepsy; the volume of the cavernoma was 4.5 cm^3; 15 Gy on a 50% isodose (turbo spin echo, T_2-weighted sequence). **b** Regression of the cavernoma 4 years after radiosurgery. **c** Increase in extent of cavernoma (rebleeding with no symptoms) observed 10 years after radiosurgery, treated conservatively. **d** 15 years after the treatment, further regression of the cavernoma.

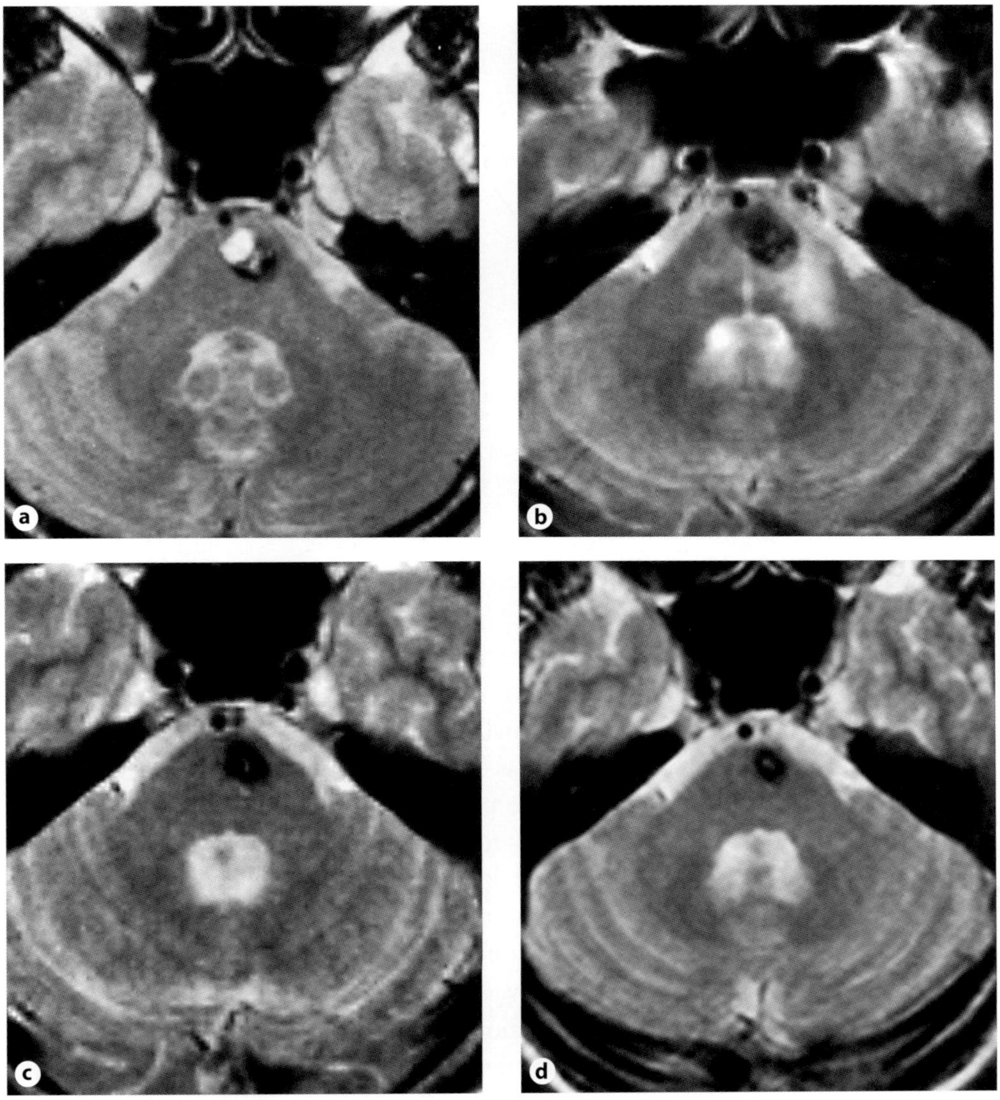

Fig. 2. **a** 45-year-old patient with cavernoma in the pons, before radiosurgery 1 bleeding, marginal dose 16.5 Gy on 55% isodose, volume 1 cm^3 (MRI, turbo spin echo 2,500/98). **b** 11 months after radiosurgery collateral oedema with impairment of hemiparesis, corticoids administered for 2 months (MRI, turbo spin echo 3,000/98). **c** 2 years after radiosurgery oedema resolved, decrease in extent of the cavernoma (MRI, turbo spin echo 3,000/98). **d** 10 years after radiosurgery further regression of the lesion.

Eleven patients underwent repeated treatment for their cavernoma: 9 patients underwent open microsurgery (1 patient for collateral oedema, 2 patients for rebleeding, 3 patients for cavernoma volume increase and 3 patients for epilepsy, which was not cured by radiosurgery). Four patients with epilepsy and cavernoma located in the region of the amigdalohippocampal complex underwent repeated radiosurgery,

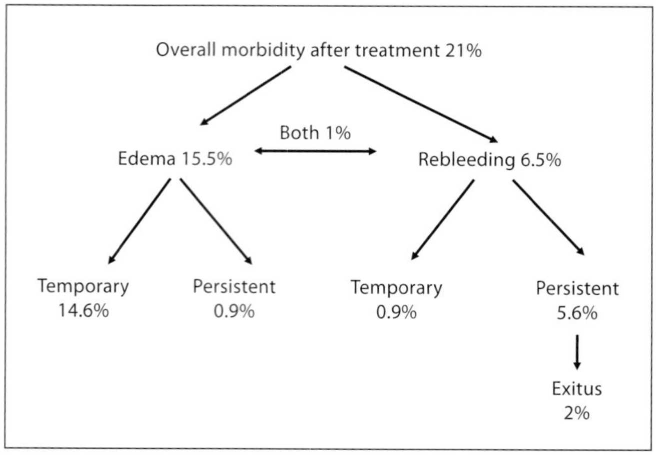

Fig. 3. Morbidity after the treatment.

but instead of selective irradiation of the cavernoma the whole amigdalohippocampal complex was the target for retreatment. This treatment was effective in 2, and the other 2 underwent later microsurgical resection.

In the whole group of patients during the follow-up, new cavernomas were detected in 2 of them – in 1 patient multiple new small cavernomas were detected after 14 years, and in another 1 new small cavernoma was detected 10 years after radiosurgery; both patients were treated conservatively. One patient with temporal medial cavernoma with secondary epilepsy, which improved and whose cavernoma regressed 8 years after radiosurgery, had a new bizzare diffuse bilateral dural AVM detected 10 years after radiosurgery with several haemorrhages in different localizations in the brain. Beside that, multiple organ angiomatosis (liver, kidney, lung, spleen) and carcinoma uteri were diagnosed. This patient underwent 5 endovascular embolizations of her new dural malformation, and 14 years after the initial radiosurgery she was in a poor condition.

Statistical analysis showed that cavernoma rebleeding after Gamma Knife radiosurgery can be expected more frequently in middle-aged patients (between 30 and 45 years), in patients with a previous history of haemorrhage, and in patients where the dose to the cavernoma margin was less than 14 Gy. Oedema occurrence after Gamma Knife treatment was more frequent for patients who had undergone prior surgery, for patients with a larger cavernoma volume and where the dose to the cavernoma margin was higher than 13 Gy.

Discussion

Over the last 18 years, the indicative criteria for radiosurgery of cavernomas in our centre have become stricter as they have evolved hand in hand with advances in microsurgery, which have changed the view of the operability of cavernomas, together with our increasing knowledge about the natural course of the disease. Cavernomas, which are considered as easily operable nowadays, two decades ago without neuronavigation or the support of stereotactic localization were not frequently found, and the view of what was operable was different.

Unlike AVMs, which are usually indicated for the treatment even in cases of incidental diagnosis, the cavernomas in the same situation are nowadays treated conservatively. However, cavernomas with no history of bleeding did not have the indolent behaviour one might have expected. In the presented group of 112 patients, 53 had no bleeding before the treatment and the reason to treat them was mainly due to secondary epilepsy. Rebleeding after the radiosurgery was observed in 4 of them (table 1). However, from the comparison of the protective effect, which is pronounced only in bleeding cavernomas, we have abandoned radiosurgery for cavernomas that have not bled before the treatment.

We have calculated the risk of bleeding before treatment as the number of haemorrhages divided by the risk years from the birth of patients, although other authors prefer to calculate the number of risk years from the time of the first haemorrhage [9–11] and the annual risk is consequently higher in such cases. The reasons given by them are mainly the absence or low incidence of haemorrhage from cavernoma in children and de novo appearance of cavernomas in familial cases [9, 11]. We considered patients with cavernoma to be at risk of bleeding from their birth for the following reasons. The age of the clinical manifestation of cavernomas does not differ from that of AVMs, which is in both our series (cavernoma and AVMs) between 30 and 45 years, but children are represented in both of them [8, 12]. Although we are more reserved in performing radiosurgery for cavernomas in children, this selection bias does not eliminate cavernomas from childhood, and the youngest patient with cavernoma treated at our centre was a 4.5-year-old boy treated in 2008. Before radiosurgery he had 2 bleedings from cavernoma in the right thalamus, the first at the age of 31 months. De novo appearance of cavernoma is possible, but very rare; in our series, this happened in 2 patients during the follow-up, which is less than 2%. Therefore we cannot presume that the cavernoma developed 1 day before the first bleeding and there was no risk before that date. The risk from birth seems to be closer to reality, although our current knowledge does not answer all questions about the natural course of the disease. The discussed topic about the variation of the risk of bleeding during the different periods of life has no definitive conclusion so far. Different methods of evaluation of the risks of bleeding before the treatment and moreover the selection bias of different published groups of patients does not allow an exact comparison of the risks before and after the treatment in different series. However, it is possible to compare the tendency for decreased risks of rebleeding, especially after the latent period of 2 or more years after radiosurgery. Lunsford et al. [10] reported an annual risk of rebleeding of 1.06% (mean follow-up 5.65 years) after the latency period of 2 years (the risk before the treatment was 32.5% from the time of the first symptomatic haemorrhage). Karlsson and his group based on their experience in the Karolinska Institute [9, 13, 14] do not support the treatment of cavernomas with the Gamma Knife since they consider the treatment results to be limited. They noted a tendency toward a decrease in the risk of rebleeding after a period of 4 years following radiosurgery. The risk of complications was higher than in AVMs, and lower rather than higher doses for cavernoma were recommended [9]. Along with the 2-year latency period, a decrease in the risk of rebleeding was observed in the group of patients treated by Amin-Hanjani et al. [15]. Using a cyclotron, radiosurgery achieved morbidity in 16% of cases. Chang et al. [16] observed a decrease in the risk of rebleeding after the treatment of cavernomas 3 years after radiosurgery that was connected with morbidity in 11% of cases. Protection from rebleeding after Gamma Knife radiosurgery of cavernomas was also observed by Mitchell et al. [17]. Liu et al. [18] observed an annual rebleeding rate after surgery of 10.3% for the first 2 years and 3.3% thereafter (mean follow-up 5.4 years).

Another important effect of cavernoma radiosurgery can be observed in cases of secondary epilepsy. Improvement of epilepsy was observed in 45% of affected patients. In his multicentric study, Régis et al. [6] observed even better results – 53% of 49 patients were seizure free after radiosurgery and a decrease in the number of seizures was achieved in another 20% of patients. The same chance for epilepsy improvement (53%) was also observed by Liu et al. [18].

One of the detectable effects after radiosurgery is regression of the cavernoma, which was observed in 53% of cases usually 2 years after the treatment. The spontaneous regression of the cavernoma could be expected as a resorption of the haematoma after previous bleeding. In the case of bleeding, radiosurgery in our group of patients was postponed for at least 3 months, but usually 6 months after the bleeding. Therefore we rate a decrease in cavernoma volume after radiosurgery to be a positive result of the treatment. Some authors have also observed a regression of the cavernoma after radiosurgery as much as in 57.3% [10, 13, 19], although others saw little change [16].

Cavernomas are considered to represent a higher risk of complications after radiosurgery compared to AVMs [9, 13, 20]. In our experience, the risk of oedema on follow-up MRI after radiosurgery of AVM was 21.3% [12], for cavernoma it was 27.3%. Oedema was associated with temporary morbidity in 7.7% in AVMs and 14.6% in cavernomas, permanent morbidity was found in 2.7% in AVMs and 0.9% in cavernomas. We do not consider this morbidity as unacceptably high, and complications from rebleeding were the main risk (fig. 3). Eventually the higher risk of temporary complications after radiosurgery of cavernomas compared to AVM was caused by our tendency to apply similarly high doses as for AVMs, which seems nowadays not adequate, because in cases of cavernoma doses higher than 13 Gy significantly increased this risk [8]. The median marginal dose in the studied group of patients with cavernoma was 16 Gy, the same as in the series published by Lunsford et al. [10]. They have observed a 13.5% risk of morbidity, which is similar to the 14.6% from our experience. Pollock et al. [20] observed complications in 59% of cases and their marginal dose was a median 18 Gy. Analysis of our results changed our treatment strategy and such high marginal doses for cavernomas are not used nowadays, so the risk of radiosurgery is further decreased and does not stand out from the risks observed in other diagnoses treated with radiosurgery. In a group of 125 patients with cavernoma and a mean margin dose of 12.1 Gy, Liu et al. [18] observed symptomatic complications in only 3 of them. We suspected that higher doses led to an increased release of vascular endothelial growth factor, which is a potent inducer of vascular permeability, whose presence in vessel malformations has been proven [21]. The appearance of new cavernomas and their increase can justify our opinion, that expression of endothelial vascular factor is pronounced more in cavernomas compared to AVMs and consequently the risk of oedema is higher. Marginal doses between 14 and 15 Gy in our current practice represent a compromise between the higher risk of oedema with the increasing marginal dose and the higher risk of rebleeding with the lower marginal dose.

In case of AVM, Gamma Knife radiosurgery was repeated in 23% of patients because complete obliteration was not achieved within 3 years of the first treatment [12]. Unfortunately we have no tool for identifying those patients in whom, after the proper latent interval from the radiosurgery of cavernoma, the treatment has had insufficient effect. This treatment failure revealed in some of them just rebleeding or increase in size. Therefore it seems advisable to consider repeated radiosurgery of cavernomas, where rebleeding occurs after the latent interval similar to AVM.

Conclusion

A decreased risk of rebleeding after the latent interval of 2 years was observed after radiosurgery of cavernomas. The risk of permanent complications after radiosurgery was lower than 1%, and temporary morbidity can be reduced by lower marginal doses. Controversial issues (incomplete knowledge of the natural course of disease and the absence of diagnostic tools, which could confirm the elimination of the risk of rebleeding) led us gradually to reserve radiosurgery for a selected group of patients with repeated bleeding or progressive impairment of neurodeficit, where alternative treatment (microsurgical resection) represents an unacceptable risk. Till now the only proof of treatment failure after radiosurgery is rebleeding or cavernoma increase after the latent interval of 2 or more years after the radiosurgery. Future studies should evaluate, if in such a case repeated radiosurgery might further decrease the risks from the natural course of the disease.

References

1 Clatterbuck RE, Moriarity JL, Elmaci I, Lee RR, Breiter SN, Rigamonti D: Dynamic nature of cavernous malformations: a prospective magnetic resonance imaging study with volumetric analysis. J Neurosurg 2000;93:981–986.
2 Pozzati E, Acciarri N, Tognetti F, Marliani F, Giangaspero F: Growth, subsequent bleeding, and de novo appearance of cerebral cavernous angiomas. Neurosurgery 1996;38:662–670.
3 Scott RM, Barnes P, Kupsky W, Adelman LS: Cavernous angiomas of the central nervous system in children. J Neurosurg 1992;76:38–46.
4 Zabramski JM, Wascher TM, Spetzler RF, Johnson B, Golfinos J, Drayer BP, Brown B, Rigamonti D, Brown G: The natural history of familial cavernous malformations: results of an ongoing study. J Neurosurg 1994;80:422–432.
5 Moran NF, Fish DR, Kitchen N, Shorvon S, Kendall BE, Stevens JM: Supratentorial cavernous hemangiomas and epilepsy: a review of the literature and case series. J Neurol Neurosurg Psychiatry 1999;66: 561–568.
6 Régis J, Bartolomei F, Kida Y, Kobayashi T, Vladyka V, Liscàk R, Forster D, Kemeny A, Schröttner O, Pendl G: Radiosurgery for epilepsy associated with cavernous malformation: retrospective study in 49 patients. Neurosurgery 2000;47:1091–1097.
7 Kondziolka D, Lunsford LD, Kestle JRW: The natural history of cerebral cavernous malformations. J Neurosurg 1995;83:820–824.
8 Liščák R, Vladyka V, Šimonová G, Vymazal J, Novotný J Jr: Gamma knife surgery of brain cavernous hemangiomas. J Neurosurg 2005;102(suppl): 207–213.
9 Karlsson B, Soderman M: Stereotactic radiosurgery for cavernomas; in Lunsford LD, Sheehan JP (eds): Intracranial Stereotactic Radiosurgery. New York, Thieme, 2009, pp 48–57.
10 Lunsford LD, Khan AA, Niranjan A, Kano H, Flickinger JC, Kondziolka D: Stereotactic radiosurgery for symptomatic solitary cerebral cavernous malformations considered high risk for resection. J Neurosurg 2010;113:23–29.
11 Steiner L, Karlsson B, Yen CP, Torner JC, Lindquist C, Schlesinger D: Radiosurgery in cavernous malformations: anatomy of a controversy. J Neurosurg 2010;113:16–22.
12 Liščák R, Vladyka V, Šimonová G, Urgošík D, Novotný J Jr, Janoušková L, Vymazal J: Arteriovenous malformations after Leksell gamma knife radiosurgery: rate of obliteration and complications. Neurosurgery 2007;60:1005–1016.
13 Karlsson B, Kihlstrom L, Lindquist C, Ericson K, Steiner L: Radiosurgery for cavernous malformations. J Neurosurg 1998;88:293–297.
14 Mathiesen T, Edner G, Kihlstrom L: Deep and brainstem cavernomas: a consecutive 8-year series. J Neurosurg 2003;99:31–37.
15 Amin-Hanjani S, Ogilvy CS, Candia GJ, Lyons S, Chapman PH: Stereotactic radiosurgery for cavernous malformations: Kjellberg's experience with proton beam therapy in 98 cases at the Harvard cyclotron. Neurosurgery 1998;42:1229–1238.
16 Chang SD, Levy RP, Adler JR, Martin DP, Krakovitz PR, Steinberg GK: Stereotactic radiosurgery of angiographically occult vascular malformations: 14-year experience. Neurosurgery 1998;43:213–221.
17 Mitchell P, Hodgson TJ, Seaman S, Kemeny AA, Forster DMC: Stereotactic radiosurgery and the risk of haemorrhage from cavernous malformations. Br J Neurosurg 2000;14:96–100.
18 Liu KD, Chung WY, Wu HM, Shiau CY, Wang LW, Guo WY, Pan DH: Gamma knife surgery for cavernous hemangiomas: an analysis of 125 patients. J Neurosurg 2005;102(suppl):81–86.
19 Kim DG, Choe WJ, Paek SH, Chung HT, Kim IH, Han DH: Radiosurgery of intracranial cavernous malformations. Acta Neurochir 2002;144:869–878.
20 Pollock E, Garces YI, Stafford SL, Foote RL, Schomberg PJ, Link MJ: Stereotactic radiosurgery for cavernous malformations. J Neurosurg 2000;93: 987–991.
21 Rothbart D, Awad IA, Lee J, Kim J, Harbaugh R, Criscuolo GR: Expression of angiogenic factors and structural proteins in central nervous system vascular malformations. Neurosurgery 1996;38:915–925.

Roman Liscak, MD
Hospital Na Homolce
Roentgenova 2
CZ-15030 Prague (Czech Republic)
Tel. +420 2 5727 2552, E-Mail roman.liscak@homolka.cz

Niranjan A, Kano H, Lunsford LD (eds): Gamma Knife Radiosurgery for Brain Vascular Malformations.
Prog Neurol Surg. Basel, Karger, 2013, vol 27, pp 157–165 (DOI: 10.1159/000341785)

Radiosurgical Treatment for Epilepsy Associated with Cavernomas

Marc Lévêque · Romain Carron · Fabrice Bartolomei · Jean Régis

Service de Neurochirurgie Fonctionnelle et Stéréotaxique, Assistance Publique des Hôpitaux de Marseille, Marseille, France

Abstract

Cavernous malformations (CMs) are congenital vascular malformations of the brain, which often present with drug-resistant epilepsy. Microsurgical excision remains the preferred approach for cortical-subcortical epileptogenic CMs that are not located in functional cortex. For patients presenting with seizures arising from eloquent cortex surrounding the lesion, radiosurgery appears to be a suitable alternative. We evaluated the effectiveness of Gamma Knife (GK) surgery in the management of drug-resistant seizures associated with CMs in a retrospective multicenter study. Forty-nine patients with cortical or subcortical CMs with severe long-term drug-resistant epilepsy underwent radiosurgery. The mean duration of epilepsy before these GK procedures was 7.5 (±9.3) years. The mean frequency of seizures was 6.9/month (±14). The mean marginal radiation dose was 19.17 Gy. At the last follow-up examination, 53% were seizure free. A highly significant decrease in the number of seizures was achieved for another 20%. The remaining 26% of patients showed little or no improvement. The morbidity was low. Radiosurgery is a promising management modality for epilepsy associated with CMs. The determination of the extent of the epileptogenic zone in CMs and dose selection are the critical steps towards successful radiosurgical outcome. Further prospective work is necessary to validate our data.

Radiosurgery is, by definition, a neurosurgical procedure that uses stereotactically focused converging narrow ionizing beams to induce a desired biological effect in a predetermined target through the intact skull; the steep fall-off of dose outside the target enables an optimal sparing of the surrounding tissues. Lars Leksell, a Swedish neurosurgeon, was the first to introduce the concept of radiosurgery in 1951 [1]. His goal in performing stereotactic procedures was to avoid the risk associated at that time, with craniectomy notably bleeding and infection. The increased worldwide use of Gamma Knife radiosurgery (GKRS) to treat various pathologies, has rendered the side effect profile of radiosurgery rare, generally transient and quite easily predictable [2]. Once it is established that resection of a small deeply seated lesion carries a significant risk of surgical complications and/or functional worsening, GKRS must be discussed as an alternative. For these indications, GKRS compares favorably with microsurgical removal in terms of safety/efficacy and cost-effectiveness in the treatment of cavernomas associated with epilepsy.

History

The first radiosurgical attempts for epilepsy surgery were performed by Talairach et al. [3] in the fifties. Unlike Leksell, they already had expertise in epilepsy surgery and led one of the first large comprehensive programs for epilepsy surgery. As early as 1974, Talairach reported on the use of radioactive yttrium implants in patients with mesial temporal lobe epilepsy without space-occupying lesions, and showed a high rate of seizure control in patients with epilepsies confined to the mesial structures of the temporal lobe [3]. In 1980, Elomaa [4] promoted the idea of the use of focal irradiation for the treatment of temporal lobe epilepsy, based on the preliminary reports of Baudouin et al. [5] and Von Wieser [6]. Furthermore, clinical experience data gathered from the use of GK and linear accelerator-based radiosurgery in arteriovenous malformations and corticosubcortical tumors (mostly metastases and low-grade glial tumors) revealed an anticonvulsive effect of radiosurgery in the absence of tissue necrosis [7–9]. A series of experimental studies in small animals confirmed this effect [10, 11] and emphasized a relationship to the dose delivered [12, 13]. Barcia Salorio et al. [14], and later Lindquist et al. [15, 16], reported on a small and heterogeneous group of patients treated by GKRS with the purpose of seizure cessation. However, their data was poor [14–16] and was unfortunately never published in peer-reviewed papers; precise data are to date unavailable.

Epileptogenicity of Cavernous Malformations

Cavernous malformations (CMs) are congenital vascular malformations of the brain. They may cause hemorrhage and repetitive neurological deficits, but the most frequent presenting symptom is epilepsy [17]. The epileptogenicity of these lesions results from the ongoing deposition of iron and blood products at the margin of the lesion [18]. The incidence of drug-resistant epilepsy is not well known. However, in one large recent series, 40% of patients with a supratentorial CM presented with drug-resistant epilepsy [19]. Since 1994, the idea was promoted that seizure cessation may be generated by a specific neuromodulatory effect of radiosurgery, without induction of a significant amount of histological necrosis [20–24]. The selection of the appropriate technical parameters (dose, volume target etc.) allowing us to accurately obtain the desired functional effect without histological damage remains an important challenge. The review of these cases, as well as other clinical and experimental data, suggests that the use of radiosurgery is beneficial only to those patients in whom a strict preoperative definition of the extent of the epileptogenic network has been achieved, and where strict rules of dose planning have been followed. The strategy is to define the niche (small groups) of patients in whom the safety/efficacy ratio makes radiosurgery advantageous or at least comparable with craniotomy and cortectomy. CM patients with a longer duration of epilepsy are thought to have a more widespread epileptogenic zone involving distant cortical structures [25–27]. For patients presenting with seizures arising from eloquent cortex surrounding the lesion, GK treatment appears to be a suitable alternative. It is essential that electroclinical correlation be established for this strategy to work. Microsurgical excision remains the preferred approach for cortical-subcortical epileptogenic CMs that are not located in functional cortex.

Radiosurgery versus Lesionectomy

GK treatment of CMs is controversial [28] and the few available studies have reported conflicting results concerning its ability to decrease the bleeding rate and provide protection from hemorrhage [29–32]. The role of radiosurgery in the treatment of CMs remains controversial, in part because of the absence of neuroimaging criteria to gauge their successful obliteration as well as its higher complication rates. Radiosurgery is recommended only for symptomatic lesions that are surgically inaccessible or located in eloquent brain. In view of the previously observed relatively high rate of radiation-induced side effects [29] and the safety and efficacy of microsurgical excision [18], the latter technique is usually recommended when the aim of the treatment is to rule out bleeding potential. Nevertheless, the low risk of clinical bleeding [33] associated with CMs located in cortical/subcortical sites, unlike the expectation with deep-seated lesions, has been clearly demonstrated. These findings explain why seizure control is often the main indication for surgery in this condition. Microsurgery is considered as the best treatment in patients with intractable epilepsy. However, in some series, a beneficial effect on the course of epilepsy was reported for supratentorial CMs [30] treated by GKRS. Since GKRS is usually associated with a minimal risk of injury to the surrounding nontarget neural tissue, this technique could be a good alternative for this indication, particularly when the CM is located in a brain region associated with a high surgical risk. The management strategy for CM is complex, but the general consensus is that microsurgical resection of the lesion is the best treatment in patients with intractable epilepsy. Two surgical strategies can be applied, depending on the date of onset and features of the seizures [34]. For patients with seizures of recent onset in whom correlation between symptoms and location of the CM is good, resection of the lesion (lesionectomy) seems to be the best method. Epilepsy surgery strategies should be preferred for patients with a long history of chronic epilepsy in whom correlation of clinical and electroencephalographic findings is lacking. In these cases, a multimodal approach including invasive techniques should be considered. In this context, the aim of surgery should be to control epilepsy rather than to remove the lesion. The appropriate use or nonuse of these criteria probably explains why the success rate for surgical excision of CM varies from 20 to 80% in the literature [18, 19, 25, 27, 33–39]. The effect of GKRS on epilepsy is probably distinct from that which could eventually account for the prevention of bleeding. Of the 11 patients presenting with intractable epilepsy before GKRS in the series of Kida et al. [30], 7 patients (65%) achieved good seizure control after GKRS even though there was no apparent change in the size of the CM. The apparent size of a CM seems to fluctuate and depend on the production and absorption of blood pigments. Although a reliable prospective study with long-term follow-up is still needed, this retrospective series indicates that GK surgery can be effective for this indication and that morbidity can be low. It should be emphasized that the GK procedure is a treatment of the lesion and immediate surrounding tissue. The results observed in this study were comparable with those reported in the recent literature for lesionectomy [18, 19, 25, 27, 33–39]. The most valuable prognostic factor for outcome after GKRS was lesion location. A probable explanation for this finding is that the relationship between the lesion and the epileptogenic zone is particularly direct in certain regions. This is especially true for simple motor partial seizures associated with CMs in the rolandic region. In contrast, when a CM is located in the mediotemporal region, a more complex organization probably accounts for the extended epileptogenic zone, and epilepsy surgery strategies should be preferred. This probably explains why patients with complex partial seizures have a less favorable evolution than patients with simple partial seizures in our study.

Efficiency of the Gamma Knife Radiosurgery

The effectiveness of GKRS in the management of drug-resistant seizures associated with CMs was evaluated in a retrospective multicenter study (Marseille, France; Graz, Austria; Komaki, Japan; Sheffield, UK; Prague, Czech Republic) [40]. Forty-nine patients with cortical/subcortical CMs with severe long-term drug-resistant epilepsy were included and followed for longer than 1 year after GKRS. The mean duration of epilepsy before these GK procedures was 7.5 (±9.3) years. The mean frequency of seizures was 6.9/month (±14). The mean marginal radiation dose was 19.17 ± 4.4 Gy. Among the 49 patients, 35% had a CM located in or involving a highly functional area. At the last follow-up examination, 53% were seizure free (Engel's class I), including 49% in class IA and 4% of the patients with occasional auras. A highly significant decrease in the number of seizures was achieved for 20% (class IIB). The remaining 26% of patients showed little or no improvement. The mesiotemporal site was associated with a higher risk of failure. One patient bled during the observation period, and another experienced radiation-induced edema with transient aphasia. Postradiosurgery excision was performed in 5 patients, and a second radiosurgical

Table 1. Comparative analysis of the seizure-free group versus the non-seizure-free group

Seizure type and location	Number in Engel's class IA (seizure-free)	Number of others (non-seizure-free)	p value
Seizure type			
GTCS	5	7	n.s.
SPS ± GS	10	3	0.025
CPS ± GS	5	13	0.0378
ND	2	4	n.s.
Location			
Mesiotemporal	2	12	0.0069
Polar temporal	1	1	n.s.
Laterotemporal	6	1	0.0048
Laterofrontal	3	6	n.s.
Basofrontal	3	1	n.s.
Mesiofrontal	2	0	n.s.
Central	4	0	0.052
Parietal	1	4	n.s.
Occipital	2	0	n.s.

GTCS = Generalized tonic-clonic seizure; SPS = simple partial seizure; GS = secondary generalization; CPS = complex partial seizure; ND = seizure type not classified; n.s. = not statistically significant.

treatment was carried out in 1 patient. Type of seizure and location of the CM are important prognostic factors (for details on p values, see table 1). The outcome was better for patients with simple partial seizures than for those with complex partial seizures. Location of the CM, which is probably related to the type of seizure, appeared to be the most valuable prognostic factor (fig. 1). Location in the mesiotemporal region was associated with a poor outcome (12 of 14 patients), whereas location in the laterotemporal region was associated with a good outcome (6 of 7 patients). Location in the central region was also associated with an excellent outcome; all 4 patients in this group were seizure free. For other locations, results were unpredictable. The morbidity was low. Radiologically, 7 patients presented major reactional edema during the first year after GKRS. In 2 of these patients, neuroradiological alterations were associated with clinical manifestations which included severe hemiparesis and speech impairment, but both patients fully recovered during the follow-up period.

What about the Bleeding Risk?

Convincing data concerning the efficacy of GKRS in the prevention of bleeding risk associated with CMs are lacking. Early authors reported no effect [29, 30, 32]. Recently, some authors have reported a decrease in bleeding 2 years after GKRS

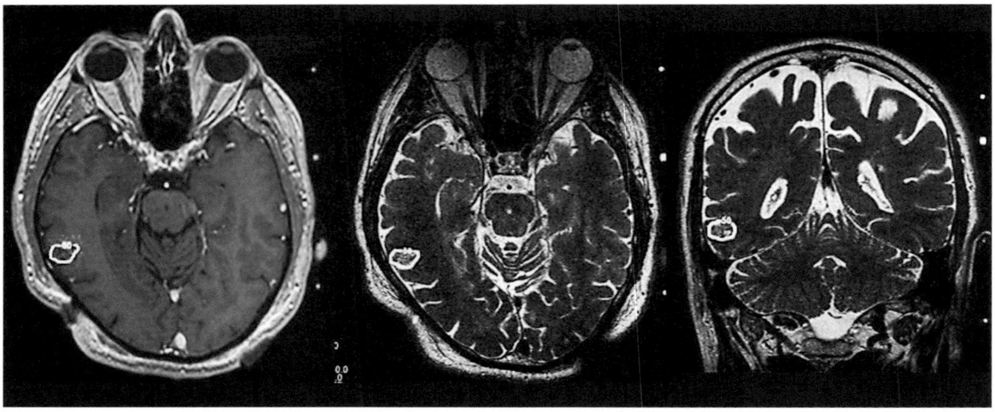

Fig. 1. A series of magnetic resonance images obtained from a 55-year-old man who experienced severe seizure from a right posterior temporal cavernoma. The patient was treated with GKRS (margin dose 14 Gy, 50% isodose at the lesion margin represented by the yellow line). The patient became seizure free without medication after 16 months. Five years after GKRS, seizures are still controlled without medication.

[31, 41], but the majority reported no effect. Thus, the role of radiosurgery in the management of these lesions remains controversial [31]. Moreover, in some studies, the incidence of radiation-induced complications was particularly high after radiosurgery of the CM [29, 42]. This is perhaps explained by poor radiological localization and the dose planning software available at that time. This problem was countered by the use of a lower radiation dose than is usually applied for other vascular targets.

Technical Questions

Target Definition

Some articles reporting microsurgical resection of occult malformations suggest that resection of the hemosiderin-stained tissue surrounding the lesion is critical for eliminating seizures [43]. Obviously, the reason for seizure cessation is not the dose received by the margin of the target (even if defined generously) but the ionizing radiation received by the epileptogenic zone located close to the CM. The aim of management of patients with cavernomas who present with a major hemorrhage is to control and prevent future hemorrhages, and the best method is usually microsurgery. However, for patients presenting with seizures arising from eloquent cortex surrounding the lesion, GK treatment appears to be a suitable alternative. It is essential that close electroclinical correlation be established for this strategy to work. Microsurgical excision remains the preferred approach for cortical-subcortical epileptogenic CMs that are not located in the functional cortex. Considering that image-guided microsurgical excision can be performed safely for the majority of patients, a comparative prospective trial is necessary to establish the possible role of GK surgery for this indication.

Dose Selection

Various doses have been tested in experimental studies on animals [23, 44, 45] and clinical experience with GKRS on epileptic lesions [46–48]. There is clearly a relationship between dose and effectiveness on seizures. Depending on the dose, animals undergo seizure cessation, seizure reduction, no change or worsening of epilepsy [45]. Dose selection is obviously crucial for the clinical control of seizures. We believe that, at present, compelling satisfactory evidence is lacking for recommendation of the systematic use of GKRS for this indication (cortical-subcortical CM associated with drug-resistant epilepsy). Although this series is very encouraging, the aim of this publication is not to promote a widespread use of GKRS. Our main interest is to gain insight into the relationships between dose selection, target volume, and effectiveness on epilepsy in this unique population. All patients treated worldwide have been treated with comparable doses (around 20 Gy peripheral dose) and volumes, which may explain the absence of a statistical correlation between these two parameters and outcome. Similarly, all patients have had a long history of epilepsy (mean duration of epilepsy before GK surgery, 7.5 ± 9.3 years), which prevented us from correlating the duration of the epilepsy with the probability of seizure cessation.

Conclusions

The field of epilepsy surgery is a new and promising one for radiosurgery. The determination of the extent of the epileptogenic zone in CMs requires specific expertise, which is crucial in order to achieve a reasonable rate of seizure cessation. In addition, the huge impact of fine technical detail on the efficacy and eventual toxicity of the procedure means that, at present, its use for these indications remains under investigation, and further prospective work is necessary.

References

1 Leksell L: The stereotaxic method and radiosurgery of the brain. Acta Chir Scand 1951;102:316–319.

2 Flickinger J, Kondziolka D, Lunsford L: Clinical applications of stereotactic radiosurgery. Cancer Treat Res 1998;93:283–297.

3 Talairach J, Bancaud J, Szikla G, Bonis A, Geler S, Vedrenne C: Approche nouvelle de la neurochirurgie de l'épilepsie. Méthodologie stéréotaxique et résultats thérapeutiques. Neurochirurgie 1974;20:92–98.

4 Elomaa E: Focal irradiation of the brain: an alternative to temporal lobe resection in intractable focal epilepsy? Med Hypotheses 1980;6:501–503.

5 Baudouin M, Stuhl L, Perrard A: Un cas d'épilepsie focale traité par la radiothérapie. Rev Neurol 1951; 84:60–63.

6 Von Wieser W: Die Roentgentherapie der traumatischen Epilepsie. Monatsschr Psychiatr Neurol 1939;101:422–424.

7 Heikkinen ER, Konnov B, Melnikow L: Relief of epilepsy by radiosurgery of cerebral arteriovenous malformations. Stereotact Funct Neurosurg 1989;53: 157–166.
8 Rogers L, Morris H, Lupica K: Effect of cranial irradiation on seizure frequency in adults with low-grade astrocytoma and medically intractable epilepsy. Neurology 1993;43:1599–1601.
9 Rossi G, Scerrati M, Roselli R: Epileptogenic cerebral low grade tumors: effect of interstitial stereotactic irradiation on seizures. Appl Neurophysiol 1985;48:127–132.
10 Barcia Salorio JL, Roldan P, Hernandez G, Lopez Gomez L: Radiosurgery treatment of epilepsy. Appl Neurophysiol 1985;48:400–403.
11 Gaffey C, Monotoya V, Lyman J, Howard J: Restriction of the spread of epileptic discharges in cats by means of Bragg peak intracranial irradiation. Int J Appl Radiat Isotope 1981;32:779–787.
12 Chen ZF, Kamiryo T, Henson SL, Yamamoto H, Bertram EH, Schottler F, et al: Anticonvulsant effects of gamma surgery in a model of chronic spontaneous limbic epilepsy in rats. J Neurosurg 2001;94:270–280.
13 Maesawa S, Kondziolka D, Dixon C, Balzer J, Fellows W, Lunsford L: Subnecrotic stereotactic radiosurgery controlling epilepsy produced by kainic acid injection in rats. J Neurosurg 2000;93: 1033–1040.
14 Barcia Salorio JL, Garcia JA, Hernandez G, Lopez Gomez L: Radiosurgery of epilepsy: long-term results. European Society for Stereotactic and Functional Neurosurgery, Stockholm, 1993.
15 Lindquist C, Hellstrand E, Kilström L, Abraham-Fuchs K, Jernberg B, Wirth A: Stereotactic localisation of epileptic foci by magnetoencephalography and MRI followed by gamma surgery. International Stereotactic Radiosurgery Symposium, Pittsburgh, 1991.
16 Lindquist C, Kihlström L, Hellstrand E, Knutsson E: Stereotactic radiosurgery instead of conventional epilepsy surgery. European Society for Stereotactic and Functional Neurosurgery, Stockholm, 1993.
17 Maraire J, Abdulrauf S, Berger S, Knisely J, Awad I: De novo development of cavernous malformation of the spinal cord following spinal axis radiation. J Neurosurg 1999;90:234–238.
18 Marraire JN, Awad IA: Intracranial cavernous malformations: lesion behavior and management strategies. Neurosurgery 1995;37:605.
19 Casazza M, Broggi G, Franzini A, Spreafico R, Bracchi M, Valentini M: Supratentorial cavernous angiomas and epileptic seizures: preoperative course and post-operative outcome. Neurosurgery 1996;39: 26–34.
20 Regis J, Semah F, Bryan R, Levrier O, Rey M, Samson Y, et al: Early and delayed MR and PET changes after selective temporomesial radiosurgery in mesial temporal lobe epilepsy. AJNR Am J Neuroradiol 1999;20:213–216.
21 Regis J, Roberts D: Gamma Knife radiosurgery relative to microsurgery: epilepsy. Stereotact Funct Neurosurg 1999;72(suppl 1):11–21.
22 Régis J, Peragut JC, Rey M, Samson Y, Levrier O, Porcheron D, et al: First selective amygdalohippocampic radiosurgery for mesial temporal lobe epilepsy. Stereotact Funct Neurosurg 1994;64:191–201.
23 Regis J, Kerkerian-Legoff L, Rey M, Vial M, Porcheron D, Nieoullon A, et al: First biochemical evidence of differential functional effects following Gamma Knife surgery. Stereotact Funct Neurosurg 1996;66(suppl 1):29–38.
24 Regis J, Bartolomei F, Hayashi M, Chauvel P: Gamma Knife surgery, a neuromodulation therapy in epilepsy surgery! Acta Neurochir Suppl 2002;84: 37–47.
25 Cohen D, Zubay G, Goodman R: Seizure outcome after lesionectomy for cavernous malformations. J Neurosurg 1995;83:237–242.
26 Kahane P, Tassi L, Hoffmann D, Francione S, Gratadou-Jery G, Pasquier B, et al: Crises dacrystiques et hamartome hypothalamique: à propos d'une observation vidéo-stéréo-EEG. Epilepsies 1994;6: 259–279.
27 Zevgaridis D, Van Velthoven V, Ebelling U, Reulen H: Seizure control following surgery in supratentorial cavernous malformations: a retrospective study in 77 patients. Acta Neurochir 1996;138:672–677.
28 Yomo S, Hayashi M: Stereotactic radiosurgery for intracranial cavernous malformations. Brain Nerve 2011;63:41–49.
29 Karlsson B, Kihlström L, Lindquist C, Ericson K, Steiner L: Radiosurgery for cavernous malformations. J Neurosurg 1998;88:293–297.
30 Kida Y, Kobayashi T, Tanaka T: Radiosurgery of symptomatic angiographically occult vascular malformations with Gamma Knife; in Kondziolka D (ed): Radiosurgery. Basel, Karger, 1995, pp 207–217.
31 Kondziolka D, Lunsford L, Flickinger J, Kestle J: Reduction of hemorrhage risk after stereotactic radiosurgery for cavernous malformations. J Neurosurg 1995;83:825–831.
32 Seo Y, Fukupka S, Takanashi M, Nakagawara J, Suematsu K, Nakamura J, et al: Gamma Knife surgery for angiographically occult vascular malformations. Stereotact Funct Neurosurg 1997;64:98–109.

33 Porter P, Willinsky R, Harper W, Wallace M: Cerebral cavernous malformations: natural history and prognosis after clinical deterioration with or without hemorrhage. J Neurosurg 1997;87:190–197.
34 Kahane P, Munari C, Hoffmann D, Tassi L, Gallina P, Francione S, et al: Approche chirurgicale multimodale des angiomes caverneux épileptogènes. Epilepsies 1994;6:113–130.
35 Engel J, Van Ness P, Rasmussen T, Ojemann L: Outcome with respect to epileptic seizures; in Engel J (ed): Surgical Treatment of the Epilepsies, ed 2. New York, Raven Press, 1993, pp 609–622.
36 Dodick D, Cascino G, Meyer F: Vascular malformations and intractable epilepsy: outcome after surgical treatment. Mayo Clin Proc 1994;69:741–745.
37 Acciari N, Giulioni M, Padovani R, Galssi E, Gaist G: Surgical management of cerebral cavernous angiomas causing epilepsy. J Neurosurg Sci 1995; 39:13–20.
38 Giulinoni M, Acciari N, Padovani R, Galassi E: Results of surgery in children with cerebral cavernous angiomas causing epilepsy. Br J Neurosurg 1995; 9:135–141.
39 Schroeder H, Gaab M, Runge U: Supratentorial cavernous angiomas and epileptic seizures: preoperative course and post-operative outcome. Neurosurgery 1996;12:1271.
40 Régis J, Bartolomei F, Kida Y, Kobayashi T, Vladyka V, Liscàk R, et al: Radiosurgery of epilepsy associated with cavernous malformation: retrospective study in 49 patients. Neurosurgery 2000;47:1091–1097.
41 Kondziolka D, Lunsford D, Flickinger J: Stereotactic radiosurgery for cavernous malformations; in Lunsford D (ed): Gamma Knife Brain Surgery. Basel, Karger, 1998, pp 78–88.
42 Amin-Hanjani S, Ogilvy CS, Candia GJ, Lyons S, Chapman PH: Stereotactic radiosurgery for cavernous malformations: Kjellberg's experience with proton beam therapy in 98 cases at Harvard cyclotron. Neurosurgery 1998;42:1229–1238.
43 Kraemer D, Griebel M, Lee N, Friedmann A, Radtke R: Surgical outcome in patients with epilepsy with occult vascular malformations treated with lesionectomy. Epilepsia 1998;39:600–607.
44 Barcia Salorio JL, Vanaclocha V, Cerda M, Roldan P: Focus irradiation in epilepsy. Experimental study in the cat. Appl Neurophysiol 1985;48:152.
45 Kondziolka D, Mori Y, Blazer J, Thulborn K: Stereotactic radiosurgery for the treatment of epilepsy evaluated in the rat kainic acid model. 8th Int Leksell Gamma Knife Soc Meet, Marseille, 1997.
46 Regis J, Bartolomei F, Metellus P, Rey M, Genton P, Dravet C, et al: Radiosurgery for trigeminal neuralgia and epilepsy. Neurosurg Clin North Am 1999; 10:359–377.
47 Regis J, Bartolomei F, de Toffol B, Genton P, Kobayashi T, Mori Y, et al: Gamma knife surgery for epilepsy related to hypothalamic hamartomas. Neurosurgery 2000;47:1343–1351, discussion 1351–1352.
48 Régis J, Bartolomei F, Rey M, Hayashi M, Genton P, Dravet C, et al: Role of Gamma Knife surgery in the treatment of severe epilepsies; in Wyllie E (ed): The Treatment of Epilepsy: Principle and Practice, ed 3. Baltimore, William & Wilkins, 2000.

Jean Régis, MD
Assistance Publique des Hôpitaux de Marseille
264, boulevard Saint-Pierre
FR–13008 Marseille (France)
Tel. +33 4 91 38 91 65 64, E-Mail jregis@ap-hm.fr

Niranjan A, Kano H, Lunsford LD (eds): Gamma Knife Radiosurgery for Brain Vascular Malformations.
Prog Neurol Surg. Basel, Karger, 2013, vol 27, pp 166–175 (DOI: 10.1159/000341792)

Stereotactic Radiosurgery Guidelines for the Management of Patients with Intracranial Cavernous Malformations

Ajay Niranjan · L. Dade Lunsford

Department of Neurological Surgery, University of Pittsburgh, Pittsburgh, Pa., USA

Abstract

Treatment options for cavernous malformations (CMs) have expanded with the application of stereotactic radiosurgery. In this report, we provide guidelines about the use of stereotactic radiosurgery in CM patients who had 2 documented symptomatic hemorrhages. We reviewed the evidence-based medicine and clinical experience with radiosurgery for CM of the brain and developed guidelines and provided a scientific foundation for patients and physicians. We also reviewed the controversy surrounding CM radiosurgery and discussed its origin and validity. Our recommendations include the selection of CM patients suitable for various management strategies ranging from observation to surgical excision and stereotactic radiosurgery. Radiosurgery is an effective management strategy that reduces the risk of additional hemorrhages from CMs that repeatedly bleed. The marginal dose ranges from 12 to 18 Gy (median 16 Gy). A clinical algorithm for the potential role of stereotactic radiosurgery for CM patients with 2 or more symptomatic hemorrhages is defined. These guidelines provide a framework for professional judgment and assessment of management alternatives for selected intracranial CMs.

Intracranial cavernous malformations (CMs) are angiographically occult developmental malformations of the vascular bed. These abnormal vascular connections may enlarge over time usually as a result of bleeding events. CMs represent approximately 1% of intracranial vascular lesions and 15% of cerebrovascular malformations although the actual incidence may be underestimated [1–4]. With the advent of magnetic resonance imaging (MRI), CMs are currently the most commonly identified brain vascular malformations. Multiple lesions are common in the familial form. The familial form of the disorder is inherited as an autosomal dominant trait with variable expression. Associated developmental venous anomalies (DVAs) are present in approximately 10–30% of patients with CMs [5, 6].

CMs may be detected at any age, but they are most likely to become clinically apparent in patients aged 20–40 years. Patients with CMs may remain asymptomatic, but they most often present with headache or neurological symptoms after a hemorrhage or repeated hemorrhage. Because of the extruded blood products and the fact that some malformations can enlarge slowly, the lesions may also produce seizures and a variety of neurological findings similar to those expected of intracranial tumors. The intracranial hemorrhage rate is estimated to be 0.1–2.5% per lesion-year and 0.25–16.5% per patient-year [5]. This risk is increased in patients with established prior hemorrhages. For patients who have had 2 prior hemorrhages, the subsequent annual risk of hemorrhage may be as high as 30% [7]. Women are at a slightly higher risk for hemorrhage, especially those in the first trimester of pregnancy. CM hemorrhages are rarely life-threatening. Hemorrhages in critical locations are more likely to result in significant neurological symptoms or signs.

Management strategies for CMs include observation for asymptomatic patients, microsurgical removal of symptomatic and accessible lesions, or stereotactic radiosurgery for symptomatic but surgically high-risk malformations.

The successful management of cerebral AVMs with stereotactic radiosurgery prompted the exploration of its role in the management of cavernous malformations. A significant decrease in the symptomatic hemorrhage rate following stereotactic radiosurgery of cerebral CM suggests that this technique is an effective management strategy for patients with hemorrhagic malformations in high-risk brain locations. The reduced hemorrhage rate achieved after a 2-year latency from radiosurgery (1%) approaches the low risk (0.6%) identified in many natural history studies for non-hemorrhagic CMs [2, 7–11]. The lack of options for surgically inaccessible CMs has made radiosurgery the only alternative to conservative management for lesions with a high risk of symptomatic bleeding.

Methods

Computerized searches of published literature (primary sources), hand searches of published literature (secondary sources) and searches of electronic clinical databases were performed. Medline and Pubmed searches were completed for the years 1971 to March 2011. Search terms included 'cavernous malformations', 'CCM' and 'stereotactic radiosurgery'. Bibliographies from recently published reviews were reviewed, and relevant articles were retrieved.

Outcomes Considered

Reduction in hemorrhage rate was the primary end point of interest. Additional outcome end points included resolution or an improvement in symptoms and improvement in the existing neurological deficits, maintenance of quality of life, and prevention of adverse radiation effects.

Major Recommendations

Diagnosis

- MRI is the modality of choice for the diagnosis and follow-up of patients as well as the assessment of family members in whom similar lesions are suspected.
- MRI findings of parenchymal CMs demonstrate typical, popcorn-like, well-circumscribed, well-delineated lesions. The core is formed by multiple foci of mixed signal intensities, which represents hemorrhage in various stages of evolution. Acute hematoma is shown by a deoxyhemoglobin signal that is isointense on T_1-weighted images and markedly hypointense on T_2-weighted images. Subacute hematoma, which contains extracellular methemoglobin, displays hyperintensity on both T_1- and T_2-weighted images because of the paramagnetic effect of the methemoglobin. The interspersed fibrous-containing elements demonstrate mild hypointensity on both T_1- and T_2-weighted images because they contain a combination of calcification and hemosiderin. The heterogeneous core is typically surrounded completely by a low-signal-intensity hemosiderin rim on T_1-weighted images. The hypointensity of this rim becomes more prominent on T_2-weighted images.
- Typically, CMs are not associated with mass effect or edema and do not demonstrate a feeding artery or draining vein, except when associated with other vascular malformations.
- CMs can be associated with DVAs, which typically demonstrate a prominent medullary vein with the *classic caput medusae* pattern of drainage.
- When the lesions occur in combination with other types of vascular malformations, as they do in as many as 30% of patients, angiography can help further define the lesions. Most CMs are avascular masses on conventional angiograms.

Management Options

- Asymptomatic low-risk CMs may not need any active management. Symptomatic CMs are considered for treatment.
- In older patients with lesions which are difficult to reach surgically, observation with periodic imaging may be appropriate.
- For patients with recurrent hemorrhages, progressive neurological deterioration, or intractable epilepsy surgery or radiosurgery should be considered.
- The management option for a patient with a CM must be based on the exact location of the lesion and its surgical accessibility.
- Surgery has the advantage of immediate elimination of the lesion with stabilization of symptoms if a complete resection can be performed. However, attempted resection of deep-seated lesions may be associated with serious morbidity.
- For younger patients with more accessible lesions, surgical removal may help control epilepsy, improve neurological deficits and prevent any subsequent hemorrhage.

- Radiosurgery is a minimally invasive option for patients presenting with recurrent hemorrhages from deep-seated CMs.
- Radiosurgery alone may be the choice for patients with a high risk of intracranial hemorrhage (patients with 2 or more prior hemorrhages, deep location).
- It is important to ascertain the presence of associated DVAs, as these are composed of functional venous channels that should not be resected or undergo radiosurgery because of the risk for venous infarction.

Patient Selection

- The selection of patients suitable for radiosurgery is dependent on prior bleeding history, age of the patient, existing comorbidities, anatomical location of CM and severity of clinical symptoms.
- Some CM patients will have previously undergone attempted resection. The optimal time between prior surgery and radiosurgery is not known, but generally waiting for a period of several weeks is considered optimal.

Target Definition

- The malformation is defined as the region characterized by a mixed signal intensity within an outer hemosiderin ring, typified by a low signal intensity. Hematoma eccentric from the malformation is excluded from dose planning.
- Targeting within the MRI-defined T_2-weighted signal hemosiderin rim is very important because radiation delivered to the iron-impregnated gliotic brain surrounding the CM may increase the risk of adverse radiation effects.

Dose Planning Technique

- All patients must have stereotactic MRI in order to target the CM. Contrast-enhanced MRI using gradient-recalled acquisitions (1–2 mm slice thickness) supplemented with T_2-weighted (2–3 mm) sequences is preferred.
- The prescription isodose should include the mixed signal intensity malformation but not the high T_2-weighted signal intensity region surrounding it. Single or multiple isocenter dose plans are used to construct a conformal and highly selective radiosurgical volume that matches the 3-dimensional malformation margin [8]. The 50% or greater isodose is used to prescribe the margin dose (fig. 1).
- Associated DVAs are excluded from dose planning.

Dose Selection

- The dose selection for volumetric conformal stereotactic CM radiosurgery is largely based on prior radiosurgery experience. Typically, the dose is less than that used for arteriovenous malformations of similar volumes.
- The doses depend on location and volume of the CMs. Doses at the margin of the CMs typically range from 12 to 18 Gy (median 16 Gy) in a single radiosurgical procedure [8].

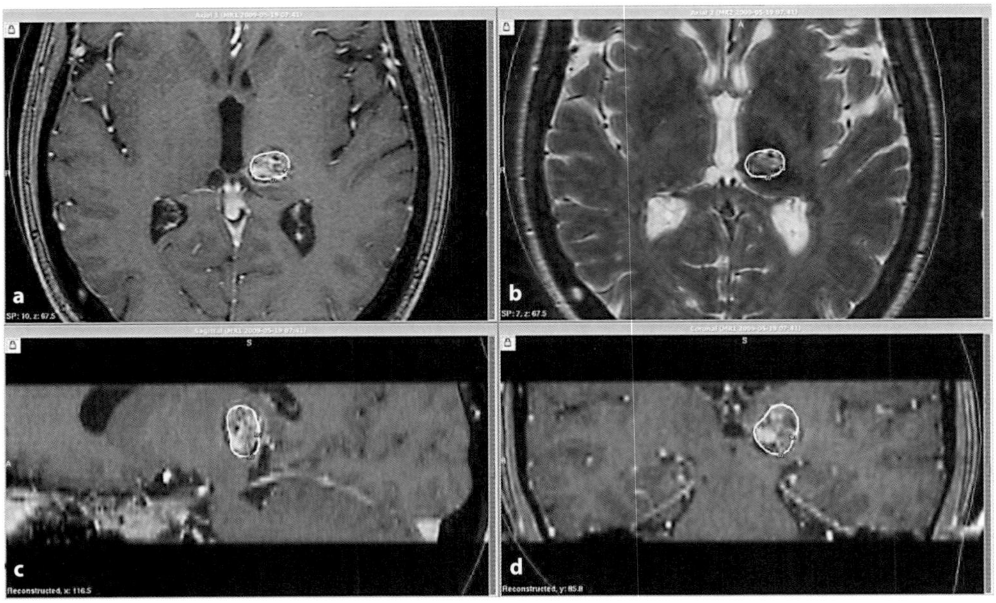

Fig. 1. A 51-year-old female presented with 2 symptomatic intracranial hemorrhages. MRI showed a left thalamic CM. A conformal radiosurgery dose plan was designed using contrast-enhanced spoiled gradient-recalled acquisition in steady state (**a**) and T_2-weighted (**b**) images with sagittal (**c**) and coronal reconstruction (**d**). A margin dose of 15 Gy (maximum dose = 30 Gy) was prescribed to the 50% isodose line.

- The margin of the CM dose is usually 50–70% of the central target dose. A sharp fall-off of the radiation dose outside of the target volume is required.

Medical Management
- Patients usually receive a single dose (40 mg) of methylprednisolone at the conclusion of the radiosurgery procedure. They can continue to take their other medications (e.g. antiepileptics, analgesics) during and after the procedure as recommended by their physicians.
- Those patients who are maintained on antiepileptic drugs to manage seizures should have their blood levels of antiepileptic drugs checked on the day of radiosurgery to make sure that a therapeutic level is maintained at the time of radiosurgery.

Follow-Up Evaluations
- Postradiosurgical clinical examinations and MR studies are requested at 6-month intervals for 2 years and then yearly to assess the effect of radiosurgery on CMs and detect any adverse radiation effect (fig. 2).
- Patients are requested to report symptoms such as severe headache, and MRI is requested to document the evidence of hemorrhage.

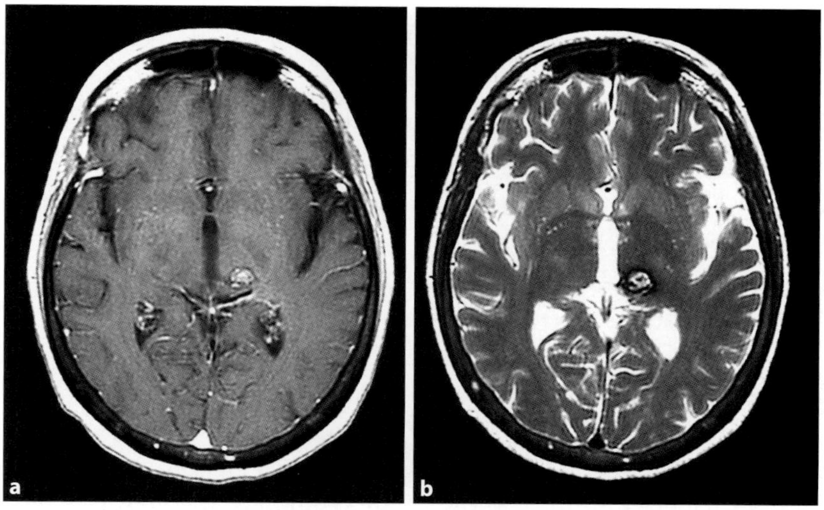

Fig. 2. One-year follow-up MRI after radiosurgery showing stable appearance of the CM on T_1- (**a**) and T_2- weighted (**b**) MRI, without evidence of new hemorrhage.

Patient Counseling

- Patients should be informed that all reports on CM radiosurgery are based on clinical outcome because CM obliteration cannot be documented using any of the available imaging modalities. Without this documentation, patients cannot be declared as 'cured' after radiosurgery. Although patients may be encouraged by a reduction in hemorrhage risk, they cannot be told that this risk is eliminated.
- Although radiosurgery significantly lowers the risk of subsequent hemorrhages, especially after a latency interval of approximately 2 years, patients should be monitored to detect potential complications or rebleeding after radiosurgery.
- These risks and benefits must be carefully balanced against the natural history of untreated lesions if the use of radiosurgery is considered.

Postradiosurgery Imaging Changes

- The probability of developing postradiosurgery imaging changes compatible with adverse radiation effects depends on the CM marginal dose and treatment volume. The volume of tissue receiving 12 Gy or more (the 12-Gy volume) provides predictive information about the probability of developing such imaging changes.

Potential Benefits of Radiosurgery

- Published studies have shown a significant reduction in hemorrhage rate after stereotactic radiosurgery for CMs and a satisfactory (10–18%) rate of adverse radiation effects.

- Potential successful outcomes include absence of new neurological deficit and long-term prevention of further bleeding events.

Subgroups Most Likely to Benefit

Radiosurgery may be especially suitable for the following group of patients:

- patients with 2 or more prior hemorrhages (a subgroup that has an increased risk of further bleeding events);
- patients with excessive medical comorbidity risk factors for surgical excision;
- patients with CMs in locations where surgery may result in severe neurological deficits;
- patients with CMs considered unsuitable for resection.

Clinical Algorithm

The treatment of CMs depends on the severity of the symptoms, the perceived risk for intracranial hemorrhage, and their location. Most high-risk CMs (those with 2 or more documented bleeding events) warrant consideration of treatment because they carry a high probability (30% per year) of additional intracranial hemorrhages or neurological deterioration. When a patient is diagnosed with a CM, the reason that led to the detection of the lesion must be factored into the final decision as to what, if any, treatment should be offered. Neurological complication risks are increased in patients whose CM lies in critical locations in the brain and brainstem. The rate of these complications must be carefully balanced against the natural history of the lesion itself. It is important to ascertain the presence of DVAs, as these are composed of functional venous channels that should not be resected or undergo radiosurgery because of the risk for venous ischemia or infarction. Increasingly, DVAs are identified in association with CMs [3].

A number of factors are considered in making a recommendation. These factors include:

1 the patient's age;
2 the perceived risk for intracranial hemorrhage;
3 history of prior bleed;
4 location of CM;
5 feasibility of successful resection.

A broad outline of the management algorithm is shown in figure 3; however, the final recommendation is usually influenced by the recommending neurosurgeon's training, experience and patient preference (fig. 3).

Is CM Radiosurgery Still Controversial?

There are several published reports from centers of excellence that discuss the role of radiosurgery for patients with CMs based on a documented significant reduction in hemorrhage rate [2, 7–11]. Still, CM radiosurgery is considered controversial by some physicians who consider radiosurgery to be ineffective and associated with a

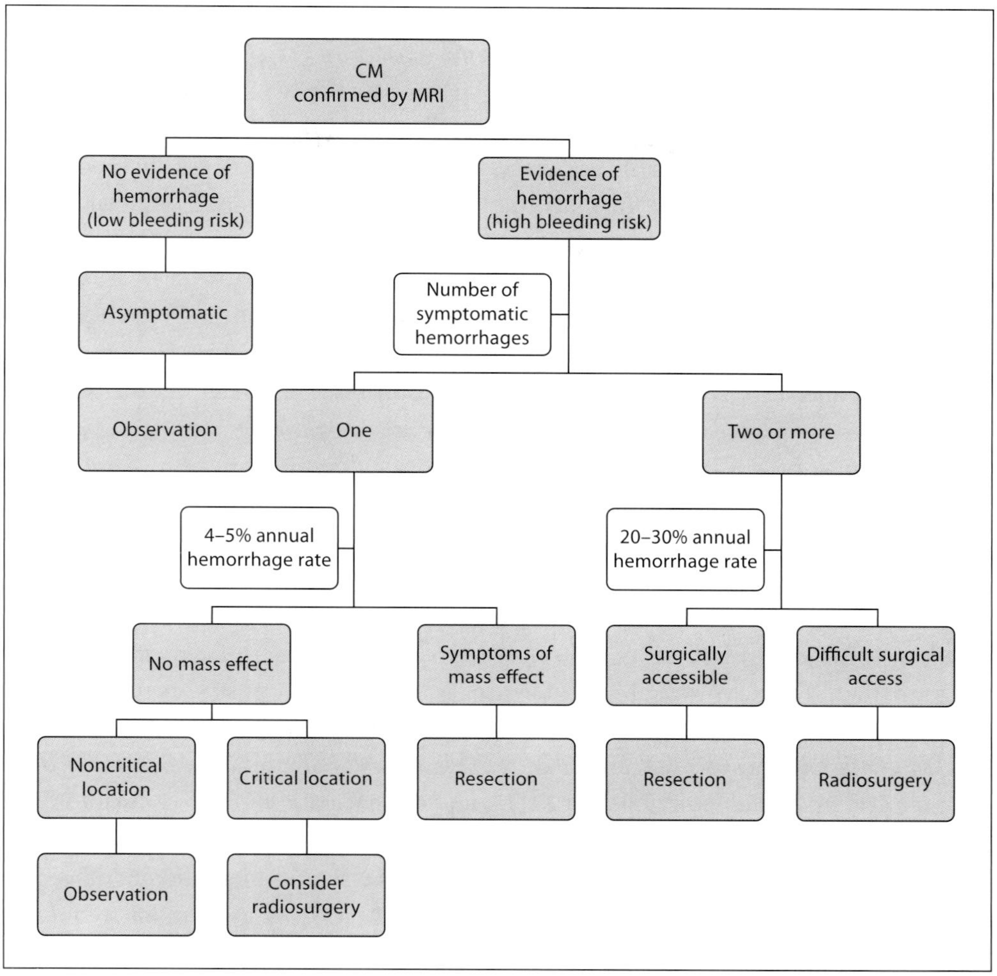

Fig. 3. Proposed management algorithm for patients with intracranial CMs.

high rate of complications [12]. We believe that this variance in the assessment of the role of radiosurgery is due to differences in radiosurgical techniques, experience, and selection and training bias.

The controversy also arises in part from the absence of an imaging modality that can clearly demonstrate response to radiosurgery. Unlike arteriovenous malformation radiosurgery (wherein follow-up angiography can demonstrate complete obliteration of the nidus), follow-up MRI of CMs rarely shows major lesion volume reduction or disappearance. In fact, the purpose of follow-up MRIs is to detect adverse radiation effects, resolution of a prior hemorrhage or a new bleeding event. The poorly understood natural history of CMs and the heterogeneity of the patient population (solitary vs. multiple, congenital vs. de novo) further complicate assessment of the hemorrhage prevention benefits of radiosurgery.

Opponents of radiosurgery for CMs argue that patient outcome following radiosurgery remains unsatisfactory. This opinion is based on the poor outcome in their own CM radiosurgery experience. Such experience bias may be related to variations in the quality of imaging needed to define the target and the radiosurgery technique itself. Appropriate definition of the target volume (exclusion of venous anomalies and hemosiderin staining the normal brain around the malformation) is needed. The radiosurgical technology itself must be able to deliver a highly conformal radiation volume with sharp selectivity that reduces the radiation dose to the hemosiderin-impregnated brain volume that surrounds the CM itself. Significant variance exists among the technologies used to deliver radiosurgery (particle beams, modified linear accelerators and the Gamma Knife®). Enhanced long-term results of radiosurgery are noted as the experience of the responsible physicians increases.

Opponents of the use of radiosurgery also suggest that the long-term hemorrhage rate (>2 years) reduction documented after radiosurgery may be part of the natural history of this disease. The intermediate period of a higher hemorrhage rate may simply be reflective of an increased hemorrhage rate following an initial hemorrhage (i.e. temporal hemorrhage clustering). Radiosurgery opponents hypothesize that observation may result in similar results as those noted after radiosurgery. Advocates of radiosurgery suggest that its availability increases the treatment options in patients who have deep-seated or high-risk CMs that are unsuitable for microsurgical removal.

CM patients who are asymptomatic warrant serial imaging studies and periodic clinical assessments. Published data suggests that patients with 2 symptomatic hemorrhages have a 32% annual risk for another symptomatic event in contrast to a 0.6% annual risk in those who have not had a prior symptomatic hemorrhage [8]. These patients are considered for intervention. Resection is used most frequently for hemorrhagic malformations or those causing symptoms when the malformation is accessible with acceptable risks [13, 14]. Radiosurgery is offered in the setting of symptomatic, hemorrhagic CMs for which resection is believed to be an unacceptable choice [2, 8, 15–19].

References

1 Aiba T, Tanaka R, Koike T, Kameyama S, Takeda N, Komata T: Natural history of intracranial cavernous malformations. J Neurosurg 1995;83:56–59.

2 Kondziolka D, Lunsford LD, Flickinger JC, Kestle JR: Reduction of hemorrhage risk after stereotactic radiosurgery for cavernous malformations. J Neurosurg 1995;83:825–831.

3 McLaughlin MR, Kondziolka D, Flickinger JC, Lunsford S, Lunsford LD: The prospective natural history of cerebral venous malformations. Neurosurgery 1998;43:195–200, discussion 201.

4 Moriarity JL, Wetzel M, Clatterbuck RE, Javedan S, Sheppard JM, Hoenig-Rigamonti K, et al: The natural history of cavernous malformations: a prospective study of 68 patients. Neurosurgery 1999;44: 1166–1171, discussion 1172–1173.

5 Labauge P, Brunereau L, Levy C, Laberge S, Houtteville JP: The natural history of familial cerebral cavernomas: a retrospective MRI study of 40 patients. Neuroradiology 2000;42:327–332.

6 Muras I, Conforti R, Scuotto A, Rinaldi F, Bernini FP: Cerebral cavernous angioma. Diagnostic considerations. J Neuroradiol 1993;20:34–41.

7 Hasegawa T, McInerney J, Kondziolka D, Lee JY, Flickinger JC, Lunsford LD: Long-term results after stereotactic radiosurgery for patients with cavernous malformations. Neurosurgery 2002;50:1190–1197, discussion 1197–1198.
8 Lunsford LD, Khan AA, Niranjan A, Kano H, Flickinger JC, Kondziolka D: Stereotactic radiosurgery for symptomatic solitary cerebral cavernous malformations considered high risk for resection. J Neurosurg 2010;113:23–29.
9 Monaco EA, Khan AA, Niranjan A, Kano H, Grandhi R, Kondziolka D, et al: Stereotactic radiosurgery for the treatment of symptomatic brainstem cavernous malformations. Neurosurg Focus 2010; 29:E11.
10 Nagy G, Razak A, Rowe JG, Hodgson TJ, Coley SC, Radatz MW, et al: Stereotactic radiosurgery for deep-seated cavernous malformations: a move toward more active, early intervention. Clinical article. J Neurosurg 2010;113:691–699.
11 Pollock BE, Garces YI, Stafford SL, Foote RL, Schomberg PJ, Link MJ: Stereotactic radiosurgery for cavernous malformations. J Neurosurg 2000;93: 987–991.
12 Steiner L, Karlsson B, Yen CP, Torner JC, Lindquist C, Schlesinger D: Radiosurgery in cavernous malformations: anatomy of a controversy. J Neurosurg 2010;113:16–21, discussion 22.
13 Mathiesen T, Edner G, Kihlstrom L: Deep and brainstem cavernomas: a consecutive 8-year series. J Neurosurg 2003;99:31–37.
14 Samii M, Eghbal R, Carvalho GA, Matthies C: Surgical management of brainstem cavernomas. J Neurosurg 2001;95:825–832.
15 Amin-Hanjani S, Ogilvy CS, Candia GJ, Lyons S, Chapman PH: Stereotactic radiosurgery for cavernous malformations: Kjellberg's experience with proton beam therapy in 98 cases at the Harvard Cyclotron. Neurosurgery 1998;42:1229–1236, discussion 1236–1238.
16 Chang SD, Levy RP, Adler JR Jr, Martin DP, Krakovitz PR, Steinberg GK: Stereotactic radiosurgery of angiographically occult vascular malformations: 14-year experience. Neurosurgery 1998;43: 213–220, discussion 220–221.
17 Kida Y, Kobayashi T, Mori Y: Radiosurgery of angiographically occult vascular malformations. Neurosurg Clin North Am 1999;10:291–303.
18 Kim DG, Choe WJ, Paek SH, Chung HT, Kim IH, Han DH: Radiosurgery of intracranial cavernous malformations. Acta Neurochir 2002;144:869–878, discussion 878.
19 Liscak R, Vladyka V, Simonova G, Vymazal J, Novotny J Jr: Gamma knife surgery of brain cavernous hemangiomas. J Neurosurg 2005;102(suppl): 207–213.

Ajay Niranjan, MCh, MBA
Department of Neurological Surgery, University of Pittsburgh Medical Center, Suite B-400
200 Lothrop Street
Pittsburgh, PA 15213 (USA)
Tel. +1 412 647 6250, E-Mail niranjana@upmc.edu

Niranjan A, Kano H, Lunsford LD (eds): Gamma Knife Radiosurgery for Brain Vascular Malformations.
Prog Neurol Surg. Basel, Karger, 2013, vol 27, pp 176–194 (DOI: 10.1159/000341793)

Intracranial Dural Arteriovenous Fistulas: Natural History and Rationale for Treatment with Stereotactic Radiosurgery

David Hung-Chi Pan[a,c] · Hsiu-Mei Wu[b,c] · Yu-Hung Kuo[a,d] · Wen-Yuh Chung[a,c] · Cheng-Chia Lee[a,c] · Wan-You Guo[b,c]

Departments of [a]Neurosurgery and [b]Radiology, Taipei Veterans General Hospital, and [c]School of Medicine, National Yang-Ming University, Taipei, Taiwan, ROC; [d]Division of Neurosurgery, Albany Medical Center, Albany, N.Y., USA

Abstract

Dural arteriovenous fistulas (DAVFs) are abnormal arteriovenous communications within the dura. The symptoms depend on their location and the pattern of the venous drainage. Patients with cavernous sinus DAVFs often present with ocular manifestations such as exophthalmos, chemosis and diplopia. Patients with transverse or sigmoid sinus DAVFs frequently experience headache and tinnitus on the affected side. DAVFs with anterograde sinus or cortical venous drainage (CVD) have been clinically regarded as benign, whereas DAVFs with retrograde CVD are considered aggressive in behavior. Similar to other cerebral arteriovenous malformations, DAVFs can hemorrhage, with an estimated annual risk of approximately 1.8%. The recommended therapeutic intervention for a DAVF is dependent on the anticipated natural history of the lesion. Management options include surgical resection, embolization and radiosurgery. Radiosurgical treatment has been used for DAVFs in various locations including the anterior cranial fossa, cavernous sinus, transverse/sigmoid sinus, superior sagittal sinus and tentorium. We present an update on 321 DAVF patients treated at the Taipei Veterans General Hospital using Gamma Knife radiosurgery. The prescribed mean margin dose was 17.2 Gy. In our series, 98% of patients had a stable or improved clinical condition after radiosurgery. Stereotactic radiosurgery using the Gamma Knife is a safe and effective alternative for the treatment of DAVFs.

Intracranial dural arteriovenous fistulas (DAVFs) are abnormal arteriovenous communications within the dura, in which meningeal arteries shunt blood directly into the dural sinus or leptomeningeal veins [1, 2]. The incidence of DAVFs has been estimated at 5–20% of all intracranial vascular malformations [3–5]. DAVFs comprise only 6% of supratentorial vascular malformations whereas they constitute 35% of infratentorial malformations [6]. The mean age of presentation for a DAVF is

50–60 years of age with no sex preference, though there is a wide range seen [7, 8]. Unlike the more common intracerebral or parenchymal arteriovenous malformations (AVMs), DAVFs are thought to be acquired in origin due to inflammation, thrombosis or trauma of the dural sinus. However, in many cases the exact etiology and underlying disease are difficult to trace and those DAVFs are considered idiopathic [9, 10]. DAVFs most commonly occur in the regions of the cavernous sinus (CS), transverse/sigmoid sinuses, tentorium/torcula, or cerebral convexities with drainage to the superior sagittal sinus [1, 11, 12].

A thorough understanding of DAVF hemodynamics requires a detailed cerebral angiographic investigation. Drainage of the venous flow from a DAVF can be antegrade or retrograde through a dural sinus, through a cortical vein or both. The pattern of the venous drainage is not necessarily static though. Gradual alternation in the venous flow from antegrade to retrograde, and delayed recruitment of arterial feeders into the nidus (sump effect) have been observed in some patients [3, 8]. This is hypothesized to occur as a result of progressive sinus hypertension with redirection of the blood flow into cortical veins [2, 11, 13]. The gradual venous hypertension and reflux of the cortical veins may eventually predispose to the risks of cerebral hemorrhage and/or other neurological deficits [1].

Not all DAVFs demonstrate such a progressive clinical course though. Although not frequently seen, some DAVFs can regress and thrombose gradually resulting in a spontaneous cure [14, 15]. The factors predisposing to DAVF progression or involution have not been clearly clarified.

Natural Course

The clinical presentation of a DAVF is dependent on its location and pattern of the venous drainage. Patients with CS DAVFs often have ocular manifestations (exophthalmos, chemosis, visual impairment and diplopia). Those with lateral tentorial (transverse/sigmoid sinus) lesions frequently complain of headache and pulse-synchronous tinnitus on the affected side. DAVFs with anterograde sinus or cortical venous drainage (CVD) have been clinically regarded as benign, whereas DAVFs with retrograde CVD are considered aggressive in behavior [8, 16, 17]. In 1990, Awad et al. [1] reported a meta-analysis of 377 DAVFs and defined 100 aggressive cases as those with hemorrhages or progressive focal neurological deficits; the other 277 DAVFs were defined as benign cases. They concluded that no location of the DAVFs was immune from the aggressive neurological behavior. The factors that predict aggressive neurological presentation included leptomeningeal venous drainage, variceal or aneurysmal venous dilation, and galenic drainage of the DAVFs.

Similar to other cerebral AVMs, DAVFs can hemorrhage, with an estimated annual risk of approximately 1.8% [7]. Van Dijk et al. [17] in 2002 reported that persistence of the cortical venous reflux in DAVFs yields an annual hemorrhage rate of 8.1% and a mortality rate of 10.4%. Duffau et al. [18] reported a high risk of early rebleeding (35% within 2 weeks) after the first episode of hemorrhage, with graver consequences from the second bleed. Söderman et al. [19] in 2008 evaluated the hemorrhage rate in their 85 cases of DAVFs with retrograde CVD. They found a lower hemorrhage rate compared to those of the other previous reports. In their patients already presenting with an intracranial hemorrhage, the annual risk for the recurrent hemorrhage was 7.4% while in those patients not presenting with a hemorrhage, the bleeding rate was approximately 1.5% per year [19].

Classifications

Two main classification systems have been proposed. The Borden-Shucart system distinguishes DAVFs depending on the site of drainage and the presence of CVD [13]. Type I DAVFs drain directly into the sinus or meningeal veins with antegrade flow, whereas type II DAVFs have retrograde flow through the sinus into the subarachnoid veins. Type III DAVFs directly drain into the subarachnoid veins in a retrograde fashion.

The system of Cognard et al. [11] similarly separates DAVFs depending on the site of drainage and the presence of CVD, but also considers the direction of flow through the draining vein as well as the presence of cortical venous ectasia. Cognard type I DAVFs have solely antegrade sinus drainage, similar to the Borden-Shucart system. Cognard type II DAVFs demonstrate retrograde drainage and are subdivided depending on whether drainage is through the sinus (IIa), cortical vein (IIb) or both (IIa + b). Cognard type III DAVFs drain directly into cortical veins similar to Borden-Shucart types, but the Cognard classification gives lesions with venous ectasia a separate designation of type IV. DAVFs that drain into spinal perimedullary veins are designated Cognard type V. The authors present their series of 258 patients and demonstrate a correlation between DAVF type and rate of aggressive clinical symptoms and risk of hemorrhage.

Therapeutic Methods

The recommended therapeutic intervention for a DAVF is dependent on the anticipated natural history of the lesion. For lesions with antegrade sinus drainage (Borden type I) and benign clinical manifestations, intervention is usually palliative or observational unless the patient's symptoms are intolerable [5, 8]. Vigilance is prudent though as conversion in flow pattern can occur in approximately 2% of patients, elevating the risks of developing new neurological deficits [8, 11]. For DAVFs with intolerable symptoms, progressive neurological deficits or elevated risk of hemorrhage, intervention is recommended [11, 13, 20].

Advances in the field of interventional neuroradiology have increased treatment options for patients with DAVFs. Obliteration of the fistula can be attempted through a transarterial or transvenous route. Transarterial embolization alone rarely leads to a complete obliteration of the DAVF, because there are usually numerous arterial feeders to the nidus. The purpose of a transarterial approach is mainly the reduction of arterial feeders and the palliative symptomatic relief [21]. For curative treatment, additional treatment through a retrograde transvenous approach may be necessary. In transvenous embolization, superselective disconnection of the refluxing vein is preferred over sacrifice of the dural sinus, although this sometimes becomes necessary to achieve a cure [21]. Endovascular therapy can also be combined with surgery or radiosurgery when it is not feasible to completely obliterate a DAVF alone.

An open surgical approach is indicated for DAVFs with aggressive features that are not amenable to comprehensive endovascular treatment. Typically, lesions involving the anterior cranial fossa or tentorial incisura are associated with hemorrhage, and surgical intervention is indicated. Surgical strategies include ligation of the fistula at the junction with the drainage vein, interruption of arterial feeders, coagulation and/or excision of the fistula in the dura, and resection of the involved sinus [22–24]. Recent studies have suggested that disconnection of the draining vein alone without resection of the sinus is equally efficacious as resection of the fistula. The former can avoid risks of venous hypertension associated with the sinus removal, particularly where the sinus is patent [25–28]. Reported morbidity and mortality of surgical intervention have ranged from 0–13% [29].

Stereotactic radiosurgery has long been used for treatment of intraparenchymal AVMs, and treatment of DAVFs would be a natural extension of this [30–32]. Radiosurgical treatment has been delivered for DAVFs in various locations including the anterior cranial fossa, CS, transverse/sigmoid sinus, superior sagittal sinus and tentorium [33–42]. Guo et al. [35] and Pollock et al. [40] have separately reported an approximately 80% obliteration rate for CS DAVFs treated by Gamma Knife alone or combined with embolization. More recently, Söderman et al. [5] reported on 49 patients with 52 DAVFs, with a 68% obliteration rate and another 24% with flow regression at 2 years. Radiosurgery is often combined with endovascular therapy to provide immediate relief of symptoms and possibly reduction in hemorrhagic risk [12, 34, 36, 37, 43–45]. Complete and partial obliteration rates are similar to those reported for radiosurgery alone, as are the rates of symptomatic improvement. While the early experience at the Taipei Veterans General Hospital using Gamma Knife radiosurgery (GKRS) to treat DAVFs have been published before [35, 39, 42], we present here an update to our experience treating DAVFs with radiosurgery with an additional 83 patients and longer length of follow-up.

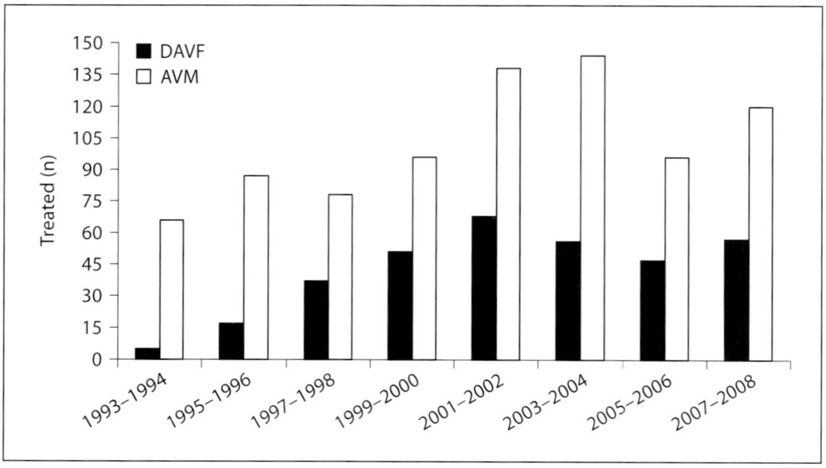

Fig. 1. Number of AVMs and DAVFs treated biennially by GKRS at the Taipei Veterans General Hospital between 1993 and 2008.

The Taipei Veterans General Hospital Experience in Treating Dural Arteriovenous Fistulas with the Gamma Knife

Patients and Classifications

Between 1993 and 2008, a total of 1,395 patients with intracranial vascular lesions were treated using GKRS at the Taipei Veterans General Hospital. 23% of these vascular malformations (321 patients) were DAVFs, a rate higher than that reported by others [4, 5, 12, 46, 47]. One possible explanation for the higher incidence at our institution is a greater awareness of the possibility of a DAVF and a higher rate of early detection of these lesions by radiological imaging [20]. This finding may thus reflect both the patient referral pattern and treatment bias at our institution. Figure 1 demonstrates the number of AVMs and DAVFs treated biennially at our institution between 1993 and 2008.

Of our 321 DAVF patients, 141 (44%) were male and 180 (56%) were female. The age at the time of GKRS ranged from 17 to 81 years (mean 57.8 years). Two potential inciting factors for DAVF formation could be traced: 31 patients (13.4%) had a history of head trauma and 14 patients (6%) had a history of head and neck surgery prior to their DAVF diagnosis. Table 1 shows the anatomical localization of the DAVFs in our patients. The most common locations are the CS (206 cases) followed by the transverse/sigmoid sinus (72 cases), which together account for 86.6% of the cases. Owing to the unique clinical characteristics of DAVFs involving the CS, we divided the DAVFs into two groups: the CS group and the non-cavernous-sinus (NCS) group. For the CS group, we applied Barrow's classification to describe the feeding arteries to the CS DAVF (table 2). All DAVFs were also classified based on their angiographic venous drainage pattern using the systems of Borden-Shucart

Table 1. Location of DAVFs in 321 patients treated by GKRS

	Number	Percentage
Cavernous sinus	206	64.2
Transverse/sigmoid sinus	72	22.4
Petrosal sinus	9	2.8
Superior sagittal sinus	8	2.5
Others		
Tentorium	9	2.8
Frontal base (anterior fossa)	6	1.9
Sphenoparietal	4	1.2
Vein of Galen	2	0.6
Jugular foramen	2	0.6
Clivus	2	0.6
Foramen magnum	1	0.3
Total	321	100.0

Table 2. Barrow classification of CS DAVFs

	Number of cases	Percentage
A (direct)	0	0.0
B (indirect, ICA feeding)	19	9.2
C (indirect, ECA feeding)	12	5.8
D (indirect, both ICA and ECA feeding)	175	85.0
Total	206	100.0

ICA = Internal carotid artery; ECA = external carotid artery.

and Cognard (table 3) [11, 13]. Of the 115 NCS DAVFs, 63 cases were Borden type I (Cognard types I and IIa) with solely dural sinus drainage, and thus considered clinically benign [8, 16, 21]. The remaining 52 cases were Borden type II or III (Cognard type IIb, III, IV, V), demonstrating retrograde CVD and thus considered clinically 'aggressive' [14, 17].

Patients with CS DAVFs frequently presented with symptoms related to ocular functions including red eyes, proptosis, chemosis, visual impairment and diplopia. The duration of clinical symptoms prior to diagnosis of CS DAVFs ranged from 1 to 38 months (median 4 and mean 6 months). Seven of the CS DAVF patients (3.4% of CS DAVFs) experienced an intracranial hemorrhage before treatment.

Table 3. Cognard and Borden classifications of 115 patients with NCS DAVFs

	Number	Percentage
Cognard type		
I	25	21.7
IIa	38	33.0
IIb	9	7.8
IIa + IIb	26	22.6
III	6	5.2
IV	8	7.0
V	3	2.6
Total	115	100.0
Borden type		
I (sinus drainage)	63	54.8
II (sinus drainage with retrograde venous filling)	35	30.4
III (retrograde drainage to cortical veins only)	17	14.8
Total	115	100.0

In the NCS DAVFs, the clinical manifestations and severity of symptoms were more varied depending on location of the fistula and pattern of the venous drainage. For the 72 patients with transverse/sigmoid sinus DAVFs, pulsatile tinnitus and headache were the most common symptoms. Hemorrhage before treatment occurred in 8 (11.1%) of the 72 patients and nonhemorrhagic neurological deficits developed in 27 (37.5%) patients. For the 9 patients with DAVFs involving the tentorium, 6 (67%) were Borden type II/III, and 2 (22.2%) had history of previous hemorrhage. Arteriovenous shunts involving the anterior skull base were all aggressive and harbored a high risk of hemorrhage (3 of 6 patients). For the 115 patients with NCS DAVFs, 16 (14%) had hemorrhagic events prior to diagnosis, and 43 (37%) suffered from persistent or slowly progressive neurological deficits (table 4).

We also analyzed the relationship between DAVF types and duration of symptoms in NCS DAVFs (table 5). The average duration of symptoms before diagnosis in Borden type I (Cognard type I and type IIa) patients was 19.2 months (range 3–168 months). For Borden type II (Cognard type IIb and type IIa + b) patients, the average duration of symptoms was 39.1 months (range 2–180 months). For Borden type III (Cognard type III, IV and type V) patients, the average duration of symptoms was 23.7 months (range 1–144 months). This longer duration of symptoms seen with a higher grade DAVFs suggests that DAVFs with retrograde CVD may be present for longer prior to diagnosis (p value <0.0001 between Borden type I and type II/III, independent t test).

Table 4. Incidence of intracerebral hemorrhage (ICH) and nonhemorrhagic neurological deficit (NHND) before GKRS in 321 patients with DAVFs

	Patients	ICH	NHND
Cavernous sinus	206	7 (3.4%)	9 (4.4%)
Transverse/sigmoid sinus	72	8 (11.1%)	27 (37.5%)
Petrosal sinus	9	1 (11.1%)	4 (44.4%)
Superior sagittal sinus	8	0 (–)	3 (37.5%)
Tentorium	9	2 (22.2%)	4 (44.4%)
Frontal base (anterior fossa)	6	3 (50%)	3 (50%)
Sphenoparietal	4	2 (50%)	0 (–)
Vein of Galen	2	0 (–)	1 (50%)
Jugular foramen	2	0 (–)	0 (–)
Clivus	2	0 (–)	0 (–)
Foramen magnum	1	0 (–)	1 (100.0%)
Total	321	23 (7.2%)	52 (16.2%)

Nonhemorrhagic neurological deficits include symptoms of hemiparesis, hemiparesthesia, cerebellar sign, dementia and mental confusion.

Table 5. Duration of symptoms before treatment in 115 patients with NCS DAVFs stratified by Borden classification

Borden type	Patients n	Average duration of symptoms months	Range months
I	63	19.2	3–168
II	35	39.1	2–180
III	17	23.7	1–144

Before radiosurgery, some of the patients had attempted other therapies for treatment of the DAVF. Thirteen of the CS DAVFs and 28 of the NCS DAVFs had undergone prior endovascular embolizations from 1 to 4 times in attempts to obliterate the lesion. Thirteen patients who suffered from intracranial hemorrhage from NCS DAVFs had undergone craniotomy for hematoma evacuation and clipping of feeding vessels. GKRS was performed as secondary treatment in these 54 patients due to their residual angiographic filling of the fistula. In 3 patients with CS DAVFs (1.5% of CS DAVFs), spontaneous remission of symptoms or angiographic regression of the DAVFs was seen and no further intervention was taken. The remaining patients underwent radiosurgery as the primary treatment. The indications for radiosurgical treatment are intolerable symptoms (ocular symptoms, headache, pulsatile tinnitus), focal neurological deficits and presence of a residual shunt after other therapeutic modalities.

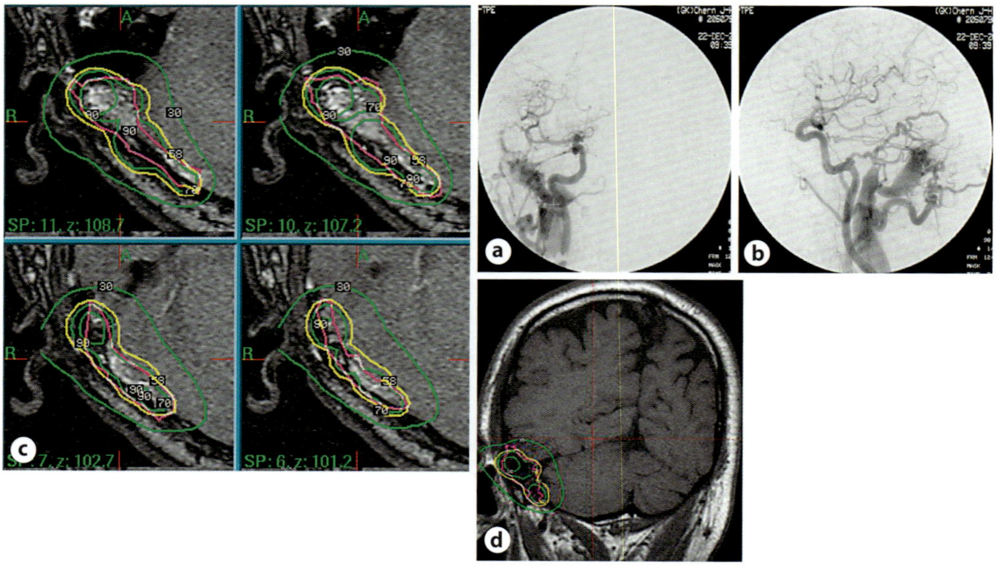

Fig. 2. A case of Borden type I DAVF at the junction of the right transverse and sigmoid sinuses, diagnosed by anteroposterior view (**a**) and lateral view (**b**) of the common carotid angiogram. The Gamma Plan® dose-planning program illustrated a 58% isodose line covering the target volume on serial transaxial time-of-flight MRA images (**c**) and coronal T_1-weighted MRI (**d**). In this case, the peripheral and maximum doses were 17.5 and 30.2 Gy, respectively, with a mean dose of 23.4 Gy. The target volume was 16.1 cm^3.

Radiosurgical Method

The standard GKRS procedure was performed using a Gamma Knife (Elekta AB, Stockholm, Sweden) either with model B (from 1993 to 2006) or model 4C (after 2007). Target localization was performed by integrating imaging data from stereotactic noncontrast magnetic resonance imaging (MRI) including thin-cut axial views time-of-flight magnetic resonance angiography (MRA), and a cerebral X-ray angiogram. Our goal of the treatment was to occlude the fistulous shunts completely. Proper delineation of the treatment target to include all abnormal arteriovenous shunts on the dural sinus wall is crucial for a successful treatment. The target volume was defined along the involved dural sinus wall where the true arteriovenous fistula occurs [2, 3, 48, 49]. The remote arterial feeders and drainage veins distal to the sinus were excluded from the treatment volume, as they were not considered part of the nidus (fig. 2). In our patients, the mean treatment target volume for CS DAVFs was 4.7 cm^3 (range 0.2–28.4 cm^3), whereas NCS DAVFs demonstrated a larger mean treatment volume of 16.9 cm^3 (range 0.8–52 cm^3).

The radiation dose profile is shown in table 6. The prescribed margin doses for both CS and NCS DAVFs were similar, with a mean dose of 17.2 Gy, although the mean maximum dose differed: 25 Gy for CS DAVFs and 30 Gy for NCS DAVFs. For the treatment of CS DAVFs, we preferred to use a large (14 or 18 mm) collimator to

Table 6. Radiation profile of GKRS for the treatment of 321 patients with DAVFs

	CS group	NCS group
Radiation volume, cm^3	4.7 (0.2–28.4)	16.9 (0.8–52)
Maximum dose, Gy	25.2 (18.1–38)	29.9 (20.6–36)
Marginal dose, Gy	17.2 (14–25)	17.2 (15–21)
Isodose level, %	68.5 (50–96)	57.7 (50–90)
Isocenters, n	3.3 (1–14)	13 (1–27)

Figures within parentheses demonstrate the range.

cover the margin of the CS. The average number of isocenters was 3. For the NCS DAVFs, a greater number of isocenters (several large and many small shots) was used to cover the treatment volume, with a mean number of isocenters of 13 (range 1–27). Care was taken to protect the adjacent critical structures such as the optic nerve and brainstem to receive radiation doses less than 8–9 Gy.

Follow-Up Program and Results

Post-GKRS follow-up studies were available in 156 (76%) of the 206 patients with CS DAVFs, and 108 (94%) of the 115 patients with NCS DAVFs. The mean follow-up period for the CS group was 20.8 months (range 1–149 months), while for the NCS group it was 28 months (range 2–141 months). After the GKRS, both a clinical neurological examination and radiographic imaging study (MRI with MRA) were performed at 6-month intervals. Cerebral X-ray angiography was usually performed between 1 and 3 years after GKRS, if complete regression of the lesion had been shown on the MRI (fig. 3). For CS DAVFs, a noninvasive color Doppler ultrasonography examined through eyeballs was performed every 3 months to evaluate flow direction and velocity in the superior ophthalmic vein [50]. Frequently, normalization of the color Doppler ultrasonography was associated with concomitant findings of complete obliteration of DAVF on MRI and cerebral angiography (fig. 4).

Patient outcomes after radiosurgery were grouped into four categories: (1) complete improvement, indicating complete symptomatic relief with complete obliteration of the DAVF on cerebral angiogram and/or MRA; (2) partial improvement, indicating partial resolution of clinical symptoms with >50% regression of the DAVF nidus on MRA; (3) stationary, indicating no change of the DAVF nidus on the follow-up MRA; (4) progression, indicating enlargement or aggressive change of the DAVF nidus on MRA.

Table 7a summarizes the clinical outcomes in our 264 DAVF patients with follow-ups. For the CS DAVFs, 109 of the 156 patients (70%) showed complete improvement, 47 (30%) were partially improved. No lesions were stationary or progressed after radiosurgery. For the NCS DAVFs, 64 of the 108 (59%) showed complete improvement, 40 (37%) were partially improved, 2 (2%) were stationary, 1 (1%) showed progression.

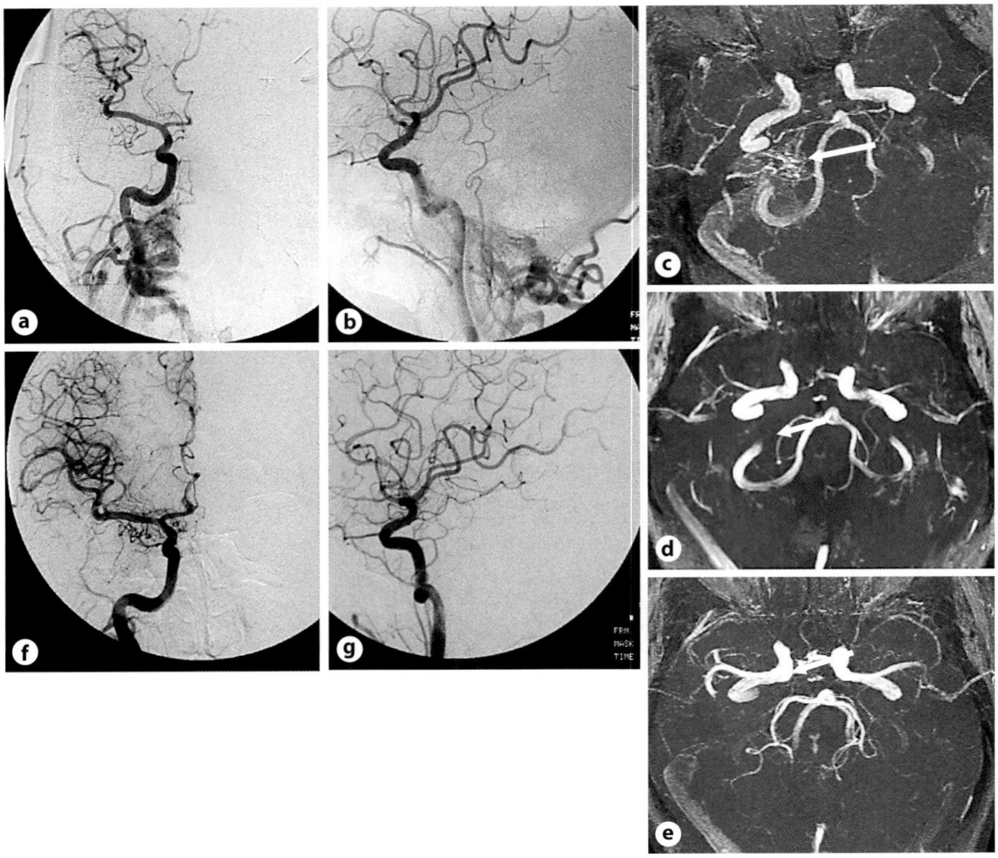

Fig. 3. A case of Borden type I DAVF in the right condylar foramen region on anteroposterior view (**a**) and lateral view (**b**) of the common carotid angiogram. A gradual decrease in the abnormal flow of the DAVF (black arrow) was noted on sequential MRA follow-up images before GKRS (**c**), 6 months after GKRS (**d**) and 20 months after GKRS (**e**). Two years after radiosurgery, the angiogram showed complete obliteration on anteroposterior view (**f**) and lateral view (**g**).

One patient died due to a new intracerebral hemorrhage after treatment. This was a 70-year-old man, with a Borden type III DAVF involving the tentorial region. GKRS was performed in 2002 and the patient had an initially stable course. However, in 2006 (59 months after GKRS), the patient developed a sudden loss of consciousness with intracerebral hemorrhage. Despite emergency craniotomy for evacuation of the hematoma, the patient expired. Thus, the mortality rate for the entire series is 0.4% (1 of 264 with follow-up available). Postradiosurgical hemorrhage due to uncontrollable venous hypertension was found in another patient with an extensive, aggressive DAVF (Borden type II) involving the transverse/sigmoid sinus. This patient recovered from the hemorrhage and improved after further combined treatment with endovascular embolization and repeated radiosurgery.

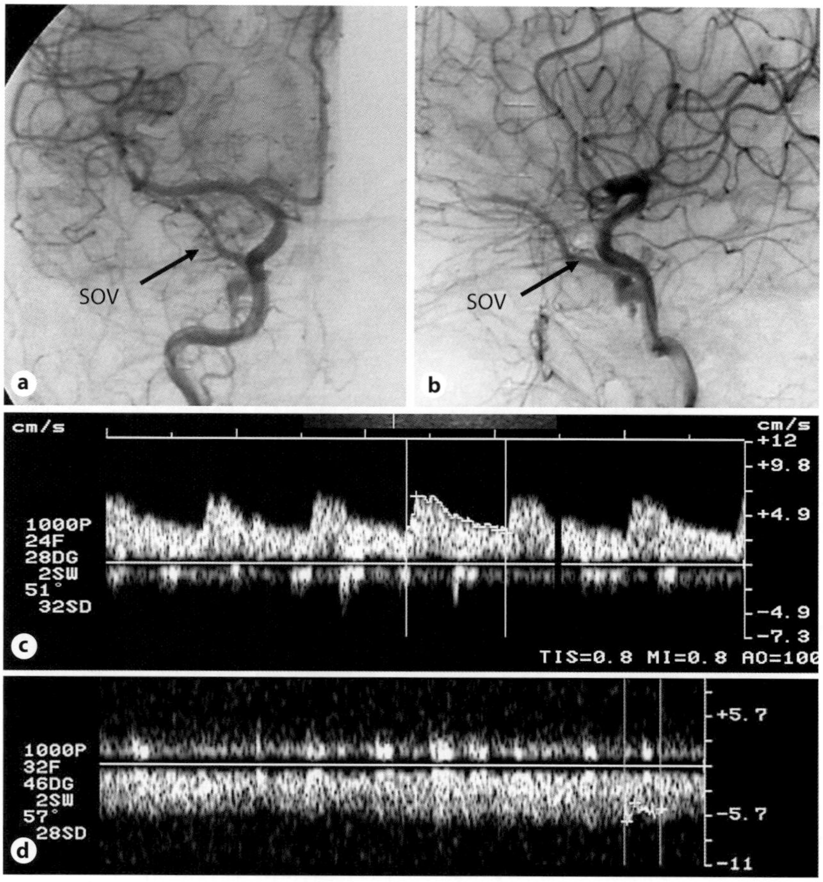

Fig. 4. Color Doppler ultrasound can be used to assess flow patterns of CS DAVF before and after treatment. A case of indirect DAVF at the right cavernous sinus with engorged superior ophthalmic vein (SOV) showing on AP (**a**) and lateral views (**b**) of the common carotid angiogram. (**c**) Color Doppler ultrasonography revealed pulsatile reverse flow of the SOV before radiosurgery. (**d**) Eight months after the treatment, the flow of the SOV returned to normal.

In this series, 98% (260 of 264 patients) had a stable or improved clinical condition after radiosurgery. For the assessment of adverse reactions to radiation on MR images, there was only 1 patient who developed radiation-induced brain edema 6 months after radiosurgery. The edema subsided gradually after steroid treatment.

In order to evaluate the response to GKRS in DAVFs with different venous drainage patterns, we further analyzed treatment results of the 108 patients with NCS DAVFs based on the Borden classification (table 7b). The results show that radiosurgery was effective in treating Borden type I lesions with a 72% complete obliteration rate, while another 28% had partial improvement. However, for Borden type II and III lesions, a lower cure rate was observed. Of the 48 Borden type II and III patients, complete obliteration was observed in 21 (44%), with another 48% showing partial

Table 7. Clinical outcomes after GKRS

a In 264 patients with DAVFs available for neurological and imaging follow-ups

	CS	NCS
Complete improvement	109 (70%)	64 (59%)
Partial improvement	47 (30%)	40 (37%)
Stationary (no change)	–	2 (2%)
Progression	–	1 (1%)
Death	–	1 (1%)
Total	156	108

b In 108 patients with NCS DAVFs stratified by Borden classification

Borden type	Complete improvement	Partial improvement	Stationary	Progression	Death	Total
I	43	17	0	0	0	60
II	12	18	1	1	0	32
III	9	5	1	0	1	16
Total	64	40	2	1	1	108

improvement, 4% stationary lesion and 2% progression. There was 1 mortality as previously described (2%).

For some DAVFs with extensive involvement of dural sinuses and cortical veins, repeated radiosurgery might be necessary for the complete obliteration of the DAVFs. In this current series, a total of 5 CS DAVFs and 14 NCS DAVFs had required repeated radiosurgery 1–3 years after the first treatment. The method and dose selection during the second radiosurgery were similar to the first treatment. Figure 5 shows one such case of repeated radiosurgery for an extensive DAVF involving the transverse/sigmoid sinus.

Discussion

Efficacy of Radiosurgery for DAVF

Due to the greater frequency of intraparenchymal AVMs, the efficacy of radiosurgery for treatment of these lesions has been well established [31, 51–53]. While most case series of DAVFs treated with radiosurgery are smaller than those for intraparenchymal AVMs, sufficient data now exist to support radiosurgical therapy for DAVFs. In 1993, Chandler and Friedman [33] published the first detailed, complete case report of a DAVF treated with radiosurgery with angiographically confirmed obliteration. Since then, a number of publications have appeared which establish a role for radiosurgery in treating DAVFs.

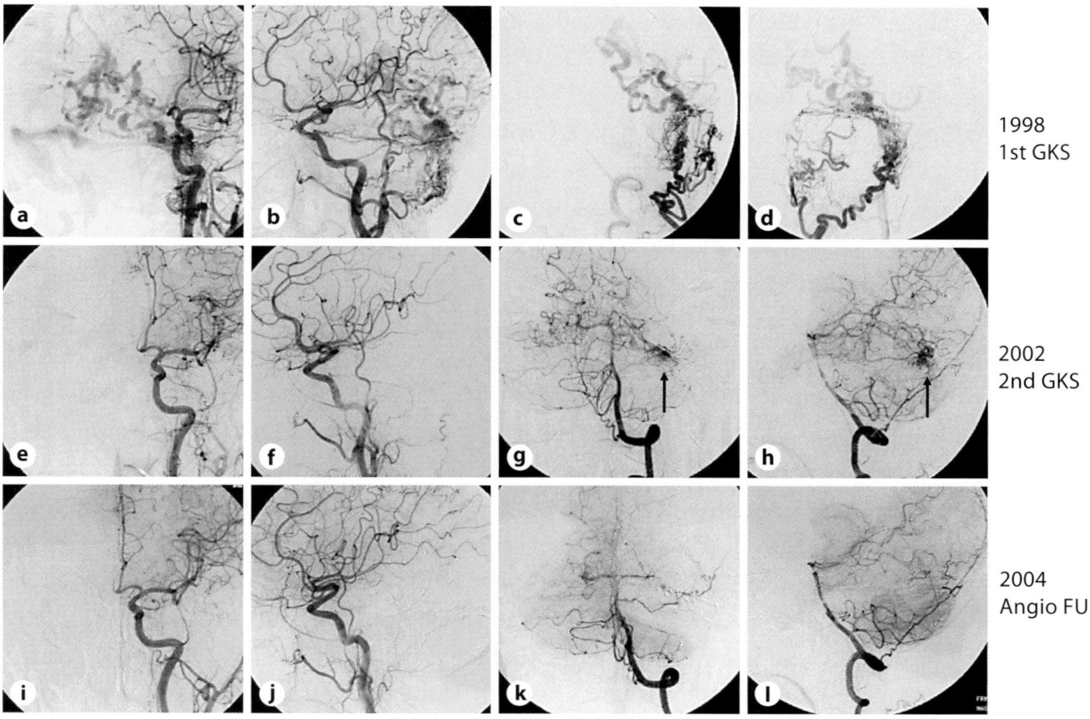

Fig. 5. Common carotid angiogram in anteroposterior (**a**) and lateral views (**b**) showed a Cognard type IIa + b DAVF at the left transverse sinus and torcular region. There were also arterial feedings from muscular branches of the left vertebral artery on anteroposterior (**c**) and lateral vertebral angiograms (**d**). Four years after GKRS, the DAVF was no longer seen on the carotid angiogram (**e**, **f**), but a small residual DAVF nidus (black arrow) supplied by the posterior meningeal artery was noted on the vertebral angiogram (**g**, **h**). A second radiosurgical treatment was performed. Complete obliteration of the DAVF on both carotid (**i, j**) and vertebral angiograms (**k, l**) was achieved 2 years after the second GKRS. Angio-FU = Angiographic follow-up.

At the Taipei Veterans General Hospital, this current study of 264 DAVF patients treated by GKRS in the past 15 years shows a 66% complete obliteration rate, with another 33% of the patients demonstrating a reduction in DAVF size with improvement in symptoms. These results are similar to those reported by other institutions. Shin et al. [41] reported on 2 patients with tentorial DAVFs treated with dosage greater than 20 Gy to the fistula, with complete obliteration obtained in both patients at 27 and 29 months. Söderman et al. [5] reported on 49 patients with 52 DAVFs, showing a 68% obliteration rate and another 24% with flow regression at 2 years. O'Leary et al. [44] achieved a 77% complete obliteration rate with improvement in another 15% of patients. In the series of Brown et al. [43], of the 50 patients with angiographic follow-up, 68% demonstrated complete obliteration, with another 14% showing near-total obliteration. In that of Koebbe et al. [12], all 18 patients had complete or near complete resolution of their presenting symptoms. Of the 8 patients with angiographic follow-up, all patients demonstrated complete obliteration. Although some of the patients in these publications had been treated with surgical resection or endovascular embolization prior to radiosurgery, they were referred for radiosurgery for further management of the residual DAVFs. From these studies we can estimate an overall success rate of complete obliteration associated with radiosurgery of DAVFs at 65–77%, with a greater number of patients gaining symptomatic relief from radiosurgical treatment. Complications directly related to the radiosurgical procedure are rare, as shown in our series.

Rationale of DAVF Radiosurgery

The management for a DAVF should be individualized, taking into consideration the clinical presentation of the patient, the anticipated natural course of the lesion based on location and angioarchitecture of the DAVFs, and the benefit and inherent risk of the treatment modality. It is widely accepted that DAVFs presenting with hemorrhage, progressive neurological deficits or increased intracranial pressure require prompt treatment by endovascular embolization, surgery, or a combination of these procedures, to provide immediate relief of the venous congestion.

For Borden type II/III lesions with a single or few CVDs, or DAVFs with an isolated dural sinus and CVDs, complete obliteration of the lesion may be achieved effectively by surgery or endovascular intervention [47, 54, 55]. However, when DAVFs involve dural sinuses with multiple complex feeders and CVDs, surgical and endovascular treatment can be technically challenging. Multisession and/or combined treatment are often needed. The rate of complete obliteration of DAVFs achieved by endovascular procedures differs from center to center, ranging from 27.3 to 81% [56]. It has been well known that partially treated DAVFs may recruit new collaterals to the fistula or redirect the venous outflow [57].

For DAVFs with antegrade sinus drainage alone (Borden type I) and no progressive focal neurological deficits, intervention may not be necessary unless the patient's symptoms (e.g. headache or pulsatile tinnitus) are intolerable. These lesions generally have a benign course and spontaneous obliteration has been reported, particularly with cavernous sinus lesions [58, 59]. Spontaneous regression of transverse/sigmoid sinus DAVFs is rare (maximum 5% of patients) [14, 15, 56]. It is noteworthy that conversion in flow pattern from antegrade to retrograde can occur in approximately 2% of patients, which leads to higher risks of developing new neurological deficits or hemorrhage [8, 11]. Interestingly, we found a significantly longer duration of nonaggressive symptoms (pulsatile tinnitus) in patients presenting with Borden type II/III DAVFs than in those with Borden type I (average 34 vs. 19 months) in our series. One may hypothesize that with a longer follow-up, the conversion rate of venous drainage from anterograde to retrograde may be higher than 2%.

When a treatment is indicated for Borden type I DAVF, its benefit should outweigh its risk. Evidence has shown that injury or increased pressure in the dural sinus could trigger the development of DAVFs or cause neurological deficits secondary to sinus hypertension [2]. Thus sacrificing a functioning dural sinus in Borden type I DAVFs by transvenous intervention or surgery may not be justified. Furthermore, it is difficult to achieve a complete obliteration of Borden type I DAVF by transarterial embolization alone due to the frequently complex and tortuous course of the arterial supply [21]. Studies have shown that persistent sinus hypertension or local ischemia caused by incomplete closure of the DAVFs after endovascular and/or surgical intervention can increase the expression of various vascular growth factors [60–65]. Thus, the use of endovascular intervention or surgery as a first-line treatment for Borden type I DAVFs with the intention of palliation rather than cure should carefully balance the risks and benefits of the procedure. Our study and those of others have shown that DAVFs with benign venous drainage can be safely treated using radiosurgery with a high angiographic complete obliteration rate with preservation of the functioning dural sinuses [19, 35, 39, 42].

Retrograde CVD had long been recognized as an angioarchitecture herald of aggressive behavior of DAVFs. However, not all DAVFs with CVDs were symptomatic. In 2009, Zipfel et al. [20] presented a modification to the existing classification scales of DAVFs based on the observation of patients' symptoms and outcome. They divided Borden type II/III patients into two subgroups: symptomatic CVD cases who present with hemorrhage or progressive neurological deficits, and those with asymptomatic CVD who present incidentally or with symptoms of tinnitus or ophthalmological phenomena with a less aggressive clinical course. According to the study of Zipfel et al., the annual rate of intracerebral hemorrhage is 7.4–7.6% for patients with symptomatic CVD, compared with 1.4–1.5% for those with asymptomatic CVD. They suggest that, for patients with asymptomatic CVD, the newly documented lower risk of subsequent hemorrhage or neurological deficits indicates that a more judicious approach toward therapeutic intervention is warranted. In many cases, endovascular or surgical intervention is still indicated, although the timing of treatment may be performed in a more elective nature. In others, particularly in patients who are elderly, medically frail or harbor complex DAVFs, radiosurgery may be a reasonable alternative.

Our results of radiosurgery support the above observation. In our 48 patients with Borden type II/III NCS DAVFs, 21 (44%) achieved a complete obliteration and 23 (48%) showed a >50% reduction of the lesion size with symptomatic improvement. This data indicates that radiosurgery is also suitable for certain DAVFs with CVD but without immediate risk of hemorrhage or focal neurological deficits.

Conclusions

Stereotactic radiosurgery using the Gamma Knife is a safe and effective alternative for the treatment of DAVFs. This method provides a minimally invasive therapeutic modality for patients who harbor less aggressive DAVFs, but who suffer from intolerable headache, bruit or ocular symptoms. For more aggressive DAVFs associated with immediate risks of hemorrhage, severe venous congestion or increased intracranial pressure, initial treatment with endovascular embolization or surgery for prompt elimination of aggressive components of DAVFs is necessary. In such cases, radiosurgery may serve as a secondary treatment for the further management of residual nidus after initial intervention. The latent period for the effects of radiation to occur and the longer time for cure compared to surgery and endovascular therapy remain a major drawback for radiosurgery. However, the gradual obliteration of a DAVF after radiosurgery can avoid the immediate risk of aggravated venous hypertension or infarction, which sometimes complicates endovascular embolization and surgery.

References

1 Awad IA, Little JR, Akarawi WP, Ahl J: Intracranial dural arteriovenous malformations: factors predisposing to an aggressive neurological course. J Neurosurg 1990;72:839–850.

2 Hamada Y, Goto K, Inoue T, Iwaki T, Matsuno H, Suzuki S, Matsushima T, Fukui M, Miyake E: Histopathological aspects of dural arteriovenous fistulas in the transverse-sigmoid sinus region in nine patients. Neurosurgery 1997;40:452–456, discussion 456–458.

3 Awad IA: The diagnosis and management of intracranial dural arteriovenous malformations. Contemp Neurosurg 1991;13:1–5.

4 Newton TH, Cronqvist S: Involvement of dural arteries in intracranial arteriovenous malformations. Radiology 1969;93:1071–1078.

5 Söderman M, Edner G, Ericson K, Karlsson B, Rahn T, Ulfarsson E, Andersson T: Gamma knife surgery for dural arteriovenous shunts: 25 years of experience. J Neurosurg 2006;104:867–875.

6 Aminoff MJ: Vascular anomalies in the intracranial dura mater. Brain 1973;96:601–612.

7 Brown RD Jr, Wiebers DO, Nichols DA: Intracranial dural arteriovenous fistulae: angiographic predictors of intracranial hemorrhage and clinical outcome in nonsurgical patients. J Neurosurg 1994;81:531–538.

8 Satomi J, van Dijk JM, Terbrugge KG, Willinsky RA, Wallace MC: Benign cranial dural arteriovenous fistulas: outcome of conservative management based on the natural history of the lesion. J Neurosurg 2002;97:767–770.

9 Chaudhary MY, Sachdev VP, Cho SH, Weitzner I Jr, Puljic S, Huang YP: Dural arteriovenous malformation of the major venous sinuses: an acquired lesion. AJNR Am J Neuroradiol 1982;3:13–19.

10 Houser OW, Campbell JK, Campbell RJ, Sundt TM Jr: Arteriovenous malformation affecting the transverse dural venous sinus – an acquired lesion. Mayo Clin Proc 1979;54:651–661.

11 Cognard C, Gobin YP, Pierot L, Bailly AL, Houdart E, Casasco A, Chiras J, Merland JJ: Cerebral dural arteriovenous fistulas: clinical and angiographic correlation with a revised classification of venous drainage. Radiology 1995;194:671–680.

12 Koebbe CJ, Singhal D, Sheehan J, Flickinger JC, Horowitz M, Kondziolka D, Lunsford LD: Radiosurgery for dural arteriovenous fistulas. Surg Neurol 2005;64:392–398, discussion 398–399.

13 Borden JA, Wu JK, Shucart WA: A proposed classification for spinal and cranial dural arteriovenous fistulous malformations and implications for treatment. J Neurosurg 1995;82:166–179.

14 Davies MA, ter Brugge K, Willinsky R, Wallace MC: The nature history and management of intracranial dural arteriovenous fistulae. 2. Aggressive lesions. Intervent Neuroradiol 1997;3:303–311.

15 Luciani A, Houdart E, Mounayer C, Saint Maurice JP, Merland JJ: Spontaneous closure of dural arteriovenous fistulas: report of three cases and review of the literature. AJNR Am J Neuroradiol 2001;22: 992–996.

16 Davies MA, ter Brugge K, Willinsky R, Coyne T, Saleh J, Wallace MC: The validity of classification for the clinical presentation of intracranial dural arteriovenous fistulas. J Neurosurg 1996;85:830–837.

17 Van Dijk JM, ter Brugge KG, Willinsky RA, Wallace MC: Clinical course of cranial dural arteriovenous fistulas with long-term persistent cortical venous reflux. Stroke 2002;33:1233–1236.

18 Duffau H, Lopes M, Janosevic V, Sichez JP, Faillot T, Capelle L, Ismail M, Bitar A, Arthuis F, Fohanno D: Early rebleeding from intracranial dural arteriovenous fistulas: report of 20 cases and review of the literature. J Neurosurg 1999;90:78–84.

19 Söderman M, Pavic L, Edner G, Holmin S, Andersson T: Natural history of dural arteriovenous shunts. Stroke 2008;39:1735–1739.

20 Zipfel GJ, Shah MN, Refai D, Dacey RG Jr, Derdeyn CP: Cranial dural arteriovenous fistulas: modification of angiographic classification scales based on new natural history data. Neurosurg Focus 2009;26:E14.

21 Sarma D, ter Brugge K: Management of intracranial dural arteriovenous shunts in adults. Eur J Radiol 2003;46:206–220.

22 Liu JK, Dogan A, Ellegala DB, Carlson J, Nesbit GM, Barnwell SL, Delashaw JB: The role of surgery for high-grade intracranial dural arteriovenous fistulas: importance of obliteration of venous outflow. J Neurosurg 2009;110:913–920.

23 Sundt TM Jr, Piepgras DG: The surgical approach to arteriovenous malformations of the lateral and sigmoid dural sinuses. J Neurosurg 1983;59:32–39.

24 Kawaguchi T, Hosoda K, Shibata Y, Kidoguchi K, Koyama J, Tamaki N: Direct surgical removal of the dural arteriovenous fistulas involving transverse-sigmoid sinuses. J Clin Neurosci 2002;9:16–18.

25 Collice M, D'Aliberti G, Talamonti G, Branca V, Boccardi E, Scialfa G, Versari PP: Surgical interruption of leptomeningeal drainage as treatment for intracranial dural arteriovenous fistulas without dural sinus drainage. J Neurosurg 1996;84:810–817.

26 Hoh BL, Choudhri TF, Connolly ES Jr, Solomon RA: Surgical management of high-grade intracranial dural arteriovenous fistulas: leptomeningeal venous disruption without nidus excision. Neurosurgery 1998;42:796–804.

27 Thompson BG, Doppman JL, Oldfield EH: Treatment of cranial dural arteriovenous fistulae by interruption of leptomeningeal venous drainage. J Neurosurg 1994;80:617–623.

28 Van Dijk JM, ter Brugge KG, Willinsky RA, Wallace MC: Selective disconnection of cortical venous reflux as treatment for cranial dural arteriovenous fistulas. J Neurosurg 2004;101:31–35.

29 Kakarla UK, Deshmukh VR, Zabramski JM, Albuquerque FC, McDougall CG, Spetzler RF: Surgical treatment of high-risk intracranial dural arteriovenous fistulae: clinical outcomes and avoidance of complications. Neurosurgery 2007;61:447–457.

30 Friedman WA, Bova FJ: Linear accelerator radiosurgery for arteriovenous malformations. J Neurosurg 1992;77:832–841.

31 Lunsford LD, Kondziolka D, Flickinger JC, Bissonette DJ, Jungreis CA, Maitz AH, Horton JA, Coffey RJ: Stereotactic radiosurgery for arteriovenous malformations of the brain. J Neurosurg 1991;75:512–524.

32 Steinberg GK, Fabrikant JI, Marks MP, Levy RP, Frankel KA, Phillips MH, Shuer LM, Silverberg GD: Stereotactic heavy-charged-particle Bragg-peak radiation for intracranial arteriovenous malformations. N Engl J Med 1990;323:96–101.

33 Chandler HC Jr, Friedman WA: Successful radiosurgical treatment of a dural arteriovenous malformation: case report. Neurosurgery 1993;33:139–141.

34 Friedman JA, Pollock BE, Nichols DA, Gorman DA, Foote RL, Stafford SL: Results of combined stereotactic radiosurgery and transarterial embolization for dural arteriovenous fistulas of the transverse and sigmoid sinuses. J Neurosurg 2001;94:886–891.

35 Guo WY, Pan DH, Wu HM, Chung WY, Shiau CY, Wang LW, Chiou HJ, Yen MY, Teng MM: Radiosurgery as a treatment alternative for dural arteriovenous fistulas of the cavernous sinus. AJNR Am J Neuroradiol 1998;19:1081–1087.

36 Lewis AI, Tomsick TA, Tew JM Jr: Management of tentorial dural arteriovenous malformations: transarterial embolization combined with stereotactic radiation or surgery. J Neurosurg 1994;81:851–859.

37 Link MJ, Coffey RJ, Nichols DA, Gorman DA: The role of radiosurgery and particulate embolization in the treatment of dural arteriovenous fistulas. J Neurosurg 1996;84:804–809.

38 Maruyama K, Shin M, Kurita H, Tago M, Kirino T: Stereotactic radiosurgery for dural arteriovenous fistula involving the superior sagittal sinus. Case report. J Neurosurg 2002;97:481–483.

39 Pan DH, Chung WY, Guo WY, Wu HM, Liu KD, Shiau CY, Wang LW: Stereotactic radiosurgery for the treatment of dural arteriovenous fistulas involving the transverse-sigmoid sinus. J Neurosurg 2002;96:823–829.

40 Pollock BE, Nichols DA, Garrity JA, Gorman DA, Stafford SL: Stereotactic radiosurgery and particulate embolization for cavernous sinus dural arteriovenous fistulae. Neurosurgery 1999;45:459–466.

41 Shin M, Kurita H, Tago M, Kirino T: Stereotactic radiosurgery for tentorial dural arteriovenous fistulae draining into the vein of Galen: report of two cases. Neurosurgery 2000;46:730–733, discussion 733–734.

42 Wu HM, Pan DH, Chung WY, Guo WY, Liu KD, Shiau CY, Wang LW, Chen SJ: Gamma Knife surgery for the management of intracranial dural arteriovenous fistulas. J Neurosurg 2006;105(suppl):43–51.

43 Brown RD Jr, Flemming KD, Meyer FB, Cloft HJ, Pollock BE, Link ML: Natural history, evaluation, and management of intracranial vascular malformations. Mayo Clin Proc 2005;80:269–281.

44 O'Leary S, Hodgson TJ, Coley SC, Kemeny AA, Radatz MW: Intracranial dural arteriovenous malformations: results of stereotactic radiosurgery in 17 patients. Clin Oncol (R Coll Radiol) 2002;14:97–102.
45 Pan HC, Sun MH, Yang DY, Wang YC, Lee SD, Chen WH, Chen CC: Multidisciplinary treatment of cavernous sinus dural arteriovenous fistulae with radiosurgery and embolization. J Clin Neurosci 2005;12:744–749.
46 Houser OW, Baker HL Jr, Rhoton AL Jr, Okazaki H: Intracranial dural arteriovenous malformations. Radiology 1972;105:55–64.
47 Van Rooij WJ, Sluzewski M, Beute GN: Dural arteriovenous fistulas with cortical venous drainage: incidence, clinical presentation, and treatment. AJNR Am J Neuroradiol 2007;28:651–655.
48 Graeb DA, Dolman CL: Radiological and pathological aspects of dural arteriovenous fistulas. Case report. J Neurosurg 1986;64:962–967.
49 Nishijima M, Takaku A, Endo S, Kuwayama N, Koizumi F, Sato H, Owada K: Etiological evaluation of dural arteriovenous malformations of the lateral and sigmoid sinuses based on histopathological examinations. J Neurosurg 1992;76:600–606.
50 Chiou HJ, Guo WY, Chou YH, WU HM, Luo CB, Lirng JF, Pan DHC, Shiau CY, Chang CY: Color Doppler ultrasonography to verify the closure of dural AV fistulae after r-knife radiosurgery. J Med Ultrasound 2004;12:107–113.
51 Pan DH, Guo WY, Chung WY, Shiau CY, Chang YC, Wang LW: Gamma knife radiosurgery as a single treatment modality for large cerebral arteriovenous malformations. J Neurosurg 2000;93(suppl 3):113–119.
52 Pan DH, Kuo YH, Guo WY, Chung WY, Wu HM, Liu KD, Chang YC, Wang LW, Wong TT: Gamma Knife surgery for cerebral arteriovenous malformations in children: a 13-year experience. J Neurosurg Pediatr 2008;1:296–304.
53 Steiner L, Lindquist C, Adler JR, Torner JC, Alves W, Steiner M: Clinical outcome of radiosurgery for cerebral arteriovenous malformations. J Neurosurg 1992;77:1–8.
54 Heros RC: Gamma knife surgery for dural arteriovenous fistulas. J Neurosurg 2006;104:861–863, discussion 865–866.
55 Jiang C, Lv X, Li Y, Zhang J, Wu Z: Endovascular treatment of high-risk tentorial dural arteriovenous fistulas: clinical outcomes. Neuroradiology 2009;51:103–111.
56 Kirsch M, Liebig T, Kuhne D, Henkes H: Endovascular management of dural arteriovenous fistulas of the transverse and sigmoid sinus in 150 patients. Neuroradiology 2009;51:477–483.
57 Cognard C, Houdart E, Casasco A, Gabrillargues J, Chiras J, Merland JJ: Long-term changes in intracranial dural arteriovenous fistulae leading to worsening in the type of venous drainage. Neuroradiology 1997;39:59–66.
58 Halbach VV, Higashida RT, Hieshima GB, Reicher M, Norman D, Newton TH: Dural fistulas involving the cavernous sinus: results of treatment in 30 patients. Radiology 1987;163:437–442.
59 Kai Y, Hamada J, Morioka M, Yano S, Kuratsu J: Treatment of cavernous sinus dural arteriovenous fistulae by external manual carotid compression. Neurosurgery 2007;60:253–257, discussion 257–258.
60 Klisch J, Kubalek R, Scheufler KM, Zirrgiebel U, Drevs J, Schumacher M: Plasma vascular endothelial growth factor and serum soluble angiopoietin receptor sTIE-2 in patients with dural arteriovenous fistulas: a pilot study. Neuroradiology 2005;47:10–17.
61 Kojima T, Miyachi S, Sahara Y, Nakai K, Okamoto T, Hattori K, Kobayashi N, Negoro M, Yoshida J: The relationship between venous hypertension and expression of vascular endothelial growth factor: hemodynamic and immunohistochemical examinations in a rat venous hypertension model. Surg Neurol 2007;68:277–284.
62 Terada T, Tsuura M, Komai N, Higashida RT, Halbach VV, Dowd CF, Wilson CB, Hieshima GB: The role of angiogenic factor bFGF in the development of dural AVFs. Acta Neurochir (Wien) 1996;138:877–883.
63 Tirakotai W, Bertalanffy H, Liu-Guan B, Farhoud A, Sure U: Immunohistochemical study in dural arteriovenous fistulas and possible role of local hypoxia for the de novo formation of dural arteriovenous fistulas. Clin Neurol Neurosurg 2005;107:455–460.
64 Uranishi R, Nakase H, Sakaki T: Expression of angiogenic growth factors in dural arteriovenous fistula. J Neurosurg 1999;91:781–786.
65 Zhu Y, Lawton MT, Du R, Shwe Y, Chen Y, Shen F, Young WL, Yang GY: Expression of hypoxia-inducible factor-1 and vascular endothelial growth factor in response to venous hypertension. Neurosurgery 2006;59:687–696.

David Hung-Chi Pan, MD
Department of Neurosurgery, Taipei Veterans General Hospital
No. 201, Sec. 2, Shi-Pai Road
Taipei, Taiwan 11217 (ROC)
Tel. +886 2 28757179, E-Mail hcpan@vghtpe.gov.tw

Niranjan A, Kano H, Lunsford LD (eds): Gamma Knife Radiosurgery for Brain Vascular Malformations.
Prog Neurol Surg. Basel, Karger, 2013, vol 27, pp 195–204 (DOI: 10.1159/000341796)

Stereotactic Radiosurgery with or without Embolization for Intracranial Dural Arteriovenous Fistulas

Huaiche Yang[a,d] · Hideyuki Kano[a,c] · Douglas Kondziolka[a,c] · Ajay Niranjan[a,c] · John C. Flickinger[a,b] · Michael B. Horowitz[a] · L. Dade Lunsford[a,c]

Departments of [a]Neurological Surgery and [b]Radiation Oncology, and [c]Center for Image-Guided Neurosurgery, University of Pittsburgh School of Medicine, Pittsburgh, Pa., USA; [d]Department of Neurosurgery, Taipei Veterans General Hospital, Taipei, Taiwan, ROC

Abstract

Treatment options for symptomatic dural arteriovenous fistulas (DAVFs) include surgery, embolization and stereotactic radiosurgery (SRS). We reviewed our DAVF experience at the University of Pittsburgh and assessed the role of SRS. We evaluated 40 consecutive patients who underwent Gamma Knife SRS for 44 DAVFs. Twenty-eight patients had upfront SRS before or after embolization performed at our institution, and 12 patients underwent delayed SRS for recurrent or residual DAVFs after initial embolization. The median SRS target volume was 2.0 cm^3, and the median marginal dose was 21.0 Gy. At a median follow-up of 45 months (range, 23–116 months), a total of 28 patients with 32 DAVFs had obliteration. The obliteration rate was 83% for patients who had upfront SRS and embolization. The obliteration rate was lower (67%) for patients managed with SRS alone. The obliteration rate was 71% for patients who had delayed SRS for recurrent or residual DAVFs following prior embolization. In our experience cavernous/carotid fistulas were associated with higher rates of obliteration and symptomatic improvement compared to transverse/sigmoid sinus region fistulas. Our experience suggests that successful DAVF obliteration is possible in most patients with upfront SRS in conjunction with embolization. SRS alone is an effective treatment for selected patients with a small-volume, low-risk DAVF.

Dural arteriovenous fistulas (DAVFs) of the brain are relatively uncommon vascular malformations and constitute approximately 10–15% of all intracranial vascular malformations [1]. DAVFs wherein dural arteries drain into venous sinuses or leptomeningeal veins may occur anywhere within the dura. The commonest sites include the transverse, sigmoid and cavernous sinus regions [1–4].

The management of DAVFs depends on several factors such as presence of symptoms, severity of the symptoms, the angiographic characteristics and the perceived risk for intracranial hemorrhage. The hemorrhage risk is higher in DAVFs associated with leptomeningeal cortical venous drainage and venous hypertension [4, 5]. DAVFs have been categorized based on venous drainage patterns seen on conventional angiography. Presence of retrograde leptomeningeal venous drainage is considered a significant risk factor for intracranial bleeding [6, 7]. Borden grade I DAVFs which are asymptomatic and low risk can be observed. Most Borden grade II or III DAVFs which are considered high risk warrant active management because they are associated with a high risk of intracranial hemorrhage [4, 8, 9]. Management strategies for DAVFs are diverse and include surgical excision [10–12], transarterial or transvenous embolization [13–15] and stereotactic radiosurgery (SRS) alone or in combination [16–22]. SRS in combination with transarterial embolization has been shown to be effective for selected patients with DAVFs [16, 19–21, 23]. We report our experience using SRS for DAVF patients, including those who had embolization before or after SRS.

Pittsburgh Experience

Forty consecutive patients with 44 intracranial DAVFs underwent Gamma Knife® SRS at the institution between 1991 and October 2006. The median age was 60 years (range, 29–90). There were 22 males and 18 females. The DAVFs were located in carotid/cavernous (n = 17, 4 bilateral), transverse/sigmoid (n = 18) and other regions (n = 9). The median follow-up interval after SRS was 45 months (range, 23–116 months).

Thirty-seven patients presented with symptoms related to the location of their DAVFs. Three patients had DAVFs detected incidentally (during an imaging evaluation for headache). Eleven of 13 patients with DAVFs located in the carotid/cavernous sinus had orbital findings including scleral injection, proptosis and chemosis. Pulsatile tinnitus was the presenting symptom in 15 of 18 patients with DAVFs located in the transverse/sigmoid sinus region. Six of 9 patients with DAVFs in other locations presented with intracranial hemorrhage. Twenty DAVFs were associated with cortical venous drainage. DAVFs were categorized using the Borden DAVF classification [6] as well as the Cognard classification [7]. Twenty-four DAVFs (55%) were Borden type I and 20 (45%) were Borden type II. Twenty-four DAVFs (55%) were Cognard type I, 6 (14%) Cognard type IIa, 6 (14%) Cognard type IIb and 8 (17%) were Cognard type IIa + b.

SRS and Embolization

Twelve patients had prior embolization at other centers and underwent delayed SRS at our center because of incomplete obliteration (n = 8) or recurrent DAVFs (n = 4). Twenty-eight patients underwent upfront DAVF management at our center. Seventeen patients were managed with SRS alone because they had either no accessible feeding vessels (n = 5), a distal location (n = 4), medical comorbidities (n = 5)

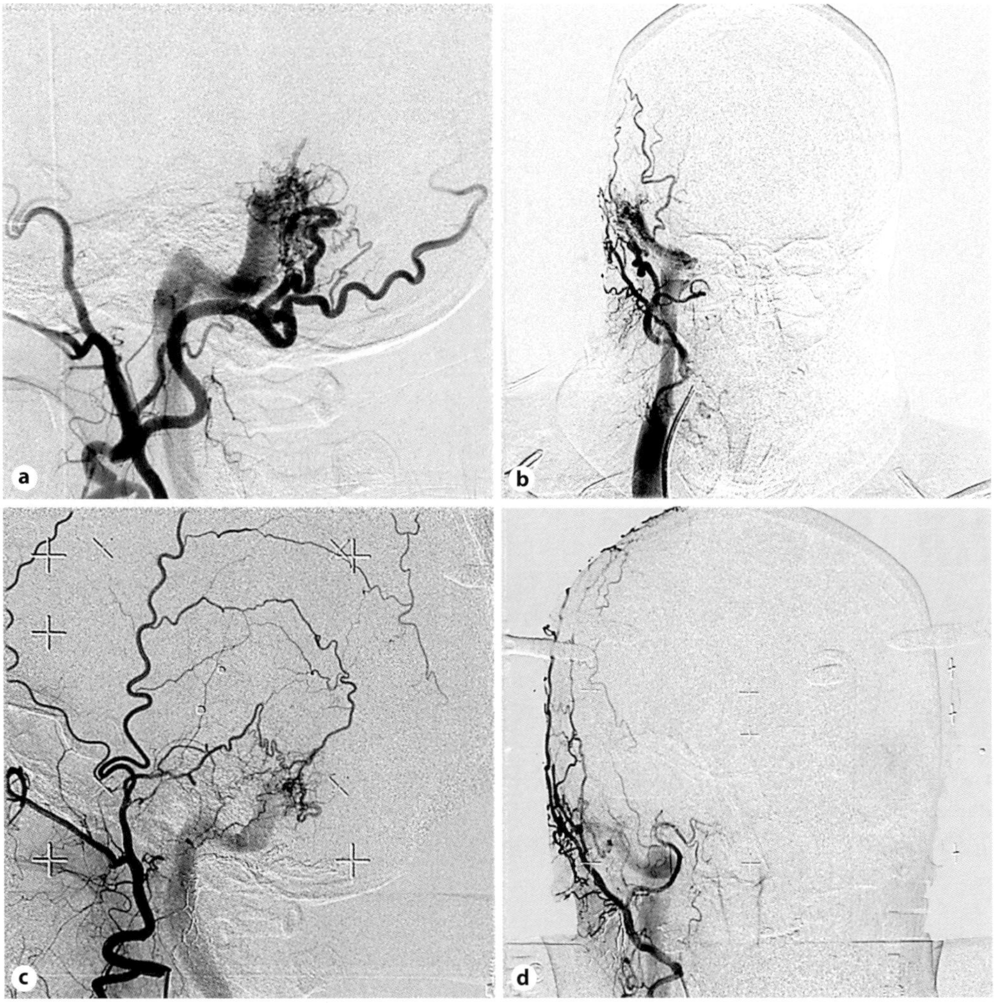

Fig. 1. A 53-year-old women presented with right-sided tinnitus. Angiograms showed a right transverse/sigmoid sinus DAVF. Lateral (**a**) and posteroanterior (**b**) views showing the DAVF. She underwent partial embolization of the right transverse/sigmoid sinus DAVF using Onyx. **c**, **d** Postembolization angiograms showing residual DAVF.

or a low bleeding risk DAVF that did not warrant early embolization (n = 3). Eleven patients had combined embolization and SRS. All patients who had combined embolization and SRS at our center had both procedures performed within 24 h. Seven patients underwent SRS immediately before embolization and 4 had embolization before SRS (fig. 1). Six patients underwent SRS after arterial embolization using polyvinyl alcohol particles. Other embolization materials included platinum coils (n = 3) and Onyx (ev3 Inc.; n = 3).

SRS was performed with a Leksell Gamma Knife (Elekta Inc., Atlanta, Ga., USA). All patients underwent application of a model G Leksell stereotactic head frame under

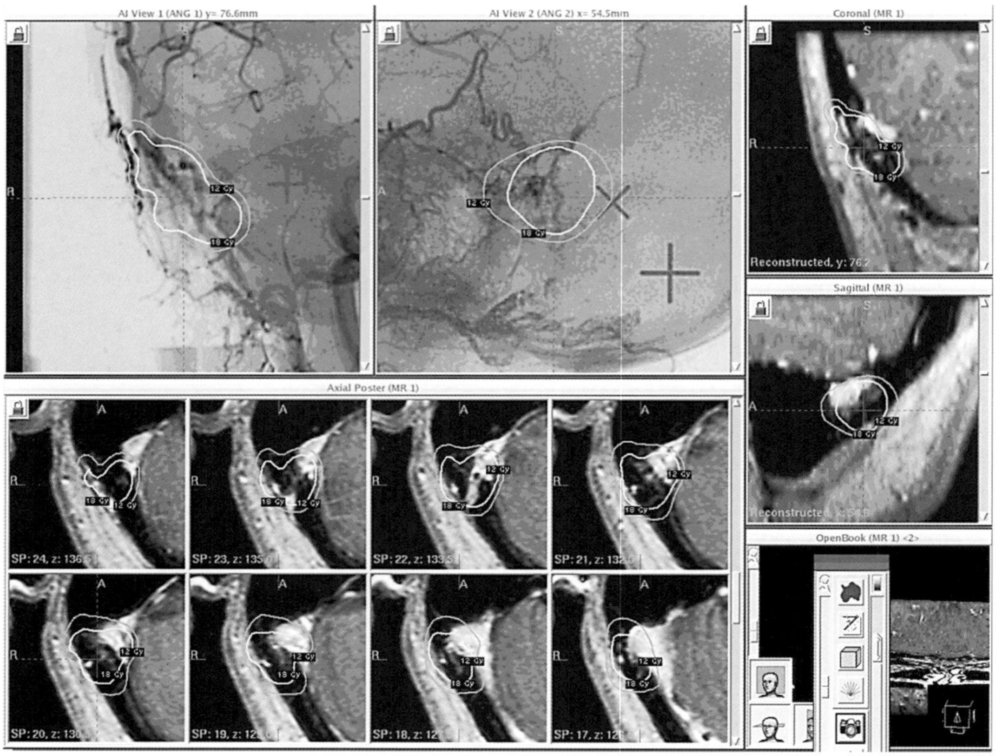

Fig. 2. A month later, this patient underwent Gamma Knife radiosurgery for residual DAVF. Radiosurgery dose planning was performed using angiograms and MR images, and a margin dose of 23 Gy was prescribed to the 50% isodose covering the DAVF.

conscious sedation and local scalp anesthesia. High-resolution magnetic resonance imaging (MRI) and high-resolution digital subtraction of conventional cerebral angiography were used for DAVF definition. Stereotactic images were exported to a computer workstation for dose planning. The median target volume was 2.0 cm^3 (range, 0.2–8.2 cm^3). The median dose prescribed to the target margin was 20 Gy (range, 15–25 Gy). The prescription isodose was 50% in 42 fistulas and 60% in 2 fistulas (fig. 2).

Follow-Up Evaluation
Clinical follow-up and MRI were performed at 6 months after SRS and then annually for 3 years. Angiography was performed to confirm obliteration patients with high-risk DAVFs.

Clinical Outcomes
Symptomatic improvement was noted in 19 (86%) of 22 patients without cortical venous drainage (low bleeding risk) DAVFs (Borden type I). Eighteen patients who had cortical venous drainage were considered to have higher-risk DAVFs (Borden

type II). One patient suffered a fatal cerebellar hemorrhage 2 months after SRS. No patient suffered an embolization-related complication or an adverse radiation effect during the follow-up period. Four patients with carotid/cavernous DAVF reported transient worsening of orbital symptoms during the first 6 months after SRS. We evaluated several different variables for their association with symptom improvement. These factors included age, sex, DAVF location, previous hemorrhage, use of embolization, cortical venous drainage, primary or secondary treatment, target volume, maximum dose and marginal dose. The DAVF location in the carotid/cavernous sinus region (as opposed to transverse sinus region) was associated with better symptom improvement ($p = 0.001$).

Imaging Outcomes
Follow-up imaging was available in 39 patients (1 died 2 months after SRS). Fourteen of 20 DAVF patients (70%) with high bleeding risk demonstrated complete fistula obliteration at the time of angiography. Eighteen of 24 DAVF patients (75%) with low bleeding risk had obliteration confirmed by MRI ($n = 11$) or angiography ($n = 7$). In our previous analysis we had reported that MRI had a 90% specificity for confirmation of obliteration compared to subsequent angiography in arteriovenous malformations following radiosurgery [24]. No patient with low-risk DAVF sustained a bleeding event or other symptoms during the follow-up interval. DAVFs of the carotid/cavernous sinus region were associated with better rates of obliteration ($p = 0.012$).

Impact of Embolization
In this series, delayed SRS was performed for 14 DAVFs that were residual or recurrent after embolization. Three of 4 DAVFs that underwent delayed SRS for recurrent fistulas had obliteration. Seven of 10 DAVFs that underwent SRS for residual fistulas had obliteration. Thirty DAVFs in 28 patients had no prior management before referral to our center. Twelve of 18 DAVFs managed by SRS alone had complete obliteration. Six of 7 DAVFs that underwent SRS followed by embolization were obliterated. Four of 5 DAVFs that underwent embolization followed by SRS had complete obliteration (fig. 3).

Discussion

The diagnosis of DAVF includes a wide spectrum of patients: asymptomatic, patients with transient symptoms followed by spontaneous thrombosis, patients with persistent symptoms, and patients with major morbidity from intracranial hemorrhage. The presentation and risk of further hemorrhage depends on DAVF location and the pattern of cortical venous drainage [3, 6]. Patients with low bleeding risk DAVF (those without cortical venous drainage) may

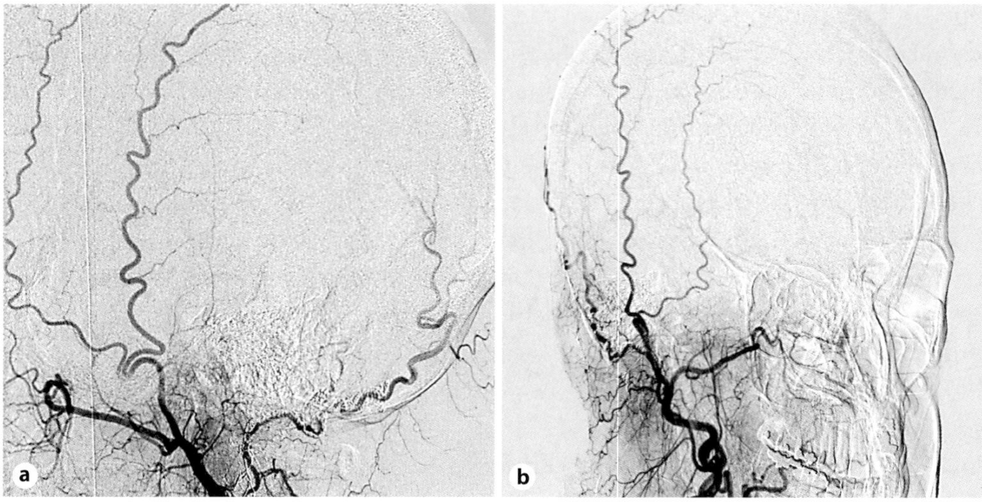

Fig. 3. Posteroanterior (**a**) and lateral (**b**) angiograms performed 2 years after radiosurgery showing complete obliteration of the DAVF.

have spontaneous thrombosis followed by symptomatic resolution [4, 25–28]. Asymptomatic low-risk DAVFs can be managed conservatively by observation and monitoring both clinically and by imaging. However, some DAVFs associated with disabling pulsatile tinnitus or ocular symptoms such as exophthalmos or acute chemosis require prompt treatment even though these are fistulas with a low hemorrhage risk.

Prompt intervention is warranted for patients with high bleeding risk DAVFs (those with cortical venous drainage). The risk of further hemorrhage may be as high as 35% in the first weeks after an initial bleed related to DAVFs [29]. In a study, van Dijk et al. [30] found an annual hemorrhage rate of 8% and an annual mortality rate of 10% from DAVFs with persistent untreated cortical venous drainage. In a recent report, Soderman et al. [9] noted that patients who presented with an intracranial hemorrhage had an annual 7.4% rebleeding risk. In contrast, patients with confirmed DAVFs with cortical venous drainage with no previous history of hemorrhage had an annual bleeding risk of 1.5% [9].

Embolization is an effective technique for symptom resolution; however, embolization fails to achieve complete and permanent obliteration of the fistula in 50% or more of cases [31, 32]. Complete obliteration can be difficult especially if not all arterial feeding vessels are seen during angiography. Superselective catheterization, which may be necessary to identify feeding vessels, can also be technically challenging. Embolization is also associated with complication resulting from inadvertent acute occlusion of feeding or adjacent vessels [33]. In some patients, delayed recanalization of the fistula is possible which restores the risk of a new bleeding event [4, 34].

Surgery is a potential management option for patients with a limited direct artery-to-vein fistula. Simple ligation or clipping may be sufficient to occlude the fistula and immediately reverse the intracranial venous hypertension characteristic of high-flow fistulas [11, 12, 14, 35]. Lucas et al. [14] described skeletonization of the venous sinus to occlude a fistula. Such an approach may not prevent recanalization [36]. However, the overall risks of direct surgical exploration may be higher than embolization plus radiosurgery, especially in elderly patients or those with medical comorbidities.

SRS is considered an effective treatment for selected patients with DAVFs [16–20, 22, 23]. In 1994, Lewis et al. [37] reported 7 patients with tentorial DAVFs who were managed with radiosurgery and embolization; 5 patients had fistula thrombosis, and 2 patients had 50% reduction in fistula flow. One patient had transient radiation injury of the brainstem 15 months after radiosurgery [37]. Several additional reports have documented potential benefits of SRS.

Pan et al. [22] managed 19 patients with transverse/sigmoid sinus DAVF with SRS alone. Fourteen DAVFs had symptom resolution and 11 patients had radiographically confirmed obliteration [22]. Soderman et al. [20] treated 52 DAVF patients with Gamma Knife radiosurgery; 43 of their 52 DAVFs were treated by SRS alone. These authors reported that 68% of DAVFs had angiographically proven obliteration and 24% had significant flow regression [20].

SRS offers the potential for complete fistula closure, especially in patients not eligible for embolization because of high medical risks or poor vascular access to the feeding fistula vasculature. We reserve SRS as a single modality of therapy for patients with no or limited cortical venous drainage, for those with only mild symptoms, and for those patients with poor vascular access for embolization. The combination of SRS and embolization seems to be an effective management strategy for DAVFs. Addition of embolization with SRS offers early symptomatic relief for symptomatic patients or those with cortical venous drainage. In the present series 23 patients underwent combined embolization and SRS. Overall, 17 of 23 patients who underwent both SRS and embolization at some time had complete fistula obliteration.

With respect to timing of embolization, we noted that 6 of 7 patients who were embolized after SRS had obliteration. Four of 5 patients who had embolization before SRS had obliteration. This study did not have large enough numbers to define a statistically significant difference between these two management approaches. Dr. Thoralf Sundt first suggested the approach of SRS followed by embolization. Friedman et al. [16] also recommended that SRS was best performed before endovascular treatment because visualization of the entire DAVF target could be reduced by previous embolization. In addition, reduction in the DAVF flow to draining cortical veins is important to achieve quickly, and thereby potentially reduce the risk of hemorrhage. Embolization is the most suited modality to accomplish this outcome quickly, if direct surgical removal is considered a high risk. Patients are best managed at a center of excellence where all therapeutic options are available: surgery, radiosurgery and embolization.

Radiosurgery in combination with embolization may represent the best overall approach as embolization provides early protection from bleeding and SRS facilitates late and long-term closure. In our data, the average latency interval until fistula closure was approximately 23 months [18]. Among 17 patients with 18 DAVFs who received only SRS, 8 were low bleeding risk DAVFs (Cognard types I and IIa), whereas 10 were high bleeding risk DAVFs (Cognard types IIb and IIa + b). Five of these DAVFs had previous DAVF-related intracranial hemorrhages. Complete obliteration was found in 12 of 18 DAVFs (67%) who had SRS alone. One patient had a second hemorrhage early after SRS. In selected patients, SRS alone may be an acceptable management strategy if their fistula does not have cortical venous drainage or has poor vascular access for embolization. High-risk DAVFs that undergo SRS alone have the potential to bleed during the latency interval until obliteration is documented, although that risk may diminish even before complete obliteration is documented. Soderman et al. [20] reported an annual bleeding rate of 2.6% for DAVFs after SRS. Other authors noted that DAVF obliteration may occur even sooner compared to obliteration of other intracranial vascular malformations [20, 22]. One of our patients had angiographically proven obliteration 7 months after SRS alone.

In our experience DAVF location was the only statistically significant factor that affected both rate of obliteration and symptom improvement. Patients with cavernous sinus region DAVFs had a better rate of obliteration and symptom improvement rate compared with patients with transverse/sigmoid sinus region fistulas. The published literature also suggests that DAVFs involving the cavernous sinus had total obliteration rates of 75–93% whereas DAVFs involving the transverse/sigmoid sinus had a 58–65% total obliteration rate [16–23]. This difference in obliteration may be related to difficulties in targeting the shunt or more complex angioarchitecture in patients with transverse sinus fistulas.

For DAVFs with good vascular access, we believe that SRS in combination with embolization has the best early and later obliteration rates. For patients with poor vascular access for embolization, SRS alone is an effective option.

Conclusion

Patients with DAVF warrant management at centers where all treatment options are available. If direct surgery is not possible or is considered high risk, embolization provides early benefit and SRS provides late benefit during the management of DAVFs. Combined SRS and embolization make an effective management strategy for DAVFs, including those that have recurred after initial embolization. In this experience no patient had embolization- or radiation-related morbidity. SRS alone is an effective treatment option for selected DAVF patients who are not eligible for embolization. DAVFs of the cavernous sinus region have higher rates of obliteration and symptom improvement. In our view embolization (performed immediately before or after) in conjunction with SRS targeting the entire fistula volume provides the best obliteration rates.

Disclosure Statement

Drs. Lunsford, Kondziolka and Niranjan are consultants with AB Elekta. Dr. Lunsford is a stockholder in AB Elekta.

References

1 Houser OW, Baker HL Jr, Rhoton AL Jr, Okazaki H: Intracranial dural arteriovenous malformations. Radiology 1972;105:55–64.

2 Malik GM, Pearce JE, Ausman JI, Mehta B: Dural arteriovenous malformations and intracranial hemorrhage. Neurosurgery 1984;15:332–339.

3 Lasjaunias P, Chiu M, ter Brugge K, Tolia A, Hurth M, Bernstein M: Neurological manifestations of intracranial dural arteriovenous malformations. J Neurosurg 1986;64:724–730.

4 Awad IA, Little JR, Akarawi WP, Ahl J: Intracranial dural arteriovenous malformations: factors predisposing to an aggressive neurological course. J Neurosurg 1990;72:839–850.

5 Biondi A, Casasco A, Houdart E, Gioino C, Sourour N, Vivas E, et al: Evolution of angiographic signs of venous hypertension and clinical signs of intracranial hypertension in intracranial dural arteriovenous fistulas. J Neuroradiol 1999;26:49–58.

6 Borden JA, Wu JK, Shucart WA: A proposed classification for spinal and cranial dural arteriovenous fistulous malformations and implications for treatment. J Neurosurg 1995;82:166–179.

7 Cognard C, Gobin YP, Pierot L, Bailly AL, Houdart E, Casasco A, et al: Cerebral dural arteriovenous fistulas: clinical and angiographic correlation with a revised classification of venous drainage. Radiology 1995;194:671–680.

8 Vinuela F, Fox AJ, Pelz DM, Drake CG: Unusual clinical manifestations of dural arteriovenous malformations. J Neurosurg 1986;64:554–558.

9 Soderman M, Pavic L, Edner G, Holmin S, Andersson T: Natural history of dural arteriovenous shunts. Stroke 2008;39:1735–1739.

10 Hugosson R, Bergstrom K: Surgical treatment of dural arteriovenous malformation in the region of the sigmoid sinus. J Neurol Neurosurg Psychiatry 1974;37:97–101.

11 Sundt TM Jr, Piepgras DG: The surgical approach to arteriovenous malformations of the lateral and sigmoid dural sinuses. J Neurosurg 1983;59:32–39.

12 Liu JK, Dogan A, Ellegala DB, Carlson J, Nesbit GM, Barnwell SL, et al: The role of surgery for high-grade intracranial dural arteriovenous fistulas: importance of obliteration of venous outflow. J Neurosurg 2009;110:913–920.

13 Halbach VV, Higashida RT, Hieshima GB, Mehringer CM, Hardin CW: Transvenous embolization of dural fistulas involving the transverse and sigmoid sinuses. AJNR Am J Neuroradiol 1989; 10:385–392.

14 Lucas CP, Zabramski JM, Spetzler RF, Jacobowitz R: Treatment for intracranial dural arteriovenous malformations: a meta-analysis from the English language literature. Neurosurgery 1997;40:1119–1130, discussion 1130–1132.

15 Shi ZS, Loh Y, Duckwiler GR, Jahan R, Vinuela F: Balloon-assisted transarterial embolization of intracranial dural arteriovenous fistulas. J Neurosurg 2009;110:921–928.

16 Friedman JA, Pollock BE, Nichols DA, Gorman DA, Foote RL, Stafford SL: Results of combined stereotactic radiosurgery and transarterial embolization for dural arteriovenous fistulas of the transverse and sigmoid sinuses. J Neurosurg 2001;94:886–891.

17 Guo WY, Pan DH, Wu HM, Chung WY, Shiau CY, Wang LW, et al: Radiosurgery as a treatment alternative for dural arteriovenous fistulas of the cavernous sinus. AJNR Am J Neuroradiol 1998;19: 1081–1087.

18 Koebbe CJ, Singhal D, Sheehan J, Flickinger JC, Horowitz M, Kondziolka D, et al: Radiosurgery for dural arteriovenous fistulas. Surg Neurol 2005;64: 392–398, discussion 398–399.

19 Link MJ, Coffey RJ, Nichols DA, Gorman DA: The role of radiosurgery and particulate embolization in the treatment of dural arteriovenous fistulas. J Neurosurg 1996;84:804–809.
20 Soderman M, Edner G, Ericson K, Karlsson B, Rahn T, Ulfarsson E, et al: Gamma knife surgery for dural arteriovenous shunts: 25 years of experience. J Neurosurg 2006;104:867–875.
21 Wu HM, Pan DH, Chung WY, Guo WY, Liu KD, Shiau CY, et al: Gamma Knife surgery for the management of intracranial dural arteriovenous fistulas. J Neurosurg 2006;105(suppl):43–51.
22 Pan DH, Chung WY, Guo WY, Wu HM, Liu KD, Shiau CY, et al: Stereotactic radiosurgery for the treatment of dural arteriovenous fistulas involving the transverse-sigmoid sinus. J Neurosurg 2002;96: 823–829.
23 Pollock BE, Nichols DA, Garrity JA, Gorman DA, Stafford SL: Stereotactic radiosurgery and particulate embolization for cavernous sinus dural arteriovenous fistulae. Neurosurgery 1999;45:459–466, discussion 466–467.
24 Pollock BE, Kondziolka D, Flickinger JC, Patel AK, Bissonette DJ, Lunsford LD: Magnetic resonance imaging: an accurate method to evaluate arteriovenous malformations after stereotactic radiosurgery. J Neurosurg 1996;85:1044–1049.
25 Davies MA, ter Brugge K, Willinsky R, Coyne T, Saleh J, Wallace MC: The validity of classification for the clinical presentation of intracranial dural arteriovenous fistulas. J Neurosurg 1996;85:830–837.
26 Fermand M, Reizine D, Melki JP, Riche MC, Merland JJ: Long term follow-up of 43 pure dural arteriovenous fistulae (AVF) of the lateral sinus. Neuroradiology 1987;29:348–353.
27 Brown RD Jr, Wiebers DO, Nichols DA: Intracranial dural arteriovenous fistulae: angiographic predictors of intracranial hemorrhage and clinical outcome in nonsurgical patients. J Neurosurg 1994;81: 531–538.
28 Satomi J, van Dijk JM, ter Brugge KG, Willinsky RA, Wallace MC: Benign cranial dural arteriovenous fistulas: outcome of conservative management based on the natural history of the lesion. J Neurosurg 2002;97:767–770.
29 Duffau H, Lopes M, Janosevic V, Sichez JP, Faillot T, Capelle L, et al: Early rebleeding from intracranial dural arteriovenous fistulas: report of 20 cases and review of the literature. J Neurosurg 1999;90:78–84.
30 Van Dijk JM, ter Brugge KG, Willinsky RA, Wallace MC: Clinical course of cranial dural arteriovenous fistulas with long-term persistent cortical venous reflux. Stroke 2002;33:1233–1236.
31 Barnwell SL, Halbach VV, Higashida RT, Hieshima G, Wilson CB: Complex dural arteriovenous fistulas. Results of combined endovascular and neurosurgical treatment in 16 patients. J Neurosurg 1989; 71:352–358.
32 Urtasun F, Biondi A, Casaco A, Houdart E, Caputo N, Aymard A, et al: Cerebral dural arteriovenous fistulas: percutaneous transvenous embolization. Radiology 1996;199:209–217.
33 Picard L, Bracard S, Islak C, Roy D, Moreno A, Marchal JC, et al: Dural fistulae of the tentorium cerebelli. Radioanatomical, clinical and therapeutic considerations. J Neuroradiol 1990;17:161–181.
34 Lalwani AK, Dowd CF, Halbach VV: Grading venous restrictive disease in patients with dural arteriovenous fistulas of the transverse/sigmoid sinus. J Neurosurg 1993;79:11–15.
35 Collice M, D'Aliberti G, Arena O, Solaini C, Fontana RA, Talamonti G: Surgical treatment of intracranial dural arteriovenous fistulae: role of venous drainage. Neurosurgery 2000;47:56–66, discussion 67.
36 Finn M, Klimo P Jr, Couldwell WT: Interpositional dural graft technique for the treatment of dural arteriovenous fistulas. Neurosurg Focus 2007;22: E10.
37 Lewis AI, Tomsick TA, Tew JM Jr: Management of tentorial dural arteriovenous malformations: transarterial embolization combined with stereotactic radiation or surgery. J Neurosurg 1994;81:851–859.

L. Dade Lunsford, MD, FACS
Lars Leksell Distinguished Professor of Neurological Surgery
University of Pittsburgh, Suite B-400, UPMC Presbyterian
200 Lothrop Street
Pittsburgh, PA 15213 (USA)
Tel. +1 412 647 6781, E-Mail lunsfordld@upmc.edu

Niranjan A, Kano H, Lunsford LD (eds): Gamma Knife Radiosurgery for Brain Vascular Malformations.
Prog Neurol Surg. Basel, Karger, 2013, vol 27, pp 205–217 (DOI: 10.1159/000341798)

Dural Arteriovenous Fistulas and the Role of Gamma Knife Stereotactic Radiosurgery: The Stockholm Experience

Michael Söderman[a,c] · Ernest Dodoo[b,c] · Bengt Karlsson[d]

Departments of [a]Neuroradiology and [b]Neurosurgery, Karolinska University Hospital, and [c]Department of Clinical Neuroscience, Karolinska Institutet, Stockholm, Sweden; [d]Division of Neurosurgery, National University Hospital, Singapore, Singapore

Abstract

We review the clinical and radiological outcomes of patients with dural arteriovenous fistulae (DAVFs), treated with the Gamma Knife® (GK) in Stockholm. During the period 1972–2008, 73 consecutive patients were treated. Eight were excluded due to lack of follow-up. Thus, the material comprises 65 patients harboring 67 DAVFs subjected to 75 treatments with GK stereotactic radiosurgery (SRS). Fifty-four cases were subjected to upfront GK SRS while 13 followed failed surgery or embolization. Nine patients had been retreated with GK SRS. One was recent and was excluded. Prescription doses varied considerably, but most commonly it was 20–25 Gy to the 40–60% isodose. Target definition was from angiography in all cases. 63 cases had an angiographic follow-up. There were 37 (59%) obliterations and 17 (27%) regressions. Nine lesions were unchanged (14%). If patients with clinical data suggestive of obliteration or magnetic resonance imaging follow-up are included, the numbers differ. Two patients are excluded. As for the 73 remaining cases, there were 46 (63%) obliterations, 17 (23%) regressions and 10 (14%) unchanged. There were 2 posttreatment hemorrhages and 5 minor adverse radiation effects. GK SRS is an effective treatment for DAVFs, with a low incidence of complications. GK SRS is a treatment alternative for patients harboring a DAVF without cortical venous reflux that causes intolerable bruit and to those not amenable to embolization or surgery.

Intracranial dural arteriovenous fistulae (DAVFs) are pathological arteriovenous shunts in the dura mater, acquired in relation to a thrombotic process in the intracranial venous system, most often in a dural sinus [1–4]. In the adult population, DAVFs are about 10 times less frequent than brain arteriovenous malformations (BAVMs) [5]. The symptoms at presentation and the prognosis depend on the location of the DAVF and in particular on the venous drainage pattern [6]. A lesion that drains, directly or indirectly, into the cortical venous system may cause intracranial hemorrhage or a nonhemorrhagic neurological deficit. Less commonly, a large arteriovenous shunt, particularly when associated with an outflow restriction, may incur increased intracranial pressure secondary to venous hypertension.

Patients at risk for bleeding or other adverse events are regularly offered treatment [7–10]. Other symptoms such as intolerable bruit, significant exophthalmos or chemosis may also prompt action.

Embolization and microsurgery are established therapeutic options for DAVF, and the indications and methods have been well described elsewhere [8, 11]. In 1972, Steiner et al. [12] published the first report on Gamma Knife stereotactic radiosurgery (GK SRS) of a patient with a BAVM. The same year the team in Stockholm treated in the GK the first patient with a DAVF. However, the Karolinska series was not reported until 2006 [13]. In 1982, Barcia-Salorio et al. [14] published their results from radiosurgery for DAVFs. These initial treatments were performed with a single cobalt-60 source. Subsequently GK SRS seems to have emerged as the preferred method [13–18]. There are a few reports on linear accelerator radiosurgery for DAVF [19–21].

Material and Methods

The Karolinska neurovascular database was searched for patients with DAVF that had been subjected to GK SRS. We found 79 consecutive adult patients with 82 DAVFs that had been treated during the period 1972–2010. These are accounted for as 82 cases. From this material were excluded 15 cases. One case had been treated with GK SRS elsewhere and was later embolized for his DAVF at the Karolinska Institute. In 1 case treated in 1983, all data have been lost. In 7 cases that had been referred from abroad, we were unable to find any information about the patients after the treatment. Finally 6 patients had been treated with GK SRS for the first time later than June 2008 and therefore still lacked a sufficient follow-up. Nine patients had been retreated once with GK SRS. One of these was recent and was excluded. Thus were included 65 patients harboring 67 DAVFs subjected to 75 treatments with GK SRS.

Locations, Venous Drainage and Presentation

Eight cavernous sinus and 1 sphenoparietal sinus DAVFs had their venous exits through the superior ophthalmic vein, occasionally in addition a petrosal sinus, and the patients consequently suffered from symptoms of orbital venous congestion. Eleven DAVFs were located in the wall of a sinus with drainage only to the sinus, i.e. type Borden I and Cognard I or IIa, and 9 of these were revealed with bruit [22, 23]. The remaining 47 patients had DAVFs with direct or indirect cortical venous reflux or venous congestion secondary to an outflow restriction (type Borden II and III or Cognard IIa + b, IIb, III and IV) [22, 23]. Thus, these were so-called aggressive DAVFs, and 22 of them had presented with hemorrhage. Details of locations, venous drainage and presentation can be found in table 1.

Events between Diagnosis and GK SRS

Prior to any treatment 1 patient experienced a first hemorrhage and a second patient rebled.

Eleven patients were subjected to surgery or embolization preceding GK SRS (table 2).

Table 1. Locations, venous drainage and presentation of the 67 DAVFs according to Borden or Cognard types

Borden:	I	II	III	III	Total	Bruit at GK
Cognard:	I, IIa	IIa + b, IIb	III	IV		
Sphenoid and cavernous sinus	9	1	0	0	10	5
Falcotentorial sinus	0	2	7	6	15	1
Transverse sinus	6	9	1	0	16	11
Sigmoid sinus	4	(also TS) 2	0	0	6	5
Superior petrosal sinus	1	2	2	1	6	1
Sagittal and straight sinus	0	3	1	2	6	1
Other locations	0	0	5	3	8	1
Total	20	19	16	12	67	25
Presentation with hemorrhage	0/20	3/19	10/16	9/12	22/67	
Bruit at presentation	14/20	10/19	3/16	9/12	36/67	

Two of the sigmoid sinus DAVFs extended into the transverse sinus, hence the Borden II classification and the added text 'also TS'. Twenty-two patients had a hemorrhage as the revealing event: 2 intraventricular, 8 intracerebral and 12 subarachnoid bleedings. Thirty-four cases had no tinnitus at the time of GK SRS, in 8 cases there is no information. The remaining 25 had an objectively verified pulse-synchronous bruit.

Table 2. The 67 cases and 8 retreatments with GK SRS including the other treatments prior to the latest irradiation

1st treatment	2nd treatment	3rd treatment	4th treatment	Retreatments
Embolization 10	Embolization 1, GK SRS 9	GK SRS 2	GKSRS 1	2
GK SRS 54	GK SRS 6			6
Surgery 3	Surgery 1, GK SRS 2	GK SRS 1		0
54	17	3	1	

Target Definition

In all cases the localization of the arteriovenous shunt was from stereotactic angiography, similar to the target definition technique in GK SRS for arteriovenous malformation [24] (fig. 1, 2). In patients treated later than 1990, there was supplementary stereotactic magnetic resonance imaging (MRI). The objective of the MRI was to outline surrounding brain tissue and to calculate radiation doses to sensitive organs such as the eyes or the brainstem [25]. The arteriovenous shunt per se could seldom be identified from the MRI.

Treatments

Fifty-four patients were subjected to upfront GK SRS while 13 were treated following failed surgery or embolization (table 2). Eight patients were subjected to a second treatment with GK SRS. Hence there are data from 75 treatments (table 3).

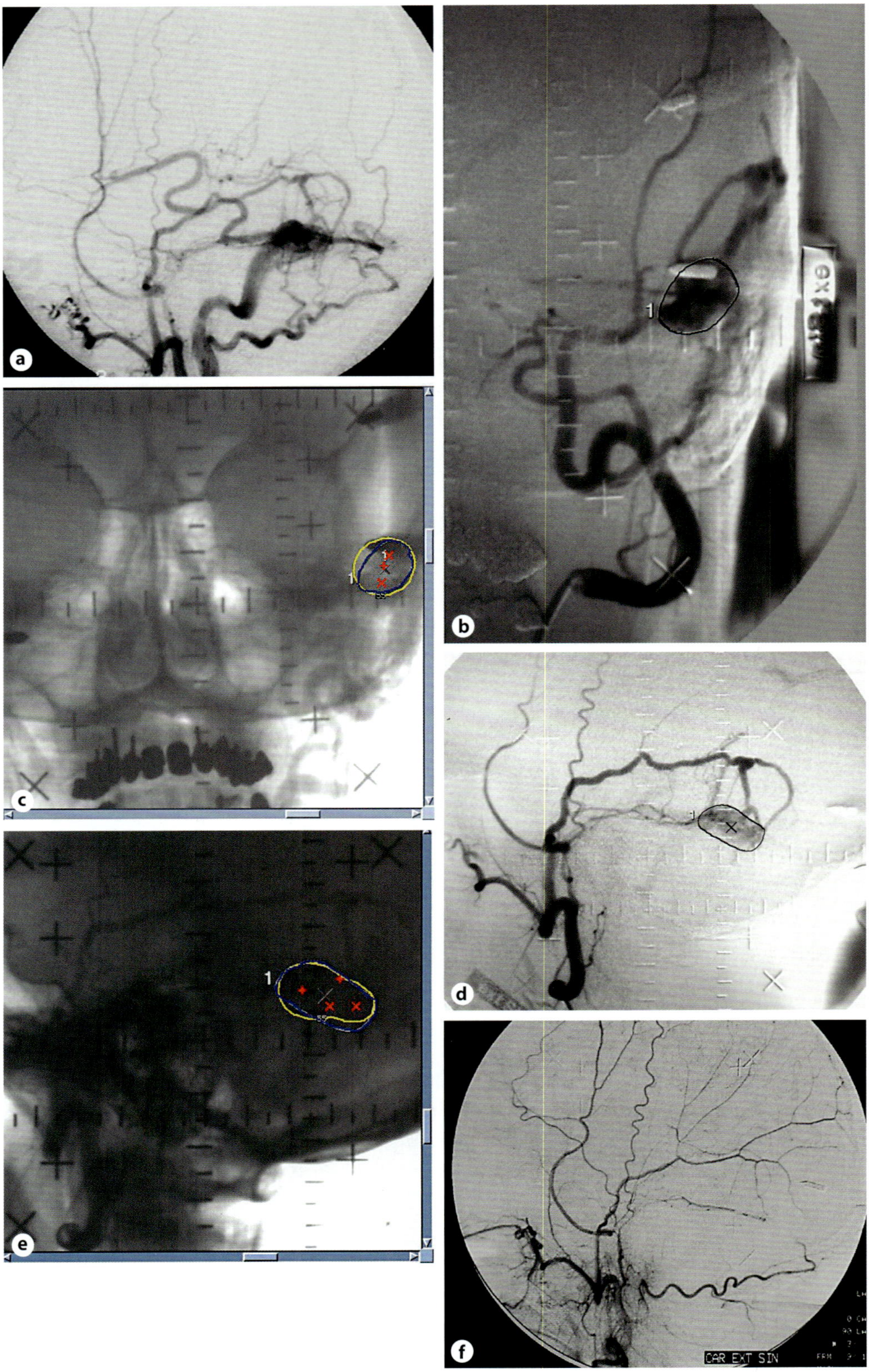
a
b
c
d
e
f
1
CAR EXT SIN

Prescription doses varied a great deal in the cases subjected to GK SRS before the introduction of the Gamma Plan® program. However, after 1990 the prescription doses were consistently 20–25 Gy to the 40–60% isodose.

Results

Obliterations

One patient bled 10 weeks after GK SRS and had the DAVF evacuated together with the hematoma. One patient was embolized 5 days after radiosurgery because of intolerable bruit partially. The control angiogram 1 year later showed obliteration. In 1 patient with a very large transverse sinus DAVF the flow in the lesion changed after the treatment and the patient worsened clinically with cerebellar edema. The DAVF was patent. Finally 1 patient with kidney insufficiency had an MRI that was suggestive of obliteration. In addition 8 patients had only a clinical follow-up; the symptoms had disappeared and the patients did not want further investigations or treatments. All 8 did well clinically and showed no symptoms of hemorrhage or adverse radiation effects (AREs) during more than 3 years after the treatment. The remaining 63 cases all had an angiographic follow-up after the GK SRS. The time varied between a few months (in cases where the bruit disappeared rapidly) and several years. There were 37 (59%) obliterations and 17 (27%) regressions. All cases with regression showed considerable flow reduction, in some cases almost obliteration. Nine lesions were unchanged (14%).

If patients with clinical data suggestive of obliteration (the bruit ceased) or MRI follow-up are included, the numbers differ. Two patients are excluded: 1 who did not have bruit prior to treatment and refused angiographic follow-up and 1 who was subjected to surgery because of hemorrhage. As for the 73 remaining cases, there were 46 (63%) obliterations, 17 (23%) regressions and 10 (14%) remained unchanged.

Fig. 1. DAVF located in the wall of the left transverse/sigmoid sinus. The patient had pulse-synchronous bruit well before she was first examined in 1993. She had not bled. She was subjected to GK SRS for the first time in 1996, and the bruit disappeared 14 days after the treatment. From Söderman et al. [13] with permission. **a** Angiography prior to GK SRS. Lateral view with injection into the external carotid artery. Note cortical venous drainage into a large temporal vein. **b–e** Posteroanterior and lateral views used for target delineation (in blue), which in this case was rather generous, particularly in the posteroanterior projection. Treatment was performed with a 25-Gy prescription dose (yellow 55% isodose line). The maximum dose was 42 Gy. **f** Follow-up angiography 2 years after the treatment. The DAVF had become obliterated.

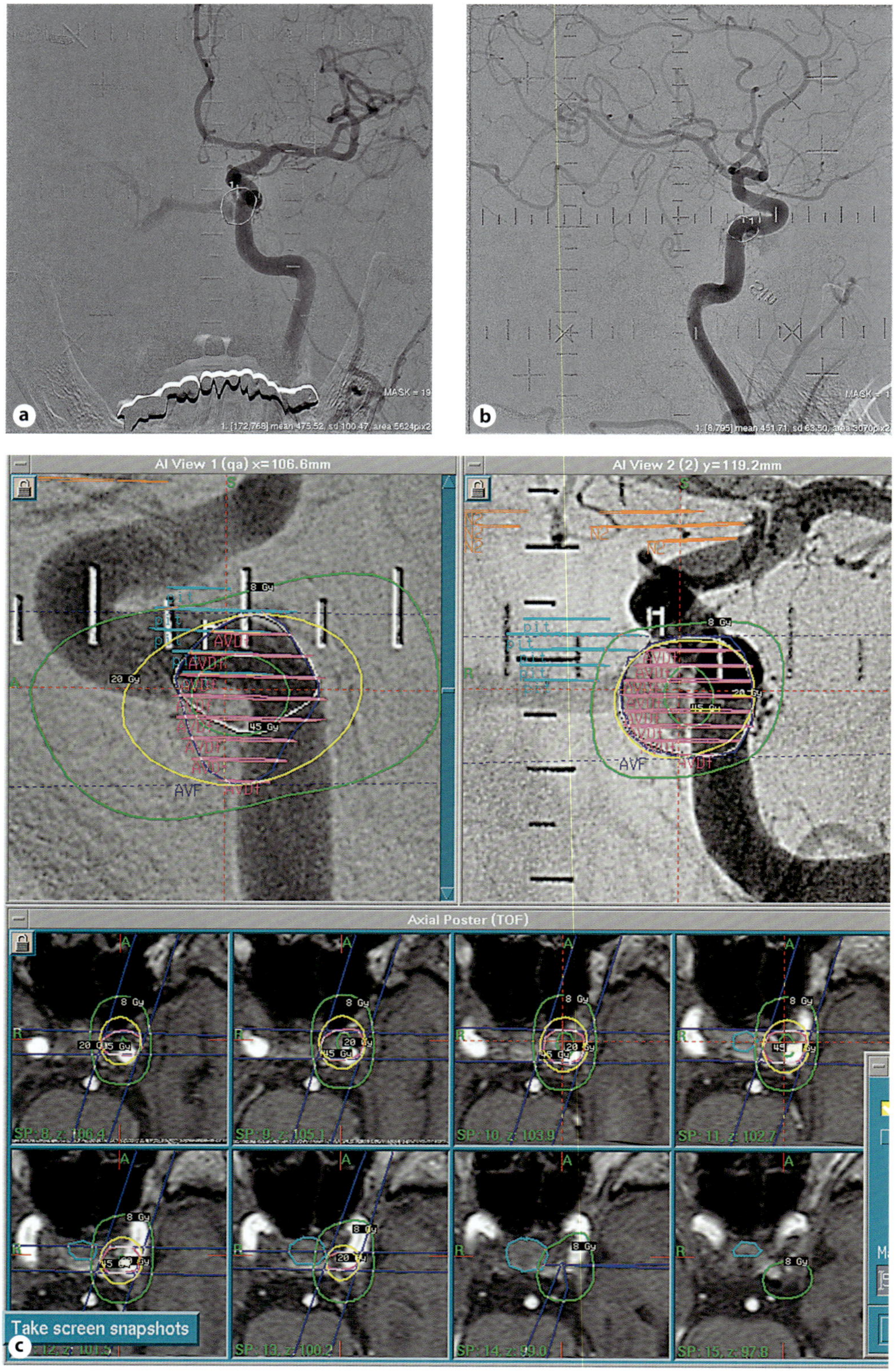
a
b
c
MASK = 19
AI View 1 (qa) x=106.6mm
AI View 2 (2) y=119.2mm
Axial Poster (TOF)
8 Gy
20 Gy
45 Gy
AVF
Take screen snapshots
SP: 8, z: 106.4
SP: 9, z: 105.1
SP: 10, z: 103.9
SP: 11, z: 102.7
SP: 13, z: 100.2
SP: 14, z: 99.0
SP: 15, z: 97.8

Fig. 2.

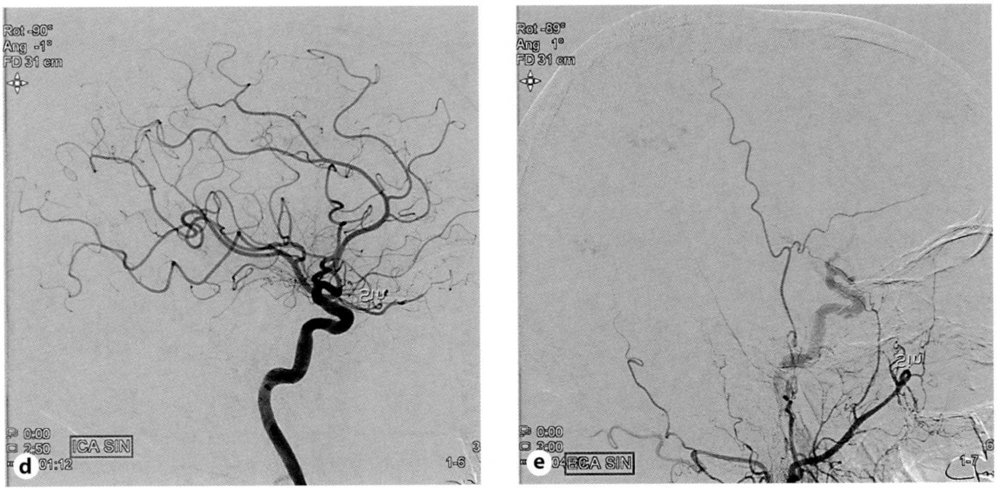

Fig. 2. An 80-year-old male with a left-sided DAVF draining over the midline towards the right cavernous sinus and secondarily into the right sylvian venous complex. A previous endovascular treatment attempt had failed as neither any petrosal sinus nor the superior ophthalmic vein on either side could be cathetherized. **a** Left internal carotid artery angiography, posteroanterior view. The target volume is delineated in white. **b** Left internal carotid artery angiography, lateral view, The target volume is delineated in white. **c** Gamma Plan® dose plan: the prescription dose was 20 Gy to the 50% isodose. The collimators were plugged and the optic nerve received less than 8 Gy as maximum dose. **d** Left internal carotid artery angiography, lateral view, 2-year follow-up. The DAVF has become obliterated. **e** Left external carotid artery angiography, lateral view, 2-year follow-up. The DAVF has become obliterated.

Complications and Hemorrhages

We noticed 3 complications from angiography. Two patients had a transient neurological sequel and 1 patient treated in 1987 had a comment in the files stating that there had been a complication. However, there was no further explanation and the patient does not remember.

Four patients had an ARE in the form of local asymptomatic edema. One patient with a cavernous sinus DAVF experienced a transient 6th-cranial nerve palsy. One patient with a tentorial DAVF (Borden III/Cognard IV) suffered a posterior fossa bleed 10 weeks after the GK SRS. It was evacuated and the fistula extirpated. The patient did clinically well with no residual deficit. However, the patient rebled 12 years later, possibly because of a very late ARE. The posthemorrhage angiogram was normal. The patient is included among the 4 with AREs, i.e. edema. One asymptomatic patient showed MRI findings consistent with asymptomatic hemorrhage. One DAVF worsened clinically during the follow-up period.

Effect on Bruit

Twenty-five cases had a pulse-synchronous bruit at the time of GK SRS (table 1).

Table 3. Irradiation parameters for all 75 treatments

	Mean prescription dose Gy	Mean isodose %	Mean target volume mm^3	Total
Sphenoid and cavernous sinus	18	58	data missing	10
Falcotentorial sinus	25	55	1,130	18
Transverse sinus	24	49	1,840	17
Sigmoid sinus	21	40	data missing	6
Superior petrosal sinus	23	56	1,650	9
Sagittal and straight sinus	23	62	4,440	7
Other locations	24	63	620	8

Prescription volume data is missing for 21 treatments. Therefore the figures given should be interpreted cautiously.

One very large falcotentorial DAVF was still patent, and the bruit was unchanged 2 years after the treatment. In 3 patients, the bruit had decreased but was still clearly audible 2 years after the treatment. The remaining 21 patients were cured from their bruit. The latency before cure was extremely variable, from 1 day(!) to about 2.5 years. Thirteen of these 21 patients had angiographically proven obliteration, while 3 showed variable degrees of regression. The remaining 5 refused follow-up angiography. In general, the bruit disappeared after 3–9 months.

Recurrence

As mentioned previously, a DAVF is a dynamic disease and therefore there are flow changes over time. However, we have not seen any recurrence of a DAVF treated with GK SRS and proven by angiography to be obliterated.

Discussion

The aims of GK SRS for DAVF are to alleviate symptoms such as bruit or orbital venous congestion and eliminate the potential risk for intracranial hemorrhage, without complications. The obvious end point is obliteration of the arteriovenous shunt, but this may not be necessary to keep the patient asymptomatic.

Natural Course of DAVF

In order to properly assess the clinical efficacy of GK SRS, the results should be compared to the natural course of the disease. Unfortunately there are only a few publications on this subject, with widely diverging figures regarding the risk for hemorrhage after disclosure [7, 9, 26–30]. To our knowledge there are no published data on the natural history of the pulse-synchronous bruit. A detailed analysis of the natural course of DAVF is outside the scope of this report, but some facts should be considered.

The presentation and prognosis of a DAVF depend on the location of the shunt and on the venous drainage pattern [2, 6, 31–37]. Classification systems combine information about anatomical location, arterial supply and venous drainage and are useful for descriptive purposes [22, 23, 38].

Thus, a DAVF without cortical venous reflux may present with externally audible pulse-synchronous bruit or symptoms related to orbital venous congestion, but will not cause a hemorrhage or elevated intracranial pressure. Conversely, a DAVF with cortical venous reflux may present with a bruit, an intracranial hemorrhage or even be an incidental finding during a neuroradiological investigation performed for an unrelated reason [9, 26].

The DAVF is a dynamic disease. Conversion from Borden I to Borden II, as well as spontaneous cure, has been reported by several authors, but the incidence is unclear [6, 26, 28, 30, 39–41]. We found clinical worsening after GK SRS in 1 case. We also found regrowth after significant regression. Most likely it was in both cases part of the natural course of the disease and not related to the treatment. In addition it may be that cavernous sinus DAVF may be more prone to occlude spontaneously than shunts in other locations [unpubl. data].

Several groups have noted that the time span between radiosurgery for DAVF and symptomatic cure, in some cases also proven obliteration, can be remarkably short [13, 16, 42–44]. It is not entirely clear to what extent obliteration after radiosurgery can be attributed to the treatment, the natural course of the disease or even to the angiography. Nevertheless, a rapid closure of the arteriovenous shunt will reduce the time that the patient suffers from orbital or other symptoms and also, in cases with cortical venous reflux, reduce the time at risk for intracranial hemorrhage.

Obliteration

The 2-year obliteration rate in our series was 59% (63%) while the regression rate was 27% (23%). These figures do not differ significantly from the 65–70% obliteration rate predicted by the Karlsson outcome model for GK SRS for BAVM treated with the same prescription dose [45]. Other studies have reported similar figures, regardless of the DAVF location and whether radiosurgery had been utilized as a single treatment or in combination with embolization [13, 16–19, 42, 46–50].

Several authors have noted the sometimes remarkably short time span between radiosurgery and symptomatic cure of DAVF, in some cases also obliteration proven by angiography [13, 16, 42, 46]. The location within the dura mater, and the usually narrow blood vessels that these transdural shunting zones represent, may be factors underlying this rapid obliteration process, with subsequent reduction of the time at risk for hemorrhage.

One might assume that there is a dose-effect relationship similar to what has been established in radiosurgery of brain arteriovenous malformations [45]. However, far more patients than in the present series are needed to create an outcome model for GK SRS for DAVF.

Complications and Hemorrhage

Cerebral angiography carries a risk for complications [51, 52]. The described complications, which were related to the stereotactic or follow-up angiograms, resolved without sequel [13, 46]. One patient had a late hemorrhagic complication probably related to a late ARE. Another 3 patients had asymptomatic radiation-induced edema, a finding similar to BAVM radiosurgery [53, 54]. The damage to the 6th cranial nerve resolved with no sequel.

The risk of intracranial hemorrhage after radiosurgery for a DAVF with cortical venous drainage persists until such leptomeningeal reflux has ceased, which is often equivalent to the closure of the arteriovenous shunt. However, this hemorrhagic risk in the latency period before occlusion may be quite low. In our material we found two such cases. If we assume a 2-year follow-up period after the GK SRS, for the 51 treatments for DAVF of the Borden II and III types, this would amount to an annual incidence of 2/102, i.e. 2%.

Effect on Bruit

The impact of GK SRS on the pulse-synchronous bruit is remarkable, and therefore we now often consider GK SRS as a primary treatment in patients plagued by the noise, if not at risk for hemorrhage.

Treatment Failure and Recurrence

In most cases where the DAVF has not been obliterated, flow regression or regression of clinical symptoms has been obvious [13, 16, 46]. Some of these patients have been retreated with subsequent obliteration. However, as pointed out previously, the disease is dynamic and we have now seen a case of regrowth after almost obliteration.

Limitations to the Technique

High-flow arteriovenous shunts seem to respond less favorably, if at all, to irradiation, possibly simply because the vessel lumina are larger [13, 42]. This corresponds with the observation in a single-center series that BAVM with plexiform nidi may respond better to radiosurgery than lesions with high-flow arteriovenous shunts [55].

Another limitation is that the patient may remain symptomatic and at risk for hemorrhage until the DAVF is obliterated.

Conclusion

GK SRS is an effective treatment for dural arteriovenous fistulae, with a low incidence of complications. In lesions with cortical venous drainage there is a possibility for intracranial hemorrhage before obliteration of the shunt. However, the risk is probably quite low.

GK SRS is a treatment alternative for patients harboring a DAVF without cortical venous reflux that causes intolerable bruit and to those not amenable to embolization or surgery.

Disclosure Statement

None of the authors have any affiliation that may cause a conflict of interest.

References

1 Chaudhary MY, Sachdev VP, Cho SH, Weitzner I Jr, Puljic S, Huang YP: Dural arteriovenous malformation of the major venous sinuses: an acquired lesion. AJNR Am J Neuroradiol 1982;3:13–19.

2 Houser OW, Baker HL Jr, Rhoton AL Jr, Okazaki H: Intracranial dural arteriovenous malformations. Radiology 1972;105:55–64.

3 Houser OW, Campbell JK, Campbell RJ, Sundt TM Jr: Arteriovenous malformation affecting the transverse dural venous sinus – an acquired lesion. Mayo Clin Proc 1979;54:651–661.

4 Mironov A: Pathogenetical consideration of spontaneous dural arteriovenous fistulas (DAVFs). Acta Neurochir 1994;131:45–58.

5 Newton TH, Cronqvist S: Involvement of dural arteries in intracranial arteriovenous malformations. Radiology 1969;93:1071–1078.

6 Lasjaunias P: Angioarchitecture and natural history of dural arteriovenous shunts. Interv Neuroradiol 1997;1997:313–317.

7 Duffau H, Lopes M, Janosevic V, Sichez JP, Faillot T, Capelle L, et al: Early rebleeding from intracranial dural arteriovenous fistulas: report of 20 cases and review of the literature. J Neurosurg 1999;90:78–84.

8 Sarma D, ter Brugge K: Management of intracranial dural arteriovenous shunts in adults. Eur J Radiol 2003;46:206–220.

9 Söderman M, Pavic L, Edner G, Holmin S, Andersson T: Natural history of dural arteriovenous shunts. Stroke 2008;39:1735–1739.

10 Van Dijk JM, ter Brugge KG, Willinsky RA, Farb RI, Wallace MC: Multidisciplinary management of spinal dural arteriovenous fistulas: clinical presentation and long-term follow-up in 49 patients. Stroke 2002;33:1578–1583.

11 Van Dijk JM, ter Brugge KG, Willinsky RA, Wallace MC: Selective disconnection of cortical venous reflux as treatment for cranial dural arteriovenous fistulas. J Neurosurg 2004;101:31–35.

12 Steiner L, Leksell L, Greitz T, Forster D, Backlund E: Stereotaxic radiosurgery for cerebral arteriovenous malformations. Report of a case. Acta Chir Scand 1972;135:459–464.

13 Söderman M, Edner G, Ericson K, Karlsson B, Rahn T, Ulfarsson E, et al: Gamma knife surgery for dural arteriovenous shunts: 25 years of experience. J Neurosurg 2006;104:867–875.

14 Barcia-Salorio JL, Hernandez G, Broseta J, Gonzalez-Darder J, Ciudad J: Radiosurgical treatment of carotid-cavernous fistula. Appl Neurophysiol 1982;45:520–522.

15 Barcia-Salorio JL, Soler F, Barcia JA, Hernandez G: Radiosurgery of carotid-cavernous fistulae. Acta Neurochir Suppl 1994;62:10–12.

16 Guo WY, Pan DH, Wu HM, Chung WY, Shiau CY, Wang LW, et al: Radiosurgery as a treatment alternative for dural arteriovenous fistulas of the cavernous sinus. AJNR Am J Neuroradiol 1998;19:1081–1087.
17 Koebbe CJ, Singhal D, Sheehan J, Flickinger JC, Horowitz M, Kondziolka D, et al: Radiosurgery for dural arteriovenous fistulas. Surg Neurol 2005;64:392–398, discussion 398–399.
18 Link MJ, Coffey RJ, Nichols DA, Gorman DA: The role of radiosurgery and particulate embolization in the treatment of dural arteriovenous fistulas. J Neurosurg 1996;84:804–809.
19 Chandler HC Jr, Friedman WA: Successful radiosurgical treatment of a dural arteriovenous malformation: case report. Neurosurgery 1993;33:139–141, discussion 141–142.
20 Kobayashi H, Hayashi M, Noguchi Y, Tsuji T, Handa Y, Caner HH: Dural arteriovenous malformations in the anterior cranial fossa. Surg Neurol 1988;30:396–401.
21 Lewis AI, Tomsick TA, Tew JM Jr: Management of tentorial dural arteriovenous malformations: transarterial embolization combined with stereotactic radiation or surgery. J Neurosurg 1994;81:851–859.
22 Borden JA, Wu JK, Shucart WA: A proposed classification for spinal and cranial dural arteriovenous fistula malformations and implications for treatment. J Neurosurg 1995;82:166–179.
23 Cognard C, Gobin YP, Pierot L, Bailly AL, Houdart E, Casasco A, et al: Cerebral dural arteriovenous fistulas: clinical and angiographic correlation with a revised classification of venous drainage. Radiology 1995;194:671–680.
24 Guo W, Lindqvist M, Lindqvist C, Ericson K, Nordell B, Karlsson B, et al: Stereotaxic angiography in gamma knife radiosurgery of intracranial arteriovenous malformations. AJNR Am J Neuroradiol 1992;13:1107–1114.
25 Guo WY: Application of MR in stereotactic radiosurgery. J Magn Reson Imaging 1998;8:415–420.
26 Brown RD Jr, Wiebers DO, Nichols DA: Intracranial dural arteriovenous fistulae: angiographic predictors of intracranial hemorrhage and clinical outcome in nonsurgical patients. J Neurosurg 1994;81:531–538.
27 Davies MA, Saleh J, ter Brugge K, Willinsky R, Wallace MC: The natural history and management of intracranial dural arteriovenous fistulae. 1. Benign lesions. Interv Neuroradiol 1997;3:295–302.
28 Satomi J, van Dijk JM, ter Brugge KG, Willinsky RA, Wallace MC: Benign cranial dural arteriovenous fistulas: outcome of conservative management based on the natural history of the lesion. J Neurosurg 2002;97:767–770.
29 Strom RG, Botros JA, Refai D, Moran CJ, Cross DT 3rd, Chicoine MR, et al: Cranial dural arteriovenous fistulae: asymptomatic cortical venous drainage portends less aggressive clinical course. Neurosurgery 2009;64:241–247, discussion 247–248.
30 Van Dijk JM, ter Brugge KG, Willinsky RA, Wallace MC: Clinical course of cranial dural arteriovenous fistulas with long-term persistent cortical venous reflux. Stroke 2002;33:1233–1236.
31 Castaigne P, Laplane D, Djindjian R, Bories J, Augustin P: Spontaneous arteriovenous communication between the external carotid and the cavernous sinus. Rev Neurol (Paris) 1966;114:5–14.
32 Castaigne P, Bories J, Brunet P, Cassan JL, Meininger V, Merland JJ: Arteriovenous fistulae of the dura mater. Clinical and radiological study of 13 cases. Ann Méd Interne (Paris) 1975;126:813–817.
33 Castaigne P, Bories J, Brunet P, Merland JJ, Meininger V: Meningeal arterio-venous fistulas with cortical venous drainage. Rev Neurol (Paris) 1976;132:169–181.
34 Djindjian R, Cophignon J, Comoy J, Rey J, Houdart R: Polymorphisme neuroradiologique des fistules carotico-caverneuses. Neurochirurgie 1968;14:881–890.
35 Djindjian R, Merland JJ: Superselective Angiography of the External Carotid Artery. Berlin, Springer, 1978.
36 Lasjaunias P, Halimi P, Lopez-Ibor L, Sichez JP, Hurth M, De Tribolet N: Endovascular treatment of pure spontaneous dural vascular malformations. Review of 23 cases studied and treated between May 1980 and October 1983. Neurochirurgie 1984;30:207–223.
37 Awad IA, Little JR, Akarawi WP, Ahl J: Intracranial dural arteriovenous malformations: factors predisposing to an aggressive neurological course. J Neurosurg 1990;72:839–850.
38 Barrow DL, Spector RH, Braun IF, Landman JA, Tindall SC, Tindall GT: Classification and treatment of spontaneous carotid-cavernous sinus fistulas. J Neurosurg 1985;62:248–256.
39 Luciani A, Houdart E, Mounayer C, Saint Maurice JP, Merland JJ: Spontaneous closure of dural arteriovenous fistulas: report of three cases and review of the literature. AJNR Am J Neuroradiol 2001;22:992–996.
40 Van Rooij WJ, Sluzewski M, Beute GN: Dural arteriovenous fistulas with cortical venous drainage: incidence, clinical presentation, and treatment. AJNR Am J Neuroradiol 2007;28:651–655.
41 Voigt K, Sauer M, Dichgans J: Spontaneous occlusion of a bilateral caroticocavernous fistula studied by serial angiography. Neuroradiology 1971;2:207–211.

42 Barcia-Salorio JL, Soler F, Barcia JA, Hernandez G: Stereotactic radiosurgery for the treatment of low-flow carotid-cavernous fistulae: results in a series of 25 cases. Stereotact Funct Neurosurg 1994;63:266–270.

43 Hasuo K, Mizushima A, Matsumoto S, Uchino A, Uehara S, Miyoshi M, et al: Type D dural carotid-cavernous fistula. Results of combined treatment with irradiation and particulate embolization. Acta Radiol 1996;37:294–298.

44 Onizuka M, Mori K, Takahashi N, Kawahara I, Hiu T, Toda K, et al: Gamma knife surgery for the treatment of spontaneous dural carotid-cavernous fistulas. Neurol Med Chir (Tokyo) 2003;43:477–482, discussion 482–483.

45 Karlsson B, Lax I, Söderman M: Can the probability for obliteration after radiosurgery for arteriovenous malformations be accurately predicted? Int J Radiat Oncol Biol Phys 1999;43:313–319.

46 Pollock BE, Nichols DA, Garrity JA, Gorman DA, Stafford SL: Stereotactic radiosurgery and particulate embolization for cavernous sinus dural arteriovenous fistulae. Neurosurgery 1999;45:459–466, discussion 466–467.

47 Shin M, Kurita H, Tago M, Kirino T: Stereotactic radiosurgery for tentorial dural arteriovenous fistulae draining into the vein of Galen: report of two cases. Neurosurgery 2000;46:730–733, discussion 733–734.

48 Friedman JA, Pollock BE, Nichols DA, Gorman DA, Foote RL, Stafford SL: Results of combined stereotactic radiosurgery and transarterial embolization for dural arteriovenous fistulas of the transverse and sigmoid sinuses. J Neurosurg 2001;94:886–891.

49 Pan DH, Chung WY, Guo WY, Wu HM, Liu KD, Shiau CY, et al: Stereotactic radiosurgery for the treatment of dural arteriovenous fistulas involving the transverse-sigmoid sinus. J Neurosurg 2002;96:823–829.

50 Maruyama K, Shin M, Kurita H, Tago M, Kirino T: Stereotactic radiosurgery for dural arteriovenous fistula involving the superior sagittal sinus. Case report. J Neurosurg 2002;97:481–483.

51 Dawkins AA, Evans AL, Wattam J, Romanowski CA, Connolly DJ, Hodgson TJ, et al: Complications of cerebral angiography: a prospective analysis of 2,924 consecutive procedures. Neuroradiology 2007;49:753–759.

52 Willinsky RA, Taylor SM, ter Brugge K, Farb RI, Tomlinson G, Montanera W: Neurologic complications of cerebral angiography: prospective analysis of 2,899 procedures and review of the literature. Radiology 2003;227:522–528.

53 Guo WY, Lindquist C, Karlsson B, Kihlstrom L, Steiner L: Gamma knife surgery of cerebral arteriovenous malformations: serial MR imaging studies after radiosurgery. Int J Radiat Oncol Biol Phys 1993;25:315–323.

54 Kihlstrom L, Guo WY, Karlsson B, Lindquist C, Lindqvist M: Magnetic resonance imaging of obliterated arteriovenous malformations up to 23 years after radiosurgery. J Neurosurg 1997;86:589–593.

55 Meder J, Oppenheim C, Blustajn J, Nataf F, Merienne L, Lefkoupolos D, et al: Cerebral arteriovenous malformations: the value of radiologic parameters in predicting response to radiosurgery. AJNR Am J Neuroradiol 1997;18:1473–1483.

Michael Söderman, MD, PhD
Department of Neuroradiology, Karolinska University Hospital
SE–171 76 Stockholm (Sweden)
Tel. +46 8 5177 4037, E-Mail michael.soderman@karolinska.se

Niranjan A, Kano H, Lunsford LD (eds): Gamma Knife Radiosurgery for Brain Vascular Malformations.
Prog Neurol Surg. Basel, Karger, 2013, vol 27, pp 218–226 (DOI: 10.1159/000341799)

Stereotactic Radiosurgery Guidelines for the Management of Patients with Intracranial Dural Arteriovenous Fistulas

Ajay Niranjan · L. Dade Lunsford

Department of Neurological Surgery, University of Pittsburgh, Pittsburgh, Pa., USA

Abstract

Treatment options for dural arteriovenous fistulas (DAVFs) have expanded with the application of stereotactic radiosurgery (SRS). Our objective was to provide guidelines about the use of SRS in symptomatic patients with imaging-identified DAVFs of the brain. The authors reviewed evidence-based medicine and clinical experience with radiosurgery for DAVFs of the brain and developed guidelines and provided a scientific foundation for patients and physicians. Major recommendations include the definition of DAVF patients suitable for various management strategies ranging from observation to surgical excision to endovascular embolization and SRS. Combined SRS and embolization is an effective management strategy for DAVFs, including those that have recurred after initial embolization. The effect of prior embolization has been evaluated. SRS before embolization facilitates the better recognition of the entire target. For selected DAVF patients who are not eligible for embolization or surgery, SRS alone is an effective treatment option. The dose range for DAVFs is similar to that of arteriovenous malformations. A clinical algorithm for the potential role of SRS for a symptomatic brain DAVF was defined. These guidelines provide a framework for professional judgment and treatment selection alternatives for the management of DAVFs.

Intracranial dural arteriovenous fistulas (DAVFs) are rare vascular malformations. DAVFs may occur anywhere within the dura mater, but develop most frequently near the transverse, sigmoid and cavernous sinuses [1, 2]. In DAVFs, dural arteries drain into venous sinuses or pial leptomeningeal veins. DAVFs with retrograde leptomeningeal venous drainage have a significantly higher risk of intracranial bleeding. The clinical presentation depends on the site and overall hemodynamics of the lesion [3, 4]. Pulsatile tinnitus commonly occurs with lesions of the transverse or sigmoid sinus and may become intolerable. With cavernous sinus lesions, double vision, impaired vision and exophthalmos may occur. Superior sagittal sinus lesions can cause papilledema, vision loss and increased intracranial pressure. Cortically based lesions can lead to hemorrhages, progressive deficits or seizures. With DAVFs, the overall risk of hemorrhage is about 2% per year and depends on the site and hemodynamics of the lesion. The hemodynamics associated with a higher risk of hemorrhage includes cortical drainage, retrograde venous drainage, presence of a venous varix, or drainage into the vein of Galen [5, 6].

DAVFs are considered suitable for 4 management strategies alone or in combination [7]: observation only, surgical excision [7–9], endovascular embolization and stereotactic radiosurgery (SRS) [10–14]. SRS in combination with transarterial embolization has been shown to be effective for patients with DAVFs [15–17]. Although there are several published reports on long-term outcome after arteriovenous malformation (AVM) radiosurgery, no guidelines are available for medical professionals to make an evidence-based decision. We developed a radiosurgery practice guideline and treatment recommendations which can be used by medical and public health professionals for patients with the diagnosis of brain or dural AVM.

Methods

Computerized searches of published literature (primary sources), hand searches of published literature (secondary sources) and searches of electronic clinical databases were performed. Medline and Pubmed searches were completed for the years 1971 to March 2011. Search terms included 'dural arteriovenous fistula', 'vascular malformation' and 'stereotactic radiosurgery'. Bibliographies from recently published reviews were reviewed, and relevant articles were retrieved.

Outcomes Considered

Total obliteration of the DAVF was the primary end point of interest. Additional outcome end points included resolution or an improvement in symptoms and prevention of bleeding risks from the DAVF. Improvement in the existing neurological deficits, maintenance of quality of life and prevention of adverse radiation effects were also considered.

Major Recommendations

Management Options

- Asymptomatic low-risk DAVFs (e.g. those without leptomeningeal drainage) may not need any active management. Symptomatic DAVFs or those found to have leptomeningeal drainage (therefore with a significantly increased risk of bleeding) are considered for treatment.

- The treatment of DAVFs depends on the severity of the symptoms, the angiographic characteristics and the perceived risk for intracranial hemorrhage. Most high-risk DAVFs warrant treatment because they carry a high probability of intracranial hemorrhage or neurological deterioration.
- DAVFs with aggressive presentation require urgent evaluation and treatment. Also, patients with intractable pulsatile tinnitus, chemosis or proptosis may be sufficiently affected by their symptoms to warrant consideration of curative or at least palliative treatment.
- Treatment strategies for DAVFs are diverse and include surgical excision [8, 9, 18], transarterial or transvenous embolization and SRS. In many instances, a multimodality management is needed.
- Direct surgery is a potential option for some patients, especially if there is a limited direct artery-to-vein fistula in a surgically accessible location.
- Although transarterial embolization is often effective for DAVFs, complete occlusion is difficult because not all arterial feeding vessels can be seen during angiography. Superselective catheterization, which may be necessary to identify the myriad of feeding vessels, can also be technically challenging (fig. 1, 2).
- Radiosurgery alone can be the choice for patients with a low risk of intracranial hemorrhage (patients with no or limited cortical venous drainage), for those with only mild symptoms, and for those patients for whom embolization proved impossible because of a difficulty to catheterize feeding vessels or the presence of significant comorbidities. Radiosurgery alone may not be the best choice for large DAVFs that are better approached by endovascular techniques.
- When possible SRS followed by embolization is preferred as embolization can provide early symptom relief, whereas SRS offers the potential for delayed complete fistula closure. Radiosurgery is better for microvasculature obliteration (a situation for which embolization techniques are deficient, e.g. when the feeding vessel is not amenable to catheterization). Radiosurgery and embolization are complementary techniques for properly selected dural fistulas.

Patient Selection

Patients with intracranial DAVF defined by cerebral angiography are considered for radiosurgery. Such patients typically present with pulsatile tinnitus, double vision, impaired vision, exophthalmos, hemorrhages, progressive deficits or seizures.

The selection of patients suitable for radiosurgery is dependent on prior bleeding history, age of the patient, existing comorbidities, anatomical location, presence of leptomeningeal drainage and severity of clinical symptoms.

Some DAVF patients initially undergo embolization for volumetric reduction or flow reduction. The optimal time between prior embolization and radiosurgery is not known, but generally waiting (to reduce the risk of posttreatment cerebral edema) for a period of several weeks is considered optimal.

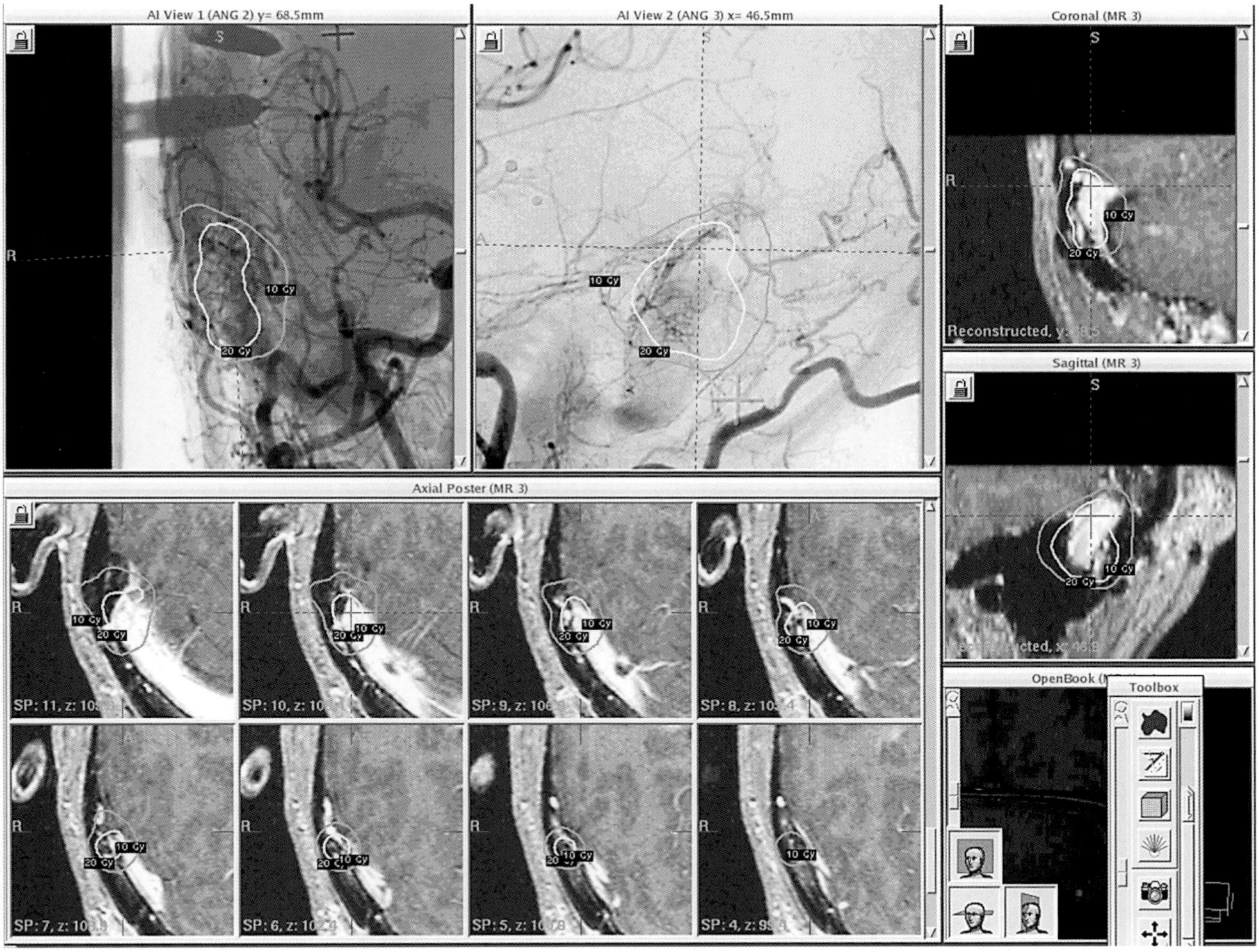

Fig. 1. A 64-year-old man presented with right-sided severe tinnitus. An angiogram showed a right transverse/sigmoid sinus DAVF. He underwent partial embolization of the right transverse/sigmoid sinus DAVF with superselective catheterization of the right posterior auricular artery and right occipital artery and embolization using Onyx [18]. Four weeks later, this patient underwent Gamma Knife radiosurgery for residual arteriovenous fistula. At the time of radiosurgery, a right common carotid artery arteriogram showed a DAVF centered around the transverse and sigmoid sinuses. Radiosurgery dose planning was performed using angiograms and MR images, and a margin dose of 22 Gy was prescribed to the 50% isodose covering the DAVF.

Imaging

Cerebral angiography supplemented by high-resolution stereotactic MR images is required for dose planning. For patients ineligible for MRI, contrast-enhanced volumetric CT should be done.

Although most small DAVFs are not visualized completely on MR images, MRI is still recommended to evaluate 3-dimensional conformity of the dose plan and to identify critical brain structures at risk. MRI also helps in selecting the optimum dose

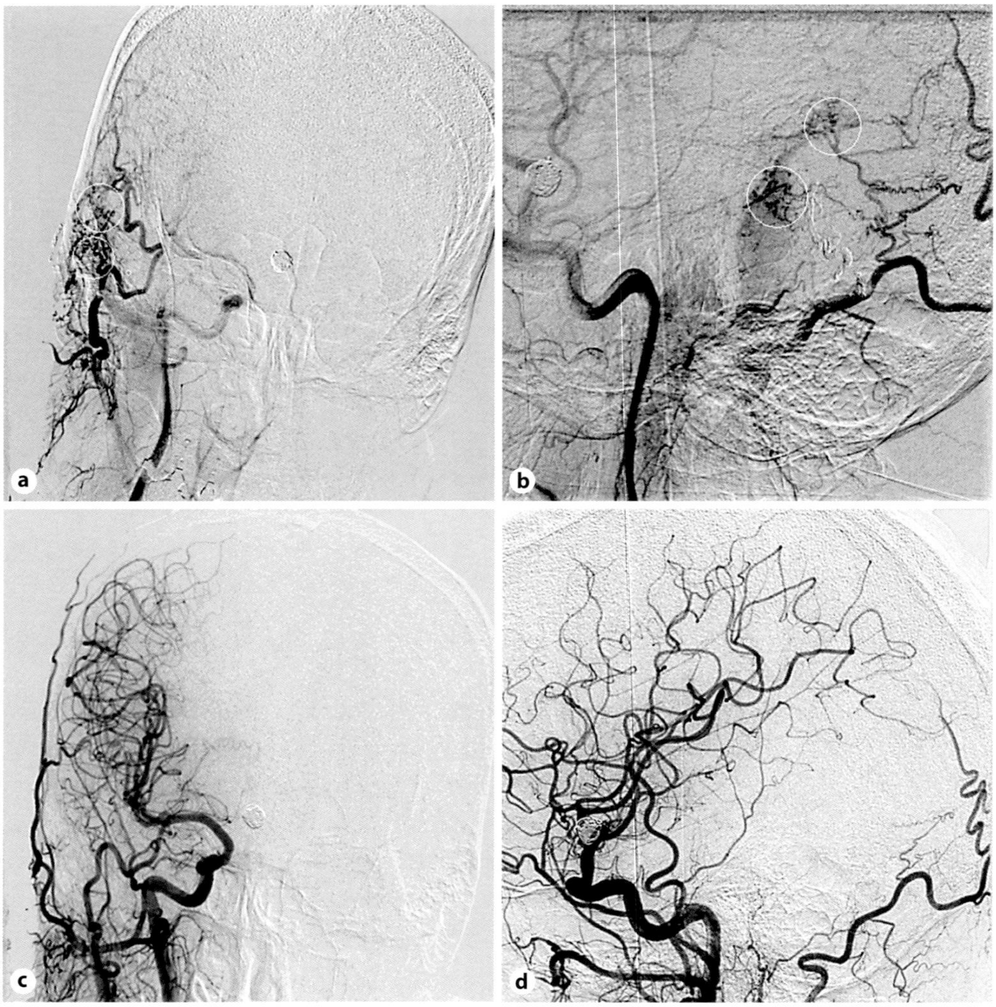

Fig. 2. Posteroanterior (**a**) and lateral (**b**) angiograms performed at radiosurgery showing residual DAVF (after embolization). **c**, **d** Two-year follow-up angiograms after radiosurgery showing complete obliteration of DAVF.

because the margin dose is selected based on the risk to surrounding critical brain structures.

High-quality digital subtraction angiography is critical for successful radiosurgery dose planning for DAVFs. Once angiography is performed and the DAVF is localized, the members of the radiosurgery team should review the images prior to removal of the angiography catheter. The radiosurgery team should ensure that the DAVF is visualized in both posteroanterior and lateral views, that all fiducial markers are visible, and adequate subtraction views are performed. The images which best visualize the DAVF should be selected and entered in the dose planning computer.

Dose Selection
The dose selection for volumetric conformal DAVF SRS is largely based on intracranial AVM radiosurgery experience. The doses depend on the location and volume of the DAVF. Doses at the margin of the DAVF typically range from 18 to 25 Gy in a single procedure. The margin of the DAVF dose is usually 50–70% of the central target dose within the AVM. A sharp fall-off of the radiation dose outside of the target volume is required.

Timing of Embolization
Embolization is a useful strategy for patients with DAVFs. Radiosurgery followed by embolization appears to be the best strategy for complete DAVF obliteration and immediate relief of symptoms, since complete visualization of the shunt is possible only before embolization is completed. Transarterial embolization, usually performed a few hours after radiosurgery, provides early palliative relief of symptoms such as pulsatile tinnitus, orbital venous congestion or diplopia when present. In addition, it may substantially reduce cortical venous drainage, thereby reducing the risk of hemorrhage during the latency interval after radiosurgery. Even if recanalization of the embolized fistula occurs, the DAVF undergoes simultaneous radiosurgery-induced obliteration. Embolization is performed after radiosurgery to avoid the pitfall of having embolization temporarily obscure portions of the nidus that would then not be targeted during the radiosurgical procedure. Thus, the combination of radiosurgery followed by transarterial embolization, when possible, provides both rapid symptom relief and facilitates the long-term cure of DAVFs.

Although the published complete obliteration rates are lower if embolization is performed prior to radiosurgery, the obliteration rate may improve with the use of newer embolization materials such as Onyx. Onyx is a nonadhesive embolic agent with lava-like flow patterns. It is possible to interrupt the injection and analyze the actual Onyx casting. For both of these reasons, it is possible to inject large volumes from one catheter position in a controlled manner and thus embolize a large part of the DAVF without filling the draining veins or leptomeningeal collaterals. Due to these properties, Onyx is thought more likely to produce permanent vascular occlusion.

Medical Management
Patients may receive a single dose (40 mg) of methylprednisolone at the conclusion of the radiosurgery procedure. They can continue to take their other medications (e.g. antiepileptics, analgesics) during and after the procedure as recommended by their physicians.

Those patients who are maintained on antiepileptic drugs to manage seizures should have their blood levels of antiepileptic drugs checked on the day of radiosurgery to make sure that a therapeutic level is maintained at the time of radiosurgery.

Follow-Up Evaluations

Postradiosurgical clinical examinations and MRI or CT (for patients ineligible for MRI) studies are requested at 6 months and then yearly for the first 3 years to assess the effect of radiosurgery on DAVF (gradual obliteration) and to detect any adverse radiation effects. An angiogram is recommended at the 3-year mark to confirm obliteration. If angiography after 3 years demonstrates that the AVM nidus is not obliterated, repeat SRS, surgery or embolization should again be considered.

Causes of failure of SRS include inadequate definition of the DAVF, insufficient dose to achieve the obliterative response, poor nidus visualization secondary to overlying vascular structures or prior embolization, or recanalization of previously embolized components.

Postradiosurgery Imaging Changes

The probability of developing postradiosurgery imaging changes related to target irradiation depends on the marginal dose and treatment volume. The volume of tissue receiving 12 Gy or more (the 12-Gy volume) is the single factor that seems to have the closest correlation with the probability of developing delayed imaging changes in the brain surrounding the target. Such imaging changes are best seen on T_2-weighted MRI and may be compatible with either edema or transient astrocytosis in the volume of brain surrounding the original target.

Late Complications after AVM Radiosurgery

Delayed complications of radiosurgery (adverse radiation effects) are similar to those discussed in AVM guidelines. The reader is referred to that guideline for further review.

Management of Residual DAVF after Radiosurgery

Repeat radiosurgery is one option for patients with residual DAVF remaining 3 years or more after initial radiosurgery. However, some patients may become eligible for surgical excision or embolization to complete the goal of complete DAVF closure.

Potential Benefits of Radiosurgery

All the published studies have shown a significant response of SRS for DAVFs, including a high rate of fistula obliteration, symptom resolution and a satisfactory (low) rate of adverse radiation effects [10–17, 19].

Potential successful outcomes include complete obliteration of DAVF, symptomatic relief, absence of new neurological deficit and sustained prevention of bleeding.

Subgroups Most Likely to Benefit

Radiosurgery may be especially suitable for the following groups of patients:

- patients in advanced age groups;
- patients with excessive medical comorbidity risk factors for surgical excision;

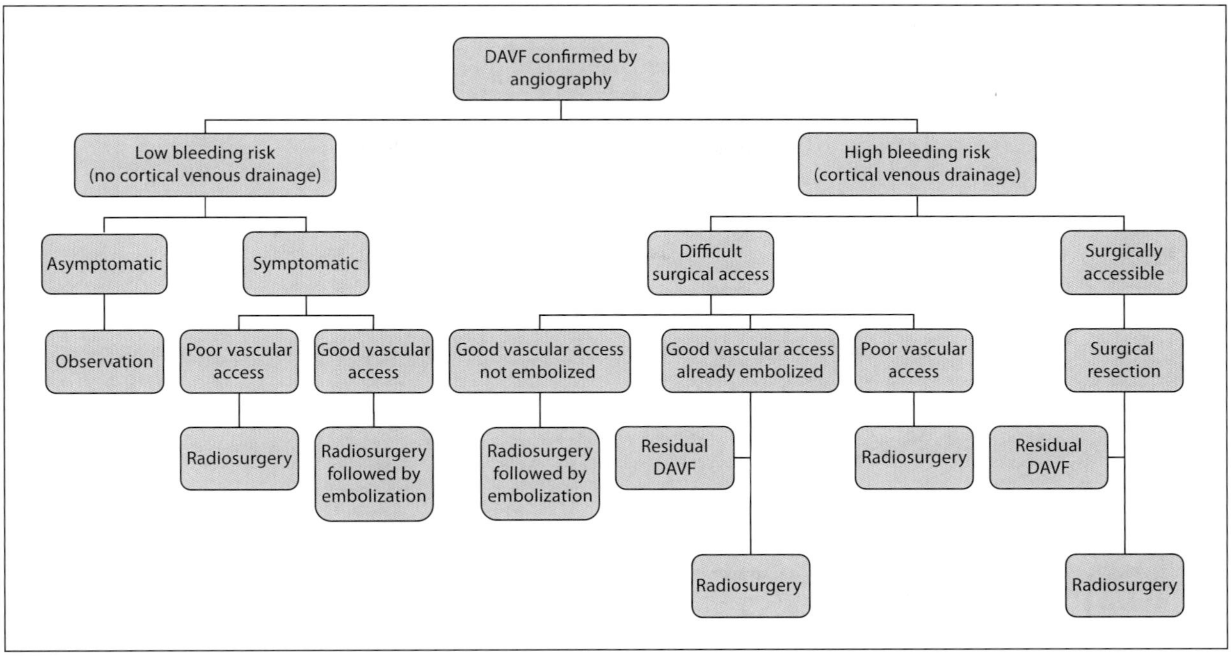

Fig. 3. Proposed management algorithm for patients with intracranial DAVF.

- patients with DAVFs in locations where surgery may result in unacceptable neurological deficits;
- patients with DAVFs considered unsuitable for complete obliteration by endovascular embolization, especially those with inadequate vascular supply to facilitate catheter placement.

Clinical Algorithm

A number of factors are considered in making a recommendation. These factors include:

1 patient's age;
2 severity of the symptoms;
3 angiographic characteristics;
4 the perceived risk for intracranial hemorrhage;
5 history of prior bleeding;
6 prior procedures (surgery or embolization);
7 volume of DAVF;
8 location of DAVF.

A broad outline of the management algorithm is shown in figure 3; however, the final recommendation is usually influenced by the treating neurosurgeon's or endovascular specialist's experience and patient preference.

References

1 Houser OW, Baker HL Jr, Rhoton AL Jr, Okazaki H: Intracranial dural arteriovenous malformations. Radiology 1972;105:55–64.

2 Söderman M, Pavic L, Edner G, Holmin S, Andersson T: Natural history of dural arteriovenous shunts. Stroke 2008;39:1735–1739.

3 Awad IA, Little JR, Akarawi WP, Ahl J: Intracranial dural arteriovenous malformations: factors predisposing to an aggressive neurological course. J Neurosurg 1990;72:839–850.

4 Malik GM, Pearce JE, Ausman JI, Mehta B: Dural arteriovenous malformations and intracranial hemorrhage. Neurosurgery 1984;15:332–339.

5 Borden JA, Wu JK, Shucart WA: A proposed classification for spinal and cranial dural arteriovenous fistulous malformations and implications for treatment. J Neurosurg 1995;82:166–179.

6 Cognard C, Gobin YP, Pierot L, Bailly AL, Houdart E, Casasco A, et al: Cerebral dural arteriovenous fistulas: clinical and angiographic correlation with a revised classification of venous drainage. Radiology 1995;194:671–680.

7 Lucas CP, Zabramski JM, Spetzler RF, Jacobowitz R: Treatment for intracranial dural arteriovenous malformations: a meta-analysis from the English language literature. Neurosurgery 1997;40:1119–1130, discussion 1130–1132.

8 Liu JK, Dogan A, Ellegala DB, Carlson J, Nesbit GM, Barnwell SL, et al: The role of surgery for high-grade intracranial dural arteriovenous fistulas: importance of obliteration of venous outflow. J Neurosurg 2009;110:913–920.

9 Sundt TM Jr, Piepgras DG: The surgical approach to arteriovenous malformations of the lateral and sigmoid dural sinuses. J Neurosurg 1983;59:32–39.

10 Guo WY, Pan DH, Wu HM, Chung WY, Shiau CY, Wang LW, et al: Radiosurgery as a treatment alternative for dural arteriovenous fistulas of the cavernous sinus. AJNR Am J Neuroradiol 1998;19: 1081–1087.

11 Koebbe CJ, Singhal D, Sheehan J, Flickinger JC, Horowitz M, Kondziolka D, et al: Radiosurgery for dural arteriovenous fistulas. Surg Neurol 2005;64: 392–398, discussion 398–399.

12 Pan DH, Chung WY, Guo WY, Wu HM, Liu KD, Shiau CY, et al: Stereotactic radiosurgery for the treatment of dural arteriovenous fistulas involving the transverse-sigmoid sinus. J Neurosurg 2002;96: 823–829.

13 Söderman M, Edner G, Ericson K, Karlsson B, Rahn T, Ulfarsson E, et al: Gamma knife surgery for dural arteriovenous shunts: 25 years of experience. J Neurosurg 2006;104:867–875.

14 Wu HM, Pan DH, Chung WY, Guo WY, Liu KD, Shiau CY, et al: Gamma Knife surgery for the management of intracranial dural arteriovenous fistulas. J Neurosurg 2006;105(suppl):43–51.

15 Friedman JA, Pollock BE, Nichols DA, Gorman DA, Foote RL, Stafford SL: Results of combined stereotactic radiosurgery and transarterial embolization for dural arteriovenous fistulas of the transverse and sigmoid sinuses. J Neurosurg 2001;94:886–891.

16 Link MJ, Coffey RJ, Nichols DA, Gorman DA: The role of radiosurgery and particulate embolization in the treatment of dural arteriovenous fistulas. J Neurosurg 1996;84:804–809.

17 Pollock BE, Nichols DA, Garrity JA, Gorman DA, Stafford SL: Stereotactic radiosurgery and particulate embolization for cavernous sinus dural arteriovenous fistulae. Neurosurgery 1999;45:459–466, discussion 466–467.

18 Hugosson R, Bergstrom K: Surgical treatment of dural arteriovenous malformation in the region of the sigmoid sinus. J Neurol Neurosurg Psychiatry 1974;37:97–101.

19 Lewis AI, Tomsick TA, Tew JM Jr: Management of tentorial dural arteriovenous malformations: transarterial embolization combined with stereotactic radiation or surgery. J Neurosurg 1994;81:851–859.

Ajay Niranjan, MCh, MBA
Department of Neurological Surgery, University of Pittsburgh Medical Center, Suite B-400
200 Lothrop Street
Pittsburgh, PA 15213 (USA)
Tel. +1 412 647 6250, E-Mail niranjana@upmc.edu

Author Index

Subject Index